AF797098

Nonprescription Products:

Formulations & Features

'96-97

A Companion to the Handbook of Nonprescription Drugs, 11th Edition

Notices

The inclusion in this book of any drug in respect to which patent or trademark rights may exist shall not be deemed, and is not intended as a grant of or authority to exercise, any right or privilege protected by such patent or trademark. All such rights or trademarks are vested in the patent or trademark owner, and no other person may exercise the same without express permission, authority, or license secured from such patent or trademark owner.

The listing of selected brand names is intended only for ease of reference. The listed brand names are a representative sampling of drug products, not a comprehensive listing. The inclusion of a brand name does not mean the editors or publisher has any particular knowledge that the brand listed has properties different from other brands of the same drug, nor should its inclusion be interpreted as an endorsement by the editors or publisher. Similarly, the fact that a particular brand has not been included does not indicate the product has been judged to be in any way unsatisfactory or unacceptable.

The nature of drug information is that it is constantly evolving because of ongoing research and clinical experience and is often subject to interpretation. Although great care has been taken to ensure the accuracy of the information presented herein, the reader is advised that the publisher, editors, and drug information analyst cannot be held responsible for the continued currency of the information or for any errors or omissions in this book or for any consequences arising therefrom. Readers are advised that decisions regarding drug therapy must be based on the independent judgment of the clinician, changing information about a drug (eg, as reflected in the literature and manufacturer's most current product information), and changing medical practices.

The editors and drug information analyst have written this book in their private capacities. No official support or endorsement by any federal or state agency or pharmaceutical company is intended or inferred.

APhA

APhA

A publication of the
American
Pharmaceutical
Association

Nonprescription Products:

Formulations & Features

'96-97

A Companion to the Handbook of Nonprescription Drugs, 11th Edition

APhA

Published by

American Pharmaceutical Association

The National Professional Society of Pharmacists

2215 Constitution Avenue, NW

Washington, DC 20037

Leroy C. Knodel, PharmD
Drug Information Analyst

Susan C. Kendall
Product Table Editor

Linda L. Young
Managing Editor

Mary Jane Hickey
Director, Art and Production

Database Development: Benjamin M. Bluml, Cygnus Systems Development Inc.

Editorial Services: Publications Professionals, Inc.

Printing: United Book Press, Inc.

ISBN 0-917330-78-1

How to Order This Book
By phone: 800-878-0729—VISA, MasterCard, and American Express cards accepted.

Contents

Introduction

Welcome to the first edition of *Nonprescription Products: Formulations & Features*. Some of you have purchased this book separately; others have received it as part of your purchase of the 11th Edition of the *Handbook of Nonprescription Drugs*. If you have opened a copy of any of the first 10 editions of the *Handbook,* you know that tables containing detailed comparative information on nonprescription products were previously incorporated in the textbook. Why have we now split the book into two publications?

The overriding reason is readers' expressed interest in receiving up-to-date nonprescription product information in today's rapidly changing market. Similar to many other comprehensive medical textbooks, a new edition of the *Handbook* is published every 3 to 4 years. In that time, however, the information in this edition of *Formulations & Features* will have become dated. To meet our readers' needs, APhA plans to publish new issues of this title once a year and to provide the most current edition of *Formulations & Features* to purchasers of the *Handbook*. The link between product and ingredient information in the two publications will be established with cross-references: Each product table contains a cross-reference to the textbook chapter that discusses the pharmacology of the ingredients and therapeutic use of the products; similarly, the textbook chapters cross-reference the appropriate product tables.

A second reason is portability. When the product tables were a part of the large—and growing—textbook, quickly extracting product information became difficult, whereas putting this material in a separate publication provides ready access to the product information. Incidentally, readers told us they preferred the hardcover binding used in editions prior to the 10th, but at the same time were concerned that the book was becoming very heavy to carry. With the 11th Edition, the textbook is once again hardbound, but the separate binding of approximately 400 pages of product tables actually makes the 11th Edition lighter than the softbound 10th Edition.

A third reason for publishing the product tables separately is simply that we believe the information in *Formulations & Features* is valuable in its own right. Creating a separate book makes this information accessible to many health care professionals whose primary interest or need is the product information.

Current changes in the U.S. health care system have made comparison of nonprescription products an invaluable tool for health care professionals. The more than 800 new product listings reflect the current rapid expansion of the nonprescription product market, which is being driven in part by sweeping changes in the U.S. health care system and the pharmaceutical industry. An increased reliance on self-care by the public and the availability of a large number of medications recently reclassified as nonprescription demand that health care professionals be on the leading edge of the self-care movement. Further, the continuing evolution of pharmacy practice from dispensing of medications to management of patients makes this type of information essential to pharmacists in making the most appropriate recommendations to their patients with regard to nonprescription drug use.

APhA's electronic database of nonprescription products—the OTC Product Database—facilitated publication of this book. This database, which is in Microsoft Access format and can be provided for computer applications in standard ASCII or other appropriate media, is available for use by system vendors, software and CD ROM developers, and health care professionals. Interested parties may call 202-429-7561 for more information about the database.

APhA welcomes your suggestions for improving its nonprescription product information and this book. Please write to *Nonprescription Products: Formulations & Features,* American Pharmaceutical Association, 2215 Constitution Avenue, NW, Washington, DC 20037.

Leroy Knodel, PharmD
Drug Information Analyst

About the Product Tables

As a result of FDA approval of new nonprescription products and reorganization of the *Handbook* chapters in the 11th Edition, 22 "new" product tables have been added to APhA's OTC Product Database. The titles of these tables are provided so that users of past editions of the *Handbook*—which included the chapters and product tables—may note the introduction of new products and the regrouping of some previously listed products.

- Adult Incontinence Garments
- Antiflatulent Products
- Asthma Auxiliary Devices
- Blood Glucose Meters
- Cholesterol Test Kits
- Emetic Products
- Feminine Hygiene Products
- First-Aid Antibiotic and Antiseptic Products
- Gastric Decontaminant Products
- Hair Regrowth Products
- Herbal and Phytomedicinal Products
- Histamine II Receptor Antagonists
- Hyperpigmentation Products
- Miscellaneous Mineral Products
- Oral Rehydration Products
- Ostomy Appliances
- Smoking Cessation Products
- Sore Throat Products
- Topical Antifungal Products
- Topical Fluoride Products
- Vaginal Antifungal Products
- Vitamin Products

Product Table Features

Some features of the product tables, such as the ingredient/formulation codes and the use of bullets and other codes, pertain to the characteristics or presentation of the product ingredient information. Other features serve as links between the product tables and the *Handbook* chapters.

Ingredient and Formulation Codes

The ingredient and formulation codes, which appear to the left of a product trade name, have been rated as "extremely useful" by past users of the product information. These codes provide guidance in selecting products for patients with special needs. The codes and their definitions are as follows:

AL = alcohol free
AF = aspirin free
CA = caffeine free
CO = cholesterol free
DY = dye free
FL = fluoride free
FR = fragrance free
GL = gluten free
LA = lactose free
PR = preservative free
PU = purine free
SO = dietetically sodium free
SL = sulfite free
SU = dietetically *sucrose* free (product may contain other sugars or artificial sweeteners)
GE = geriatric formulation
PE = pediatric formulation

These codes are supplied by the manufacturers and are not necessarily comprehensive. Because this information could not be independently verified, readers should use the codes only as a guide to help them locate products that might meet special needs. Further, product formulations change frequently; therefore, pharmacists and patients should always carefully check the ingredients listed on product packages.

Other Codes

**** = New listing**
This code, which also appears to the left of an applicable product trade name, designates products that were not listed in the *Handbook of Nonprescription Drug Product Updates* or in previous editions of the *Handbook of Nonprescription Drugs*. These products can be either new to the marketplace or new to the OTC Product Database.

· = Bullet
This graphic symbol serves to separate the ingredients listed for each product.

Blank column = No information supplied
If a column for a particular product contains no data, the product may not contain the ingredient(s) pertinent to that column, or the manufacturer may have chosen not to provide the information. In the case of the column Other Ingredients, a blank column usually means the manufacturer did not provide the information.

Cross-References to the *Handbook*

To allow *Handbook* users quick access to the product information, the tables are grouped and ordered according to the chapter discussions of the product ingredients and their therapeutic uses. Each product table contains a cross-reference to the *Handbook* chapter that discusses the product ingredients in detail.

Multisource Products

For a small number of products, the manufacturer/supplier is listed as "Multisource." This term is commonly used to designate generic or store-brand versions of trade-name products, which are available from many manufacturers/suppliers. Because of the numerous generic products available, multisource listings in this publication have been limited to products whose dosage forms or strengths differ from those of trade-name products and to widely used products for which no trade-name product is available (e.g., Ipecac, Magnesium Salicylate).

Scope

Formulations & Features presents a broad range of products in each therapeutic category, including national as well as regional products. The numerous products available in some categories preclude listing every product submitted by manufacturers. If a large number of products are available for a particular category, a representative sampling of the dosage forms, strengths, flavors, etc., is presented.

Data Accuracy and Completeness

Every effort has been made to ensure that product data are as accurate and complete as possible. The scope of the product tables, however, makes it impossible to verify all information independently. Some manufacturers listed all ingredient information for their products, whereas others concentrated on providing information for only active or significant ingredients. Pharmacists and patients are encouraged to also check product packages for ingredient information.

New Listings

The 875 products classified here as "new listings" fall into one of the following three categories:

- Products new to the market since publication of the *Handbook of Nonprescription Drugs Product Updates*;
- Existing products not recently, or never before, listed in the *Handbook of Nonprescription Drugs*;
- New dosage forms of products that became available after publication of the *Product Updates*.

Note: Some brand names of phytomedicinal products include the total weight of the solid dosage forms, not the weight of the active ingredients alone.

A and D Medicated Powder
Schering-Plough HealthCare

A-200 Lice Control for Dogs and Household aerosol spray
Hogil Pharmaceutical

A-200 Lice Killing gel
Hogil Pharmaceutical

A-200 Lice Treatment Kit shampoo/aerosol spray
Hogil Pharmaceutical

A-D_3-E with Selenium Tablets
Freeda Vitamins

Accu-Chek III
Boehringer Mannheim

Accu-Chek Instant
Boehringer Mannheim

Acerola Chewable Tablet
Goldline Labs

Acetaminophen Suspension, Children's Flavored drops
Multisource

Acid-X tablet
BDI Pharmaceuticals

Acne Treatment Cleanser liquid
C&M Pharmacal

Acne Treatment Wash liquid
C&M Pharmacal

Acne Treatment, Tinted lotion
C&M Pharmacal

Acne Treatment, Vanishing lotion
C&M Pharmacal

Actidose with Sorbitol liquid
Paddock Labs

Actidose-Aqua liquid
Paddock Labs

Active Life Drainable Pouches with Stomahesive Skin Barrier
ConvaTec

Actron caplet/tablet
Bayer Consumer

Adhesive Drainable Pouches
Hollister

Adsorbonac solution
Alcon Labs

Advanced Stress Formula Plus Zinc Tablets
Sundown

Advanced Stress Formula, with or without Iron, Tablets
Sundown

Advil gel caplet
Whitehall-Robins Healthcare

Aim Extra Strength gel
Chesebrough-Pond's

AK-NaCl ointment/solution
Akorn

Alcon Enzymatic Cleaner tablet
Alcon Labs

Alka-Seltzer Anti-Gas gelcap
Bayer Consumer

Alka-Seltzer caplet
Bayer Consumer

Alka-Seltzer gelcap
Bayer Consumer

Alka-Seltzer Plus Flu & Body Aches effervescent tablet
Bayer Consumer

Alka-Seltzer Plus Flu & Body Aches Liqui-Gels
Bayer Consumer

Aller-med caplet
Republic Drug

Alpha Glow Body Care lotion
Fischer Pharmaceuticals

ALternaGEL liquid
Johnson & Johnson·Merck

AMBI 10 Acne Medication cream
Kiwi

AMBI 10 Acne Pads
Kiwi

Ambi Cocoa Butter cream
Kiwi

Ambi Skin Discoloration Fade Cream, Dry Skin
Kiwi

Ambi Skin Discoloration Fade Cream, Normal Skin
Kiwi

Ambi Skin Discoloration Fade Cream, Oily Skin
Kiwi

Amin-Aid Instant Drink individual packet
R&D Labs

Anacin caplet
Whitehall-Robins Healthcare

Androvite for Men Tablets
Optimox

Anusol suppository
Warner Wellcome Consumer

Apatate Liquid or Tablets
Kenwood Labs

Apatate with Fluoride Liquid
Kenwood Labs

Aquanil HC lotion
Person & Covey

Aquaray lotion
Harold Pharmacal

Arm & Hammer Pure Baking Soda powder
Church & Dwight

Assess Low Range
HealthScan

Assess Standard Range
HealthScan

Asian Ginseng Complex tablet
Shaklee

Attends Briefs pad
Procter & Gamble

Attends Guards pad
Procter & Gamble

Attends Pads
Procter & Gamble

Attends Undergarments pad
Procter & Gamble

Auto-Lancet
Palco Labs

Autoject
Owen Mumford

Autoject 2
Owen Mumford

Autoject Mini
Owen Mumford

Autolet Lite
Owen Mumford

Autopen
Owen Mumford

Avanti polyurethane
London International U.S. Holdings

Avanti Super Thin polyurethane
London International U.S. Holdings

Aveeno Gentle Skin Cleanser lotion
Rydelle Labs

Aveeno Medicated Cleanser liquid
Rydelle Labs

Axid AR tablet
Whitehall-Robins Healthcare

Ayr Saline gel
B.F. Ascher

Azo-Dine tablet
Republic Drug

B 100 "11" B Factors Tablets or Timed-Release Tablets
Sundown

B 100% RDA Complex Tablets
Sundown

B 150 "11" B Factors Timed-Release Tablets
Sundown

B 50 "11" B Factors Tablets
Sundown

B 50 Complex Capsules or Tablets
Sundown

B Complex Maxi Softgels
Sundown

B Complex Maxi Tablets
Sundown

B Complex Tablets
Sundown

B Complex with C Tablets
Sundown

B-C Complex Capsules
Sundown

B-D Home Sharps Container
Becton Dickinson Consumer

B-D Lancet Device
Becton Dickinson Consumer

Baby Sunblock lotion
Goldline Labs

Bain de Soleil Mega Tan lotion
Pfizer Consumer

Bain de Soleil Orange Gelee lotion
Pfizer Consumer

Bain de Soleil Sand Buster lotion
Pfizer Consumer

Bain de Soleil Tropical Deluxe Tanning lotion
Pfizer Consumer

Banana Boat Faces Plus Sunblock, Normal/Combination Skin lotion
Sun Pharmaceuticals

Banana Boat Faces Plus Sunscreen, Normal to Oily Skin lotion
Sun Pharmaceuticals

Banana Boat Sooth-A-Caine gel
Sun Pharmaceuticals

Bayer PM Extra Strength caplet
Bayer Consumer

Beano drops
AkPharma

Beano tablet
AkPharma

Benadryl Allergy chewable tablet
Warner Wellcome Consumer

Benadryl Allergy Decongestant tablet
Warner Wellcome Consumer

Benadryl Allergy Dye-Free Liqui-gels softgel
Warner Wellcome Consumer

Benadryl Allergy/Sinus/ Headache Formula caplet
Warner Wellcome Consumer

Benadryl Itch Stopping Extra Strength gel
Warner Wellcome Consumer

Benadryl Itch Stopping Extra Strength stick
Warner Wellcome Consumer

Benadryl Itch Stopping Regular Strength cream
Warner Wellcome Consumer

Benadryl Itch Stopping Regular Strength gel
Warner Wellcome Consumer

Benadryl Itch Stopping Regular Strength spray
Warner Wellcome Consumer

Beta Carotene Softgels
Sundown

Betadine First Aid Antibiotics + Moisturizer ointment
Purdue Frederick

Bilberry 40 mg capsule
Herbal Choice-Botalia

Bilberry Extract 50 mg tablet
Source Natural

Bilberry Extract 80 mg capsule
PhytoPharmica

Bilberry-Power 440 mg capsule
Nature's Herbs

Bisacodyl, Enteric Coated tablet
Paddock Labs

Blairex Sterile Contact Lens Cleaner liquid
Blairex Labs

Blairex Sterile Contact Lens Conditioning Solution
Blairex Labs

Blanchard Karaya Wafers
Blanchard

Blistex DCT Daily Conditioning Treatment for Lips cream
Blistex

Blistex Lip Tone Lip Balm stick
Blistex

Blue Star ointment
McCue

Boost liquid
Mead Johnson Nutritionals

Boston Advance Comfort Formula Conditioning Solution
Polymer Technology

Boston Simplicity solution
Polymer Technology

Bronkaid Mist Suspension oral inhaler
Bayer Consumer

Buffered C Tablets
Sundown

Bull Frog Quik gel
Chattem

C Chewable Tablets
Sundown

C Color Free or Regular Timed-Release Capsules
Sundown

C Plus Tablets
Sundown

C Rolla Chewable Tablets
Sundown

C Tablets
Sundown

C Timed-Release Tablets
Sundown

C Vitamin Tablets
Freeda Vitamins

C Vitamin Timed-Release Tablets
Freeda Vitamins

C with Rose Hips Chewable Tablets
Sundown

Calamycin pump spray
Pfeiffer Pharmaceuticals

Calcet Plus Tablets
Mission Pharmacal

Calci-Caps tablet
Nion Labs

Calci-Caps with Iron tablet
Nion Labs

Calcium and Magnesium tablet
Sundown

Calcium Complex chewable tablet
Shaklee

Calcium Complex tablet
Shaklee

Calcium Magnesium tablet
Shaklee

Calcium tablet
Sundown

Calcium with Vitamin D tablet
Sundown

Calcium, Magnesium, and Zinc tablet
Sundown

Calel-D tablet
Rhône-Poulenc Rorer Pharmaceuticals

Caltrate 600 + D tablet
Lederle Consumer

Caltrate 600 tablet
Lederle Consumer

Caltrate Plus tablet
Lederle Consumer

Caltrate Plus, Assorted Fruit or Spearmint chewable tablet
Lederle Consumer

Carelet Safety
Gainor Medical

Carmex Lip Balm ointment
Carma Labs

Carmol 20 lotion
Doak Dermatologics

Carnation Alsoy concentrate powder, ready-to-feed
Carnation Nutritional

Carnation Follow-Up Soy powder
Carnation Nutritional

Castellani Paint, Modified liquid
Pedinol Pharmacal

Cayenne 450 mg capsule
Nature's Resource

Cayenne Extract tincture
Herb Pharm

Cecon Solution
Abbott Labs

Cepacol Maximum Strength, Mint lozenge
J. B. Williams

Cepacol Sore Throat, Cherry lozenge
J. B. Williams

Cepacol Sore Throat, Mint lozenge
J. B. Williams

Cetaphil Moisturizing Cream
Galderma Labs

Cetaphil Moisturizing Lotion liquid
Galderma Labs

ChapStick Lip Moisturizer ointment/stick
Whitehall-Robins Healthcare

ChapStick Ultra stick
Whitehall-Robins Healthcare

CharcoAid 2000 suspension
Requa

CharcoAid suspension
Requa

Charcoal Plus DS tablet
Kramer Labs

Chemstrip 2LN strip
Boehringer Mannheim

Chemstrip 4 the OB strip
Boehringer Mannheim

Chemstrip 6 strip
Boehringer Mannheim

Chemstrip 7 strip
Boehringer Mannheim

Choice dm liquid
Mead Johnson Nutritionals

CholesTrak
ChemTrak

Chromium Picolinate tablet
Mericon

Chromium Picolinate tablet
Sundown

Chromium, Organic tablet
Freeda Vitamins

Circus Chews Complete Chewable Tablets
Sundown

Circus Chews with Beta Carotene Chewable Tablets
Sundown

Circus Chews with Calcium Chewable Tablets
Sundown

Circus Chews with Extra Vitamin C Tablets
Sundown

Circus Chews with Iron
Sundown

Citracal + D caplet
Mission Pharmacal

Citrucel Sugar Free powder
SmithKline Beecham

Class Act Sensitive latex
Carter Products

Clean & Clear Invisible Blemish Treatment gel
Johnson & Johnson Consumer

Clean & Clear Invisible Blemish Treatment, Sensitive Skin gel
Johnson & Johnson Consumer

Clean & Clear Oil Controlling Astringent liquid
Johnson & Johnson Consumer

Clean & Clear Oil Controlling Astringent Sensitive Skin liquid
Johnson & Johnson Consumer

Clean & Clear Persa-Gel Extra Strength gel
Johnson & Johnson Consumer

Clean & Clear Persa-Gel Maximum Strength gel
Johnson & Johnson Consumer

Clear Cough Night Time liquid
Vetco

CareCard Medical Card
CareCard

Closed-End Adhesive Pouches
Bard

Codimal tablet
Central Pharmaceuticals

Cola syrup
Unico

Colgate Baking Soda & Peroxide Tartar Control paste
Colgate-Palmolive

ColoCARE
Helena Labs

Cool Comfort Nu-Support Belts
Nu-Hope

Coppertone Kids Sunblock lotion
Schering-Plough HealthCare

Coppertone Oil-Free Sunblock lotion
Schering-Plough HealthCare

Coppertone Protect and Tan lotion
Schering-Plough HealthCare

Coppertone Skin Selects Dry Skin Sunblock lotion
Schering-Plough HealthCare

Coppertone Skin Selects Oily Skin Sunblock lotion
Schering-Plough HealthCare

Coppertone Skin Selects Sensitive Skin Sunblock lotion
Schering-Plough HealthCare

Coricidin Cough & Cold tablet
Schering-Plough HealthCare

Correctol caplet/tablet
Schering-Plough HealthCare

Correctol Herbal Tea, Honey Lemon or Cinnamon Spice liquid
Schering-Plough HealthCare

Cortaid FastStick
Pharmacia & Upjohn

Cranberry Extract 400 mg capsule
Herbal Choice-Botalia

Creamy Dandruff Shampoo
C&M Pharmacal

Creomulsion Complete syrup
Summit

Creomulsion Cough Medicine syrup
Summit

Creomulsion for Children syrup
Summit

Creomulsion Pediatric syrup
Summit

Crest Gum Care gel/paste
Procter & Gamble

Curél Nutrient Rich Severe Dry Skin lotion
Bausch & Lomb

Cushion Grip gel
Schering-Plough HealthCare

Cutter Pleasant Protection pump spray
Spectrum

Cutter with Sunscreen lotion
Spectrum

Cystex tablet
Numark Labs

D-alpha Tocopherol Softgels
Sundown

Daily Diabetic's Case
Medport

Daily Multiple Vitamins & Minerals Tablets
Sundown

Daily Multiple Vitamins, with or without Iron, Tablets
Sundown

Dairy Ease caplet
Blistex

Dairy Ease chewable tablet
Blistex

Dairy Ease drops
Blistex

Dandruff Shampoo Maximum Strength
C&M Pharmacal

Dandruff Wash, Medicated cream
C&M Pharmacal

DayGel liquid-cap
Republic Drug

Delazinc ointment
Mericon

DentSure Denture Rinse, Peppermint liquid
Pfizer Consumer

Depend Fitted Briefs pad
Kimberly-Clark

Depend Guards for Men pad
Kimberly-Clark

Depend Poise Guards pad
Kimberly-Clark

Depend Poise pad
Kimberly-Clark

Depend Poise Shields pad
Kimberly-Clark

Depend Undergarments pad
Kimberly-Clark

Dermal Therapy Extra Strength Body lotion
Bayer Diagnostics

Desenex AF aerosol spray powder
Ciba Self-Medication

Desenex AF cream
Ciba Self-Medication

Desenex AF Spray Liquid aerosol spray
Ciba Self-Medication

DHS Sal liquid
Person & Covey

Diabetic's Travel Organizer
Medport

Diabetic's Traveler and Diabetic's Traveler II
Entry 21

Diabetic's Wallet
Medport

Diabetes Works
ITA Software

Diabetic Tussin Cough Drops, Cherry tablet
Health Care Products

Diabetic Tussin Cough Drops, Menthol-Eucalyptus tablet
Health Care Products

Diabetic Tussin DM Maximum Strength syrup
Health Care Products

DiabetiSource liquid
Sandoz Nutrition

Diabe-tuss DM syrup
Paddock Labs

DiabeVite Tablets
R&D Labs

Dia-Pak Jr.
Atwater Carey

Dia-Pak Mini
Atwater Carey

Dia-Pak Original
Atwater Carey

Diascan Partner
Home Diagnostics

DiaVite Plus Caplets
Jordan Medical

Dickinson's Witch Hazel Formula liquid
E.E. Dickinson

Digi-Voice Deluxe and Mini-DV
Science Products

Dimetapp Allergy Sinus caplet
Whitehall-Robins Healthcare

Dimetapp Allergy, Children's elixir
Whitehall-Robins Healthcare

Dimetapp Cold & Fever, Children's suspension
Whitehall-Robins Healthcare

Diphenylin Cough syrup
Schein Pharmaceutical

Diurex MPR caplet
Alva-Amco Pharmacal

Diurex PMS caplet
Alva-Amco Pharmacal

DK Organizer
Cases Plus

DML Lotion
Person & Covey

Doan's P.M. Extra Strength caplet
Ciba Self-Medication

Docusate Sodium softgel
Schein Pharmaceutical

Dr. Scholl's Advanced Pain Relief Callus Removers disc
Schering-Plough HealthCare

Dr. Scholl's One Step Callus Remover disc
Schering-Plough HealthCare

Dr. Tichenor's Antiseptic liquid
Dr. G.H.Tichenor

Dr. Tichenor's Antiseptic liquid
Dr. G.H.Tichenor

Dr. Tichenor's Toothpaste
Dr. G.H.Tichenor

Drainable Adhesive Pouches
Bard

Dri-Ear drops
Pfeiffer Pharmaceuticals

Dristan Cold & Cough Liqui-Gels softgel
Whitehall-Robins Healthcare

Duadacin capsule
Kenwood Labs

DuraScreen lotion
Schwarz Pharma

DuraScreen lotion
Schwarz Pharma

Dynafed Jr. tablet
BDI Pharmaceuticals

Dynafed Pseudo tablet
BDI Pharmaceuticals

E-Z Let
Palco Labs

early Pregancy test
Selfcare

EchinaCare tincture
PhytoPharmica

Echinacea 125 mg capsule
Herbal Choice-Botalia

Echinacea Complex tablet
Shaklee

Echinacea Extract 125 mg capsule
Botalia Gold

Echinacea-Power 550 mg capsule
Nature's Herbs

EchinaGuard 355 mg capsule
Nature's Way

Efamol Evening Primrose Oil 500 mg capsule
Nature's Way

Efferdent Plus tablet
Warner Wellcome Consumer

Efidac 24 Chlorpheniramine timed-release tablet
Ciba Self-Medication

Eldopaque cream
ICN Pharmaceuticals

Eldoquin cream
ICN Pharmaceuticals

Enfamil Next Step concentrate, powder, ready-to-feed
Mead Johnson Nutritionals

Enfamil Next Step Soy concentrate
Mead Johnson Nutritionals

Enfamil Next Step Soy powder
Mead Johnson Nutritionals

Ensure High Protein liquid
Ross Products/Abbott Labs

Ensure Light liquid
Ross Products/Abbott Labs

Esotérica Facial Formula with Sunscreens cream
Medicis

Esotérica Regular Formula cream
Medicis

ExACT Adult Medication cream
APS/Premier

ExACT Pore Treatment gel
APS/Premier

Excedrin Aspirin Free geltab
Bristol-Myers Products

Excedrin Extra Strength geltab
Bristol-Myers Products

Exfoliating Astringent for Oily Skin liquid
C&M Pharmacal

EyeSed drops
Scherer Labs

EyeSine drops
Akorn

Eyetamins Tablets
Sundown

EZ-LH
Biomerica

Facial Hydrating Fluid, Oil Free lotion
C&M Pharmacal

Facial Hydrating Gel, Oil Free gel
C&M Pharmacal

Facial Moisturizing Sunscreen cream
C&M Pharmacal

Family Medic Afterburn gel
Tender

Fe-50 Extended Release caplet
Northampton Medical

Feen-A-Mint tablet
Schering-Plough HealthCare

Fem-1 tablet
BDI Pharmaceuticals

Femaprin-Vitex 290 mg capsule
Nature's Way

Feminique Douche, Baby Powder or Spring Fresh Scent liquid
Quality Health

Feminique Douche, Extra Cleansing liquid
Quality Health

Feminique Douche, Natural Vinegar & Water liquid
Quality Health

Feminique Feminine Cloth Towelettes wipe
Quality Health

Femiron Daily Iron Supplement tablet
Menley & James Labs

Femizole-7 cream
Lake Consumer

Femstat 3 cream
Procter & Gamble

Ferrous Gluconate tablet
Upsher-Smith Labs

Ferrous Gluconate tablet
Sundown

Ferrous Sulfate tablet
Sundown

Ferrous Sulfate timed-release capsule
Sundown

Feverall Adult Strength suppository
Upsher-Smith Labs

Feverfew 125 mg capsule
Herbal Choice-Botalia

Feverfew Extract tincture
Herb Pharm

First Aid Cream
Johnson & Johnson Consumer

First Aid Medicated Powder
Johnson & Johnson Consumer

1st Sneeze tincture
Trout Lake Farm

Fish Liver Oil Softgels
Sundown

Fleet Magnesium Citrate Prep Kit 4 powder/suppository/tablet
C.B. Fleet

Fleet Magnesium Citrate Prep Kit 5 enema/powder/tablet
C.B. Fleet

Fleet Magnesium Citrate Prep Kit 6 enema/powder/tablet
C.B. Fleet

Fleet Pain-Relief pad
C.B. Fleet

Florammune tincture
Flora Laboratories

Florased tincture
Flora Laboratories

Formula for Life Tablets
Sundown

Fortel Plus
Biomerica

Fosfree Tablets
Mission Pharmacal

Fourex animal membrane
London International U.S. Holdings

Fruit C Chewable Tablets
Freeda Vitamins

Full Body Sunscreen lotion
C&M Pharmacal

Fungoid Tincture solution
Pedinol Pharmacal

Garlic 300 mg capsule
Herbal Choice-Botalia

Garlic tablet
Shaklee

Garlicin Enteric Coated 550 mg tablet
Nature's Way

Garlique Enteric Coated 400 mg tablet
Sunsource

Garlitrin 4000 Enteric Coated 320 mg tablet
PhytoPharmica

Gas-X Extra Strength softgel
Sandoz Consumer

Gaviscon Liquid suspension
SmithKline Beecham

Genasyme chewable tablet
Goldline Labs

Genasyme drops
Goldline Labs

GenTeal Lubricant drops
CIBA Vision Ophthalmics

Gentle-let 1
Ulster Scientific

Gentle-let, GP style
Ulster Scientific

Gentle-let-PC
Ulster Scientific

Ginger 250 mg capsule
Herbal Choice-Botalia

Ginger Extract tincture
Herb Pharm

Ginger Root 550 mg capsule
Nature's Resource

Ginkgo 60 mg capsule
Herbal Choice-Botalia

Ginkgo Biloba 30 mg tablet
Hudson

Ginkgo Biloba 360 mg capsule
Thompson Medical

Ginkgo Biloba Extract 420 mg capsule
NaturaLife

Ginkgo Biloba Extract 60 mg capsule
Botalia Gold

Ginkgo Biloba Leaf Extract 40 mg capsule
Nature's Resource

Ginkgo Extract tincture
Herb Pharm

Ginkgo Phytosome 80 mg capsule
PhytoPharmica

Ginkgold 260 mg tablet
Nature's Way

Ginkgolidin 40 mg capsule
PhytoPharmica

Ginsai 100 mg capsule
Lichtwer

Ginsana 100 mg capsule
Sunsource

Ginseng Root - Korean White 560 mg capsule
Nature's Resource

Ginseng-7 100 mg capsule
Herbal Choice-Botalia

Ginsun 324 mg softgel
Nature's Way

Goldware Jewelry
Goldware

Glandosane Mouth Moisturizer, Lemon Mint, or Unflavored aerosol spray
Kenwood Labs

Glover's Dandruff Control Medicine liquid
J. K. Pharmaceuticals

Glover's Medicated Dandruff Soap cleansing bar
J. K. Pharmaceuticals

Glover's Medicated for Dandruff ointment
J. K. Pharmaceuticals

Glover's Medicated shampoo
J. K. Pharmaceuticals

Glucofilm strip
Bayer Diagnostics

Glucometer M+
Bayer Diagnostics

Glucotrac
Kaufman Associates

Glutofac Caplets
Kenwood Labs

Gordofilm solution
Gordon Labs

Grape Seed Extract 25 mg tablet
Herbal Choice-Botalia

Halls Juniors Sugar Free Cough Drops, Grape or Orange lozenge
Warner-Lambert

Halls Vitamin C Lozenges
Warner-Lambert

Hawaiian Tropic Facial Sunblock lotion
Hawaiian Tropic

Hawaiian Tropic Tan Amplifier gel
Hawaiian Tropic

Hawthorn HC 160 mg softgel
Nature's Way

Heartline tablet
BDI Pharmaceuticals

Hemalet
Home Diagnostics

Hemaspan tablet
Bock Pharmacal

Hemorid for Women ointment
Thompson Medical

Hepacolin Capsules
Kenwood Labs

Herbal-Menthol lozenge
Shaklee

Herpalieve cream
PhytoPharmica

Hydrosal Hemorrhoidal ointment
Hydrosal

Hydrosal ointment
Hydrosal

Hypericum Extract 300 mg capsule
PhytoPharmica

Hytone cream
Dermik Labs

Hytone lotion
Dermik Labs

I.L.X. B_{12} Caplets
Kenwood Labs

I.L.X. B_{12} elixir
Kenwood Labs

I.L.X. B_{12} Sugar Free Elixir
Kenwood Labs

I.L.X. Elixir
Kenwood Labs

ICAPS Plus Tablets
Ciba Vision

ICAPS Timed-Release Tablets
Ciba Vision

Icy Hot Chill Stick
Chattem

Icy Hot cream
Chattem

Identifind Iron-on Labels
Identifind

Impact 1.5 liquid
Sandoz Nutrition

Infalyte
Mead Johnson Nutritionals

Insul-eze
Palco Labs

Insul-Tote
Palco Labs

Insul-Tote Junior
Palco Labs

Ipecac syrup
Multisource

Ipsatol syrup
Kenwood Labs

Ircon FA tablet
Kenwood Labs

Ircon tablet
Kenwood Labs

Iromin-G Tablets
Mission Pharmacal

Iron Plus Vitamin C tablet
Shaklee

IsoSource 1.5 liquid
Sandoz Nutrition

IsoSource VHN liquid
Sandoz Nutrition

Jergens Advanced Therapy Dry Skin Care lotion
Andrew Jergens

Jergens Advanced Therapy Dual Healing cream
Andrew Jergens

Jergens Advanced Therapy Ultra Healing, Regular or Fragrance Free lotion
Andrew Jergens

Johnson's Baby, Medicated powder
Johnson & Johnson Consumer

Johnson's Odor-Eaters aerosol spray powder
Johnson & Johnson Consumer

Johnson's Ultra Sensitive Baby Cream
Johnson & Johnson Consumer

Johnson's Ultra Sensitive Baby Lotion
Johnson & Johnson Consumer

Karaya Seal Drainable Pouches
Hollister

Kenwood Therapeutic Liquid
Kenwood Labs

Kindercal ready-to-feed
Mead Johnson Nutritionals

Korean White Ginseng 560 mg capsule
NaturaLife

Koromex Inserts suppository
Quality Health

Kwai Coated 100 mg tablet
Lichtwer

Lacri-Lube N.P. ointment
Allergan

Lacri-Lube S.O.P. ointment
Allergan

Lactaid caplet
McNeil Consumer

Lactaid drops
McNeil Consumer

Lactaid Extra Strength caplet
McNeil Consumer

Lactrase capsule
Schwarz Pharm

Lady Lite
Medicore

Lanaphilic ointment
Medco Lab

Lantiseptic Skin Protectant ointment
Summit

Lantiseptic Therapeutic cream
Summit

Legatrin PM caplet
Columbia Labs

Level
HealthWare

Licetrol shampoo
Republic Drug

Liqui Char liquid
Jones Medical

Liqui-Lea Liquid
Shaklee

Liquid Calcium + D softgel
Sundown

Listerine Toothpaste, Cool Mint gel
Warner Wellcome Consumer

Listerine Toothpaste, Cool Mint paste
Warner Wellcome Consumer

Listermint Mouthrinse liquid
Warner Wellcome Consumer

Little Noses Decongestant nasal drops
Vetco

Little Ones Active Life Drainable Pouch
ConvaTec

Little Ones Sur-Fit Drainable Pouch
ConvaTec

Little Teethers Oral Pain Relief gel
Vetco

Load-Matic
Palco Labs

Lobana Derm-ADE cream
Lobana Labs

Lobana Peri-Gard ointment
Lobana Labs

Lubricating Hand and Body cream
C&M Pharmacal

Luden's Maximum Strength Sugar Free, Cherry lozenge
Hershey

Luden's Maximum Strength, Cherry lozenge
Hershey

Luden's Maximum Strength, Menthol Eucalyptus lozenge
Hershey

Luden's Original Menthol lozenge
Hershey

Maalox Antacid Plus Anti-Gas Extra Strength tablet
Ciba Self-Medication

Maalox suspension
Ciba Self-Medication

Mag/Cal Mega tablet
Freeda Vitamins

Magnesium Salicylate caplet
Multisource

Manganese tablet
Sundown

Manganese tablet
Freeda Vitamins

Marshall Model 82 Manual Inflation B.P. Monitor
Omron

Marshall Model 92 Automatic Inflation B.P. Monitor
Omron

Mature Complete Tablets
Sundown

Maxilube jelly
Mission Pharmacal

Medic Alert Jewelry
Medic Alert

MediCheck Identification
MediCheck

Med-I-Dent Jewelry
Med-I-Dent

Medi-Lance II
Medicore

MedMaster
Generation Software

Mega Mineral tablet
Sundown

Melatonex timed-release tablet
Sunsource

Melatonin tablet
Hudson

Mellitus Manager
MetaMedix

Men's Multi Iron Free Tablets
Sundown

Mentadent Gum Care gel/paste
Chesebrough-Pond's

Mentadent Mouthwash, Cool Mint or Fresh Mint liquid
Chesebrough-Pond's

Mentadent Tartar Control gel/paste
Chesebrough-Pond's

Menthacin cream
Mentholatum

Mentholatum Lipbalm, Cherry Ice stick
Mentholatum

Metamucil Original Texture, Orange powder
Procter & Gamble

Metamucil Smooth Texture; Sugar Free, Citrus or Orange powder
Procter & Gamble

MG217 for Psoriasis Sal-Acid ointment
Triton Consumer

Midol PMS Maximum Strength Multisymptom Formula gelcap
Bayer Consumer

Milk of Magnesia suspension
Schein Pharmaceutical

Milk Thistle 100 mg capsule
Herbal Choice-Botalia

Milk Thistle 310 mg capsule
NaturaLife

Milk Thistle Extract tincture
Herb Pharm

Milk-Thistle Power 535 mg capsule
Nature's Herbs

Mini-Wright Low Range
Clement Clarke

Mini-Wright Standard Range
Clement Clarke

Minoxidil Topical Solution
Bausch & Lomb Pharmaceutical

Minoxidil Topical Solution
Lemmon

Minoxidil Topical Solution
Barre-National

Mirasept Step 1 solution
Alcon Labs

Mirasept Step 2 solution
Alcon Labs

Mission Prenatal F.A. Tablets
Mission Pharmacal

Mission Prenatal H.P. Tablets
Mission Pharmacal

Mission Prenatal Tablets
Mission Pharmacal

Moisturizing Lotion
C&M Pharmacal

Monistat 7 Prefilled Applicators cream
Advanced Care

Mosco-Cain liquid
Medtech Labs

Motrin, Children's suspension
McNeil Consumer

Muro 128 ointment
Bausch & Lomb

Muro 128 solution
Bausch & Lomb

MygraFew 152 mg tablet
Nature's Way

Mylanta Double Strength chewable tablet
Johnson & Johnson·Merck

Mylanta Gas Relief gelcap
Johnson & Johnson·Merck

Mylanta gelcap
Johnson & Johnson·Merck

Mylanta Regular Strength chewable tablet
Johnson & Johnson·Merck

Nasal-D tablet
Shaklee

Natrapel lotion/pump spray
Tender

Natural Cranberry Concentrate softgel
Herbal Harvest

Natural Feverfew 380 mg capsule
Herbal Harvest

Natural Korean Ginseng 500 mg capsule
Herbal Harvest

Natural White paste
Natural White

Natural White Tartar Control paste
Natural White

Naturalyte, Bubblegum or Unflavored liquid
Unico

Naturalyte, Fruit Flavored or Grape liquid
Unico

Neo-Synephrine Extra Moisturizing 12-Hour nasal spray
Bayer Consumer

Neoloid oil
Kenwood Labs

Nicorette DS gum
SmithKline Beecham

Nicorette gum
SmithKline Beecham

Nimbus Quick Strip
Biomerica

NiteGel liquid-cap
Republic Drug

Noncomedogenic Facial Moisturizing Cream
C&M Pharmacal

Nose Better spray
Lee Pharmaceuticals

NovoPen1.5
Novo Nordisk Pharmaceuticals

Nudit Fade Cream
Medtech Labs

Nu-Flex Adult Oval or Round Drainable Pouches
Nu-Hope

Nu-Flex Adult Oval or Round Urinary Pouches
Nu-Hope

Nu-Flex Brief or Mini Urinary Pouches
Nu-Hope

Nu-Self Adult or Brief Drainable Pouches
Nu-Hope

Nutra Start liquid
Advanced Nutrition Foods

NutraVescent Calcium effervescent tablet
Northampton Medical

OcuHist drops
Pfizer Consumer

Off! Skintastic for Kids pump spray
S. C. Johnson

Off! Deep Woods for Maximum Protection pump spray
S. C. Johnson

Off! Deep Woods Formula for Sportsmen aerosol spray
S. C. Johnson

Omron Model HEM-412C Manual Inflation B.P. Monitor
Omron

Omron Model HEM-601 Wrist B.P. Monitor
Omron

Omron Model HEM-602 Wrist B.P. Monitor with Memory
Omron

Omron Model HEM-605 Compact Wrist B.P. Monitor
Omron

Omron Model HEM-703CP Measurement Print-out B.P. Monitor
Omron

Omron Model HEM-704C Self-Storing B.P. Monitor
Omron

Omron Model HEM-705CP Memory, Print-out, and Graph B.P. Monitor
Omron

Omron Model HEM-706 Fuzzy Logic B.P. Monitor
Omron

Omron Model HEM-711 Smart-Inflate B.P. Monitor with Fuzzy Logic
Omron

Omron Model HEM-712C Automatic Inflation B.P. Monitor
Omron

Omron Model HEM-806F Deluxe Finger B.P. Monitor
Omron

Omron Model HEM-808F Travel Finger B.P. Monitor
Omron

Omron Model HEM-815F Finger B.P. Monitor
Omron

One Touch Profile
LifeScan

One-A-Day Calcium Plus chewable tablet
Bayer Consumer

One-A-Day Extras Garlic 600 mg softgel
Bayer Consumer

Opti-Free Express liquid
Alcon Labs

Opti-Soak Conditioning solution
Alcon Labs

Opti-Soak Daily Cleaner liquid
Alcon Labs

Opti-Soak Soothing drops
Alcon Labs

Optimox Prenatal Tablets
Optimox

Optimum Bilberry 300 mg capsule
Nature's Way

Optimum Cranberry 530 mg capsule
Nature's Way

Oragesic solution
Parnell Pharmaceuticals

Orajel Baby Tooth & Gum Cleanser gel
Del Pharmaceuticals

Orajel CoverMed, Tinted Light or Medium cream
Del Pharmaceuticals

Orazinc 110 tablet
Mericon

Orazinc 220 capsule
Mericon

Ornex Maximum Strength caplet
Menley & James Labs

Ornex Regular Strength caplet
Menley & James Labs

Orudis KT caplet/tablet
Whitehall-Robins Healthcare

Os-Cal 500 tablet
SmithKline Beecham

Os-Cal Fortified Tablets
SmithKline Beecham

Ostiderm paste
Pedinol Pharmacal

Ostiderm Roll-on lotion
Pedinol Pharmacal

Oxi-Freeda Tablets
Freeda Vitamins

Oyster Shell Calcium tablet
Sundown

Oyster Shell Calcium with Vitamin D tablet
Sundown

Pain Doctor cream
E. Fougera

PainBreak cream
Stevens Skin

Palmer's Skin Success cream
E.T. Browne

Palmitate-A 5,000 Tablets
Akorn

Palmitate-A Tablets
Akorn

Panax Ginseng Extract 100 mg capsule
Botalia Gold

Panaxin 100 mg capsule
PhytoPharmica

Parvacal tablet
Freeda Vitamins

PCO Phytosome 50 mg tablet
PhytoPharmica

Pedi-Pro powder
Pedinol Pharmacal

PediaCare Infants' Decongestant Plus Cough drops
McNeil Consumer

Pedialyte
Ross Products/Abbott Labs

PediApap solution
Central Pharmaceuticals

Pepcid AC tablet
Johnson & Johnson·Merck

Pepto-Bismol caplet
Procter & Gamble

Perfect Antioxidant Caplet
Sundown

Perfect Iron tablet
Sundown

Permathene Maximum Strength Chromium Picolinate softgel
CCA Industries

Permathene with Calcium tablet
CCA Industries

Phazyme Gas Relief drops
Block Drug

Phazyme Gas Relief Maximum Strength chewable tablet
Block Drug

Phazyme Gas Relief Maximum Strength softgel
Block Drug

Phazyme Gas Relief tablet
Block Drug

Phillips' gelcap
Bayer Consumer

Plax Advanced Formula, Mint Sensation liquid
Pfizer Consumer

Plexo Hand cream
Alvin Last

Pliagel solution
Alcon Labs

Plus+White Anti-Stain Oral Rinse liquid
CCA Industries

Plus+White Plus Peroxide paste
CCA Industries

Plus+White with Fluoride gel
CCA Industries

Plus+White with Fluoride paste
CCA Industries

Polytar cleansing bar
Stiefel Labs

Polytar shampoo
Stiefel Labs

Porcelana Original Formula cream
Dep

Porcelana Sunscreen Formula cream
Dep

Precision Q·I·D
MediSense

Pregestimil nursette bottle, ready-to-feed
Mead Johnson Nutritionals

Pre-Natal Multi Vitamin-Mineral Complex Tablets
Sundown

PreSun 21 lotion
Westwood-Squibb Pharmaceuticals

Primatene tablet
Whitehall-Robins Healthcare

Privine nasal solution
Ciba Self-Medication

Procto Foam
Schwarz Pharma

Prominicol Cough syrup
Republic Drug

Prompt Relief ointment
Goldline Labs

Prompt Relief suppository
Goldline Labs

Pronto Lice Killing aerosol spray
Del Pharmaceuticals

Propa pH Astringent Cleanser lotion
Del Pharmaceuticals

Propa pH Astringent Cleanser Maximum Strength lotion
Del Pharmaceuticals

Propa pH Peel-off mask
Del Pharmaceuticals

Propa pH Perfectly Clear Cleansing, Oily Skin lotion
Del Pharmaceuticals

Propa pH Perfectly Clear Cleansing, Sensitive Skin lotion
Del Pharmaceuticals

Protac DM liquid
Republic Drug

Protective Barrier ointment
C&M Pharmacal

Psoriasin gel
Alva-Amco Pharmacal

Psoriasis Tar lotion
C&M Pharmacal

Pure Eyes 1 Cleaner/Rinse liquid
Ciba Vision

Pure Eyes 2 Disinfectant/ Soaking solution
Ciba Vision

Pycnogenol 25 mg tablet
Agrolabs

Ramses Extra with Spermicide latex
London International U.S. Holdings

Ramses Personal Spermicidal Lubricant gel
London International U.S. Holdings

Ramses Ultra Thin latex
London International U.S. Holdings

Red Cross Canker Sore Medication ointment
Mentholatum

Refresh P.M. ointment
Allergan

Rehydralyte
Ross Products/Abbott Labs

Rembrandt Mouth Refreshing Rinse liquid
Den-Mat

Rembrandt Whitening Baking Soda paste
Den-Mat

Rembrandt Whitening Natural paste
Den-Mat

Repel Family Formula Scented IPF 15
Wisconsin Pharmacal

Repel Scented IPF 7
Wisconsin Pharmacal

Repel Scented IPF 18
Wisconsin Pharmacal

Repel Sportsmen Formula Unscented IPF 27
Wisconsin Pharmacal

Repel Unscented IPF 20
Wisconsin Pharmacal

Resinol Diaper Rash ointment
Mentholatum

Resinol Medicated ointment
Mentholatum

ReSource Fructose Sweetened/ ReSource Diabetic liquid
Sandoz Nutrition

ReSource Fruit Beverage liquid
Sandoz Nutrition

ReSource Just for Kids liquid
Sandoz Nutrition

ReSource Shake Plus (Frozen) liquid
Sandoz Nutrition

ReSource Shake Thickened (Frozen) liquid
Sandoz Nutrition

Rest Easy tincture
Trout Lake Farm

Revital Ice Freezer Pops
Clear Mountain Labs

Ricola Throat Drops, Honey-Herb lozenge
Ricola

RID Lice Control for Dogs and Household aerosol spray
Pfizer Consumer

RID Lice Elimination Kit aerosol spray/shampoo
Pfizer Consumer

Rid-a-Pain Dental Drops liquid
Pfeiffer Pharmaceuticals

Rid-a-Pain HP cream
Pfeiffer Pharmaceuticals

Rid-a-Pain with Codeine tablet
Pfeiffer Pharmaceuticals

Robitussin Night-Time Cold Formula softgel
Whitehall-Robins Healthcare

Robitussin Pediatric drops
Whitehall-Robins Healthcare

Rogaine for Men solution
Pharmacia & Upjohn

Rogaine for Women solution
Pharmacia & Upjohn

Royal Brittany Evening Primrose Oil 500 mg capsule
American Health

RV Paque cream
ICN Pharmaceuticals

SandoSource Peptide liquid
Sandoz Nutrition

Saw Palmetto 160 mg; 320 mg softgel
NaturaLife

Saw Palmetto 80 mg capsule
Herbal Choice

Saw Palmetto Extract 80 mg capsule
Botalia Gold

Saw Palmetto Extract tincture
Herb Pharm

Scalpicin Maximum Strength foam
Combe

Scalpicin Maximum Strength liquid
Combe

Scalpmycin liquid
Pfeiffer Pharmaceuticals

Schamberg's Anti-itch lotion
C&M Pharmacal

Scot-Tussin Senior liquid
Scot-Tussin Pharmacal

Selenium tablet
Sundown

Selenium, Oceanic tablet
Freeda Vitamins

Senokot Children's syrup
Purdue Frederick

Sensitive Eyes Plus Lubricating drops
Bausch & Lomb

Sensitive Eyes Redness Reliever Lubricant drops
Bausch & Lomb

Sensitive Eyes Redness Reliever Lubricant Maximum Strength drops
Bausch & Lomb

Sheer Plus Drainable Pouches
Smith & Nephew

Sheik Classic latex
London International U.S. Holdings

Sib-150 150 mg capsule
PhytoPharmica

Siberian Ginseng 100 mg capsule
Herbal Choice-Botalia

Siberian Ginseng 410 mg capsule
NaturaLife

Siberian Ginseng 500 mg capsule
Herbal Harvest

Siberian Ginseng Extract tincture
Herb Pharm

Singlet caplet
SmithKline Beecham

Sinutol Maximum Strength tablet
Republic Drug

Slimer paste
Perio

SLT Lotion
C&M Pharmacal

Smart Dot
Pharmacy Counter

Sof·lax gelcap
C.B. Fleet

Sof·lax Overnight gelcap
C.B. Fleet

Soft Sense Alpha Hydroxy Moisturizing lotion
Bausch & Lomb

Soft Touch II
Boehringer Mannheim

Softclix
Boehringer Mannheim

Softlips, Sparkle Mint stick
Mentholatum

Softlips, UV stick
Mentholatum

Solaquin cream
ICN Pharmaceuticals

Solarcaine Aloe Extra Burn Relief cream
Schering-Plough HealthCare

Solarcaine Aloe Extra Burn Relief Gel or Mist gel/pump spray
Schering-Plough HealthCare

Solbar PF 50 cream
Person & Covey

Sport Sunblock lotion
Goldline Labs

St. John's Wort 150 mg capsule
Herbal Choice

St. John's Wort 545 mg capsule
Nature's Way

St. John's Wort Extract 150 mg capsule
Botalia Gold

St. John's Wort Extract tincture
Herb Pharm

Standardized Feverfew Extract 125 mg capsule
Botalia Gold

Stayfree Serenity Curved Pads
McNeil Consumer

Stayfree Serenity Guards
McNeil Consumer

Stayfree Serenity Pads
McNeil Consumer

Stevens Baby cream
Stevens Skin

Stevens Skin Softener cream
Stevens Skin

Stevens Sun Block cream
Stevens Skin

Stoma Urine Bags
Bard

Stye Sterile Lubricant ointment
Del Pharmaceuticals

Sudafed Children's Cold & Cough liquid
Warner Wellcome Consumer

Sudafed Children's Nasal Decongestant liquid
Warner Wellcome Consumer

Sudafed Pediatric Nasal Decongestant drops
Warner Wellcome Consumer

Sudafed Sinus Non-Drying Non-Drowsy Maximum Strength liquid-cap
Warner Wellcome Consumer

Sulfoam Medicated Antidandruff shampoo
Doak Dermatologics

Sulpho-Lac cream
Doak Dermatologics

Sulpho-Lac Soap cleansing bar
Doak Dermatologics

Sulray Acne Treatment cream
Alvin Last

Summer's Eve Douche, Extra-Cleansing Vinegar & Water liquid
C.B. Fleet

Summer's Eve Feminine Powder
C.B. Fleet

Summer's Eve Feminine Wash Cleansing Cloths wipe
C.B. Fleet

Sunbeam Model 7684 Digital Wrist Unit B.P. Monitor
Sunbeam-Oster

Sunkist Vitamin C Caplets
Ciba Self-Medication

Sunkist Vitamin C Chewable Tablets
Ciba Self-Medication

Sunvite Multi Vitamin-Mineral Formula Tablets
Sundown

Sunvite Platinum Multi Vitamin-Mineral Formula Tablets
Sundown

Super A&D$_3$ Tablets
Freeda Vitamins

Super C Tablets
Sundown

Super Calci-Caps tablet
Nion Labs

Super Echinacea Extract Tablets 500 mg tablet
Herb Pharm

Super Echinacea Liquid Extract tincture
Herb Pharm

Super Multiple 33 with Minerals Tablets
Sundown

Super Multiple 42 with Beta Carotene Softgels
Sundown

Super Multiple 50 Tablets
Sundown

Super Multiple Minus Iron Tablets
Sundown

Super Saw Palmetto-160 160 mg capsule
PhytoPharmica

Supreme strip
Chronimed

Sure latex
Aladan

Sure with Spermicide latex
Aladan

Sur-Fit Drainable Pouches
ConvaTec

Surgel
Ulmer

Sustacal individual packet
Mead Johnson Nutritionals

Sustained Effect Hydrating Lotion
C&M Pharmacal

Swish, Cool Mint liquid
Unico

Swish, Peppermint liquid
Unico

Tagamet HB tablet
SmithKline Beecham

Tanacet 125 mg tablet
Herbal Laboratories

Tar Scalp Solution
C&M Pharmacal

Tar Shampoo Maximum Strength shampoo
C&M Pharmacal

Tegrin-LT Lice Treatment shampoo/conditioner
Block Drug

Terumo Syringe
Terumo

Tetrahist tablet
Republic Drug

TheraFlu Maximum Strength Flu & Cold Medicine For Sore Throat individual packet
Sandoz Consumer

TheraFlu Maximum Strength Sinus Non-Drowsy caplet
Sandoz Consumer

Therapeutic M Multi Vitamins Plus Minerals Tablets
Sundown

Theraplex Hydrolotion
Medicis

Thermakit
Jordan Medical

Thisilyn 310 mg capsule
Nature's Way

Tom's Natural Baking Soda with Propolis & Myrrh paste
Tom's of Maine

Tom's Natural with Calcium & Fluoride paste
Tom's of Maine

Torbot Belts
Torbot

Torbot Foam Pads
Torbot

Torbot Plastic Pouches, Opaque White
Torbot

Torbot Plastic Pouches, Transparent
Torbot

Torbot Plastic Urinary Pouches, Opaque White
Torbot

Torbot Plastic Urinary Pouches, Transparent
Torbot

Torbot Rubber Pouches
Torbot

Torbot Rubber Urinary Pouches
Torbot

Touch latex
London International U.S. Holdings

Touch Lubricated latex
London International U.S. Holdings

Transfer-Ease
Transfer-Ease

Trans-Ver-Sal 12mm "Adult Patch" Wart Remover Kit patch
Doak Dermatologics

Trans-Ver-Sal 20mm "PlantarPatch" Wart Remover Kit patch
Doak Dermatologics

Trans-Ver-Sal 6mm "PediaPatch" Wart Remover Kit patch
Doak Dermatologics

Tri-Fed tablet
Republic Drug

Triaminic Infant, Oral Decongestant drops
Sandoz Consumer

Trojan Ultra Texture latex
Carter Products

Trojan Ultra Texture with Spermicide latex
Carter Products

Tucks Clear gel
Warner Wellcome Consumer

20/20 Lubricating & Rewetting Solution
S.S.S. Company

Tylenol Allergy Sinus Maximum Strength geltab
McNeil Consumer

Tylenol Flu NightTime Maximum Strength Hot Medication individual packet
McNeil Consumer

Tylenol Infants' Cold Decongestant and Fever Reducer drops
McNeil Consumer

Tylenol PM Extra Strength geltab
McNeil Consumer

Tylenol Severe Allergy Maximum Strength caplet
McNeil Consumer

Tylenol Sinus Maximum Strength gelcap/geltab
McNeil Consumer

Tylenol, Children's Bubble Gum Flavor chewable tablet
McNeil Consumer

Tylenol, Children's Liquid Bubble Gum Flavor suspension
McNeil Consumer

Undelenic ointment
Gordon Labs

Undelenic tincture
Gordon Labs

Unilet and Unilet G.P.
Owen Mumford

Unilet Superlite and Unilet G.P. Superlite
Owen Mumford

Unilet Universal ComforTouch
Owen Mumford

Unilife-A Gelcaps
Chronimed

Unisol Plus liquid
Alcon Labs

Uristix 4 strip
Bayer Diagnostics

Urostomy Pouches
Hollister

Vaginex Douche liquid
Quality Health

Vaginex Medicated powder
Quality Health

Vaginex, Scented or Unscented cream
Quality Health

Valer-A-Som 150 mg capsule
PhytoPharmica

Valerian 150 mg capsule
Herbal Choice-Botalia

Valerian Extract 150 mg tablet
Botalia Gold

Valerian Extract tincture
Herb Pharm

Valerian Nighttime Tablets 495 mg tablet
Nature's Way

Valerian Plus tablet
Shaklee

Vasocon-A drops
CIBA Vision Ophthalmics

Vicks Cough Drops, Cherry lozenge
Procter & Gamble

Vicks Cough Drops, Menthol lozenge
Procter & Gamble

Visine Lubricating drops
Pfizer Consumer

Vita-Cal chewable tablet
Shaklee

Vita-Lea for Children Tablets
Shaklee

Vita-Lea for Infants & Toddlers Powder
Shaklee

Vita-Lea, with or without Iron, Tablets
Shaklee

Vivonex Pediatric powder
Sandoz Nutrition

VPI Non-Adhesive Colostomy Systems
VPI

VPI Non-Adhesive Ileostomy Systems
VPI

VPI Non-Adhesive Urostomy Systems
VPI

Women's One Daily Multiple Vitamin Tablets
Sundown

Wyanoids Relief Factor suppository
Wyeth-Ayerst Labs

Yeast-X cream
C.B. Fleet

Yeast·Guard Advanced Sensitive Formula cream
Lake Consumer

Yeast·Guard Disposable Douche Premix liquid
Lake Consumer

Yeast·Guard Disposable Douche solution
Lake Consumer

Yeast·Guard Douche Concentrate liquid
Lake Consumer

Yeast·Guard Maximum Strength cream
Lake Consumer

Zantac 75 tablet
Warner Wellcome Consumer

Zilactin B gel
Zila Pharmaceuticals

Zinc 15 tablet
Mericon

Zinc lozenge
Goldline Labs

Zinc tablet
Goldline Labs

Zinc tablet
Freeda Vitamins

Zinc, Elemental tablet
Freeda Vitamins

Zostrix Sports cream
GenDerm

FECAL OCCULT BLOOD TEST KITS

	Product [a] Manufacturer/Supplier	No. of Tests	Comments
**	**ColoCARE** Helena Labs	3	use for three consecutive bowel movements · flush toilet twice before each bowel movement · pad is floated in toilet bowl with specimen · observe for 30 seconds · pad check area on left will turn blue and/or green, the other will not · positive result is appearance of a blue color on the test pad · flush pad away when test is complete
	EZ-Detect Stool Blood Test Biomerica	3	one step procedure · use for three consecutive bowel movements · flush toilet twice before each bowel movement · test pad is floated in toilet bowl with specimen · observe for up to 2 minutes · positive result appears as a blue-green color on test pad · no diet restrictions (vitamin C and rare meat are okay) · avoid anti-inflammatory medications and those that cause internal bleeding

** New listing
[a] Other nonprescription test kits for fecal occult blood may be obtained from physicians.

See Chapter 3, "In-Home Testing and Monitoring Products," for more information about these products.

OVULATION PREDICTION TEST KITS

	Product Manufacturer/Supplier	No. of Tests	Reaction Time (min)	Indication of Positive Result	Comments
	Answer 1-Step Ovulation Test Kit Carter Products	5	5	test line color similar to or darker than reference line color	test any time of day · reduce liquid intake 2 hrs before testing · positive result indicates ovulation should occur within 24-36 hrs
	Clearplan Easy Whitehall-Robins Healthcare	5	5	test line color in large window is similar to or darker than small window line color	test any time of day, but test at same time each day · use concentrated (at least 4 hrs) urine specimen · positive result indicates ovulation should occur within 24-36 hrs · blue line in small window indicates test is complete and performed correctly
	Conceive Ovulation Test Quidel	5	3	pink-to-purple test line color is darker than reference line color	test any time of day, but collect at same time each day · positive result indicates ovulation should occur within 24-40 hrs
**	**EZ-LH** Biomerica	6 & 10	1-5	comparison of test band to control band · pink band appears	one step procedure
	First Response 1-Step Ovulation Predictor Test Carter Products	5	5	test line color similar to or darker than reference line color	test any time of day · reduce liquid intake 2 hrs before testing · positive result indicates ovulation should occur within 24-36 hrs
	OvuKIT Quidel	6 & 9	60	blue test stick color is darker than the surge guide test	use urine collected between 10am and 8pm · do not use first morning urine · collect at same time each day · positive result indicates ovulation should occur within 24-40 hrs
	OvuQUICK Quidel	6 & 9	4	color of test result area on test pad matches or is darker than the reference spot	use urine collected between 10am and 8pm · do not use first morning urine · collect at same time each day · positive result indicates ovulation should occur within 24-40 hrs
	Q Test for Ovulation Prediction Quidel	5	35	result pad on test strip changes color from pale blue to dark blue	test any time of day · predicts ovulation within 20-44 hrs · error control pad on test strip indicates if test is performed correctly

** New listing

See Chapter 3, "In-Home Testing and Monitoring Products," for more information about these products.

PREGNANCY TEST KITS

	Product Manufacturer/Supplier	No. of Tests	Reaction Time (min)	Indication of Positive Result	Control	Comments
	Advance 1 Easy Step Stream Test Direct Access Diagnostics	1 & 2	5	appearance of "+" on test stick	appearance of "-" on test stick	use any time after missed period · one step procedure after collecting urine
	Answer Pregnancy Test Carter Products	1	3	2 pink lines appear in result window		use any time after missed period
	Answer Quick & Simple 1-Step Stick Pregnancy Test Carter Products	1 & 2	2	2 pink lines appear in result window		use any time after missed period · one step procedure · hold test stick in urine stream
	Clearblue Easy Whitehall-Robins Healthcare	1 & 2	3	blue line appears in large window	blue line in small window indicates test is complete and performed correctly	use any time after missed period · one step procedure · hold test stick in stream of concentrated (at least 6 hrs.) urine to wet tip · must hold stick downward during testing
	Conceive Pregnancy Test Quidel	1 & 2	1-3	pink-to-purple test line appears	blue control line indicates test is performing correctly	use any time after missed period
	Confirm London Int'l U.S. Holdings	1 & 2	3	appearance of blue line in both the test and control windows		use any time after missed period · one step procedure · hold test stick in urine stream
	e.p.t. Warner Wellcome Consumer	1 & 2	3	pink line appears in round results window	square control window always shows a pink line	use any time after missed period · one step procedure · hold test stick in urine stream
**	**early Pregancy test** Selfcare	1	1	pink line appears in square test window	pink line in round reference window	use any time after missed period · one step procedure · choose one of two test methods: either hold test stick in urine stream or dip test stick in a cup of collected urine
	Fact Plus One Step Direct Access Diagnostics	1 & 2	5-8	appearance of "+" on test disk	appearance of a dark "-" on test disk	use any time after missed period · one step procedure after collecting urine
	First Response 1-Step Pregnancy Test Carter Products	1 & 2	2	2 pink lines appear in result window		use any time after missed period · one step procedure · hold test stick in urine stream
	Fortel Midstream Biomerica	1 & 2	1-5	pink band appears in large test window		use any time after missed period · one step procedure
**	**Fortel Plus** Biomerica	1 & 2	1	pink band appears in test window		use any time after missed period · one step procedure
**	**Nimbus Quick Strip** Biomerica	25	1-5	pink band appears in test window		one step procedure
	Precise Becton Dickinson Consumer	1 & 2	1	end-of-test window turns pink, and blue check mark appears in result window	error control bar in result window indicates test is working correctly	use any time after missed period · one step procedure
	Q-Test For Pregnancy Quidel	1	positive results as early as 9	test strip result pad turns blue	error control pad on test strip indicates if test is performed correctly	use any time after missed period · negative results can be verified in 16 minutes

See Chapter 3, "In-Home Testing and Monitoring Products," for more information about these products.

PREGNANCY TEST KITS - continued

Product Manufacturer/Supplier	**No. of Tests**	**Reaction Time (min)**	**Indication of Positive Result**	**Control**	**Comments**
RapidVue Quidel	1	1	pink-to-purple test line appears	blue control line appears	use any time after missed period · one step procedure · add 3 drops from urine collection to test well of test cassette

** New listing

See Chapter 3, "In-Home Testing and Monitoring Products," for more information about these products.

CHOLESTEROL TEST KITS

	Product [a] Manufacturer/Supplier	No. of Tests	Reaction Time (min)	Comments
**	**CholesTrak** ChemTrak	1 & 2	12-15	can test at any time; but do not test within 4 hrs of taking 500mg or more of vitamin C, or a standard dose of acetaminophen (may cause falsely low result) · prick fingertip, according to package instructions/supplies, to obtain blood sample · apply one or more drops of blood into the blood well, to fill · wait two to four minutes, then pull tab of test device · test is complete 12 minutes later after the "OK" indicator has turned purple, and "END" indicator turns green · read test device like a thermometer, and check the result chart for cholesterol level

** New listing
[a] This product measures total cholesterol only. If a result of 200mg/dL or greater is obtained, the patient should see a physician for further evaluation.

See Chapter 3, "In-Home Testing and Monitoring Products," for more information about these products.

ELECTRONIC OSCILLOMETRIC BLOOD PRESSURE MONITOR PRODUCTS

	Product Manufacturer/Supplier	Comments
	Labtron Model 02-707 Digital B.P./Pulse Monitor Graham-Field	compact, palm-sized · inflates manually, deflates automatically · self adjusting "D"-bar cuff · pressure release valve · lcd display · minute automatic shut-off · comes complete with zippered vinyl carrying case, 9-volt battery · several cuff sizes available
	Labtron Model 02-847 Automatic Digital B.P./Pulse Monitor Graham-Field	fully automatic, portable · inflates automatically · activated by start button · self adjusting "D"-bar · automatic pressure release valve · lcd display · low battery indicator · 5-minute automatic shut-off · comes complete with zippered vinyl carrying case, 4 "AA" batteries · several cuff sizes available
	Labtron Model 02-857 Auto. B.P. Kit w/Memory & XL Display Graham-Field	memory function recalls last reading · inflates automatically with 9 preset settings · easy 3-step procedure · self adjusting "D"-bar cuff · extra-large lcd display · 2.5-minute automatic shut-off · comes complete with zippered vinyl carrying case, 4 "AA" batteries · several cuff sizes available
	Labtron Model 02-947 Automatic Digital B.P./Pulse w/Printer Graham-Field	fully automatic, portable · permanent record of time, date, systolic, diastolic, and pulse measurements · self adjusting "D"-bar cuff · built-in automatic pump · large lcd display · comes complete with 1 extra roll of chart paper, zippered vinyl carrying case, 4 "AA" batteries · several cuff sizes available
	Labtron Model 02-949 Finger B.P./Pulse Monitor Graham-Field	compact, lightweight, portable · self adjusting "D"-bar finger cuff · inflates and deflates automatically · digital display · low battery indicator · comes complete with 4 "AAA" batteries
	Lumiscope Model 1060 Blood Pressure Monitor Lumiscope	memory recall of readings · oscillometric cuff design · inflates manually and deflates automatically
	Lumiscope Model 1083 Blood Pressure Monitor Lumiscope	takes readings from finger · adjusts for correct fit · record log
	Lumiscope Model 1085M Blood Pressure Monitor Lumiscope	extra large lcd display · memory recall of readings · oscillometric cuff design · inflates and deflates automatically · one-button operation · error indicator · pre-set inflation pressure
	Lumiscope Model 1091 Blood Pressure Monitor with Printer Lumiscope	completely automatic · printout of systolic and diastolic measurements, time, and date · D-ring cuff · inflates and deflates automatically · lcd panel · operates on two "AA" batteries (not included) · includes 2 rolls of printing tape
**	**Marshall Model 82 Manual Inflation B.P. Monitor** Omron Healthcare	contoured D-ring cuff inflates manually and deflates automatically · large digital display panel
**	**Marshall Model 92 Manual Inflation B.P. Monitor** Omron Healthcare	contoured D-ring cuff inflates and deflates automatically · large digital display panel · memory feature
	Marshall Model 97 Measurement Print-out B.P. Monitor Omron Healthcare	prints systolic, diastolic, and pulse measurements · contoured D-ring cuff inflates and deflates automatically · digital display panel
	Marshall Model F-89 Finger B.P. Monitor Omron Healthcare	measures blood pressure and pulse from the finger · adjustable finger cuff inflates and deflates automatically · digital display panel
**	**Omron Model HEM-412C Manual Inflation B.P. Monitor** Omron Healthcare	contoured D-ring cuff inflates manually and deflates automatically · digital display panel
**	**Omron Model HEM-601 Wrist B.P. Monitor** Omron Healthcare	measures blood pressure and pulse from the wrist · inflates and deflates automatically · jumbo digital display panel · built-in cuff storage feature

See Chapter 3, "In-Home Testing and Monitoring Products," for more information about these products.

ELECTRONIC OSCILLOMETRIC BLOOD PRESSURE MONITOR PRODUCTS - continued

	Product Manufacturer/Supplier	Comments
**	**Omron Model HEM-602 Wrist B.P. Monitor with Memory** Omron Healthcare	displays up to 7 readings in digital and bar-graph form · cuff inflates and deflates automatically · jumbo digital display panel · built-in cuff storage feature · includes 4 "AA" batteries
**	**Omron Model HEM-605 Compact Wrist B.P. Monitor** Omron Healthcare	convenient watch-style design · measures blood pressure and pulse directly from the wrist · small, pre-formed wrist cuff · inflates and deflates automatically · easy-to-read display panel folds down when not in use · includes storage case and 2 "AA" batteries
**	**Omron Model HEM-703CP Measurement Print-out B.P. Monitor** Omron Healthcare	prints systolic, diastolic, and pulse measurements · contoured D-ring cuff inflates and deflates automatically · digital display panel
**	**Omron Model HEM-704C Self-Storing B.P. Monitor** Omron Healthcare	curved contour D-ring cuff inflates and deflates automatically · jumbo digital display panel · folds into its own carrying case
**	**Omron Model HEM-705CP Memory/Print-out/Graph B.P. Monitor** Omron Healthcare	prints in numerical and bar-graph form · curved contour D-ring cuff inflates and deflates automatically · large digital display panel · memory of 14 readings
**	**Omron Model HEM-706 Fuzzy Logic B.P. Monitor** Omron Healthcare	automatically determines ideal cuff inflation level · curved contour D-ring cuff · large digital display panel · built-in cuff storage feature
**	**Omron Model HEM-711 Smart-Inflate Fuzzy Logic B.P. Monitor** Omron Healthcare	automatically determines ideal cuff inflation level · curved contour D-ring cuff with "How To Apply" label · large digital display panel
**	**Omron Model HEM-712C Automatic Inflation B.P. Monitor** Omron Healthcare	contoured D-ring cuff inflates and deflates automatically · digital display panel · memory feature
**	**Omron Model HEM-806F Deluxe Finger B.P. Monitor** Omron Healthcare	finger cuff adjusts size automatically · digital display panel · includes carrying case and 2 "AA" batteries
**	**Omron Model HEM-808F Travel Finger B.P. Monitor** Omron Healthcare	compact, self-store design · inflates and deflates automatically · large digital display panel · includes 2 "AAA" batteries
**	**Omron Model HEM-815F Finger B.P. Monitor** Omron Healthcare	measures blood pressure and pulse from the finger · adjustable finger cuff inflates and deflates automatically · digital display panel
	Sunbeam Model 7622 Digital B.P. Monitor Sunbeam-Oster	measures heart rate · inflates manually · one-touch operation · jumbo display · memory recall of readings · carrying case
	Sunbeam Model 7650-10 Digital B.P. Monitor Sunbeam-Oster	measures heart rate · inflates automatically · over- or under-inflation indicator
	Sunbeam Model 7652 Digital B.P. Monitor Sunbeam-Oster	measures heart rate · inflates automatically · one-touch operation · jumbo display · memory recall of readings · automatic pressure setting · carrying case
	Sunbeam Model 7655-10 Digital Finger B.P. Monitor Sunbeam-Oster	measures heart rate · inflates automatically · adjustable finger cuff · over- or under-inflation indicator

See Chapter 3, "In-Home Testing and Monitoring Products," for more information about these products.

ELECTRONIC OSCILLOMETRIC BLOOD PRESSURE MONITOR PRODUCTS - continued

	Product Manufacturer/Supplier	Comments
	Sunbeam Model 7656-10 Digital Finger B.P. Monitor Sunbeam-Oster	measures heart rate · adjustable finger cuff · inflates automatically
	Sunbeam Model 7657-10 Digital B.P. Monitor with Printer Sunbeam-Oster	measures heart rate · inflates automatically · prints current display information · memory stores up to 7 blood pressure readings by date and time · graphic display of readings in memory
**	**Sunbeam Model 7684 Digital Wrist Unit B.P. Monitor** Sunbeam-Oster	measures heart rate · jumbo display · inflates automatically · fuzzy logic operation · 2-person memory (14 measurements per person) · 2.5 lbs.

** New listing

See Chapter 3, "In-Home Testing and Monitoring Products," for more information about these products.

INTERNAL ANALGESIC AND ANTIPYRETIC PRODUCTS

	Product [a] Manufacturer/Supplier	Dosage Form	Acetaminophen	Aspirin	Ibuprofen	Other Analgesics	Other Ingredients [b]
	Acetaminophen						
	Acephen G & W Labs	suppository	120mg; 325mg; 650mg				hydrogenated vegetable oil · polysorbate 80
AF CA GL SO SL	**Aceta** Century Ph'cals	elixir	160mg/5ml				alcohol, 7%
AL AF CA	**Acetaminophen Oral Solution USP, Cherry** Roxane Labs	solution	160mg/5ml				polyethylene glycol · propylene glycol · glycerin · sorbitol · methylparaben · propylparaben · FD&C red#40 · cherry flavoring · water
AF CA	**Acetaminophen Oral Solution USP, Lime** Roxane Labs	solution	160mg/5ml				polyethylene glycol · glycerin · sorbitol solution · methylparaben · propylparaben · D&C yellow#10 · FD&C blue#1 · FD&C yellow#6 · alcohol · lime flavoring · water
** AL AF PE	**Acetaminophen Suspension, Children's Flavored** Multisource	drops	80mg/0.8ml				
AF CA GL PU SO	**Acetaminophen Uniserts** Upsher-Smith Labs	suppository	120mg; 325mg; 650mg				
AF CA	**Actamin** Buffington	tablet	325mg				
AF CA	**Actamin Extra** Buffington	tablet	500mg				
AF SO	**Actamin Super** Buffington	tablet	500mg				caffeine, 65mg
** AF	**Alka-Seltzer** Bayer Consumer	caplet	500mg				calcium carbonate, 380mg · crospovidone · docusate sodium · hydroxypropyl methylcellulose · lecithin · magnesium stearate · polyvinylpyrrolidone · sodium benzoate · sodium hexametaphosphate · sodium starch glycolate · starch · stearic acid
AF CA SU	**Aminofen** Dover	tablet	324mg				
AF CA SU	**Aminofen Max** Dover	tablet	500mg				

See Chapter 4, "Internal Analgesic and Antipyretic Products," for more information about these products.

INTERNAL ANALGESIC AND ANTIPYRETIC PRODUCTS - continued

	Product [a] Manufacturer/Supplier	Dosage Form	Acetaminophen	Aspirin	Ibuprofen	Other Analgesics	Other Ingredients [b]
AF	**Anacin Aspirin Free Maximum Strength** Whitehall-Robins Healthcare	tablet	500mg				calcium stearate · croscarmellose sodium · D&C red#7 lake · FD&C blue#1 lake · hydroxypropyl methylcellulose · polyethylene glycol · povidone · propylene glycol · starch · stearic acid · titanium dioxide
AF	**APAP** Schein Ph'cal	tablet	325mg				povidone · starch · stearic acid · may also contain: croscarmellose sodium · microcrystalline cellulose · sodium starch glycolate
AF	**APAP** Schein Ph'cal	suppository	650mg				
AF	**APAP Extra Strength** Schein Ph'cal	tablet	500mg				povidone · starch · stearic acid · may also contain: croscarmellose sodium · microcrystalline cellulose · sodium starch glycolate
AF	**APAP Extra Strength** Schein Ph'cal	caplet	500mg				hydroxypropyl methylcellulose · povidone · starch · stearic acid · titanium dioxide · may also contain: croscarmellose sodium · sodium starch glycolate
AL AF PE	**APAP, Children's** Schein Ph'cal	elixir	80mg/2.5ml				benzoic acid · citric acid · corn syrup · D&C red#33 · FD&C red#40 · flavor · glycerin · methylparaben · polyethylene glycol · propylene glycol · propylparaben · purified water · sodium benzoate · sorbitol · sucrose
AF PE	**APAP, Children's** Schein Ph'cal	chewable tablet	80mg				microcrystalline cellulose · aspartame · citric acid · flavors · hydroxypropyl methylcellulose · mannitol · starch · magnesium stearate · color
AL AF CA PE	**APAP, Children's** Goldline Labs	suspension	80mg/2.5ml				
AL AF PE	**APAP, Infants'** Schein Ph'cal	drops	80mg/0.8ml				
AL AF CA PE	**APAP, Infants' Suspension** Goldline Labs	drops	80mg/0.8ml				
AF PE	**APAP, Pediatric** Schein Ph'cal	suppository	120mg				
AF DY GL PR SO SU	**Arthriten** Alva-Amco Pharmacal	tablet	250mg			magnesium salicylate, 250mg	caffeine, 32.5mg · magnesium carbonate · magnesium oxide · calcium carbonate

See Chapter 4, "Internal Analgesic and Antipyretic Products," for more information about these products.

INTERNAL ANALGESIC AND ANTIPYRETIC PRODUCTS - continued

	Product [a] Manufacturer/Supplier	Dosage Form	Acetaminophen	Aspirin	Ibuprofen	Other Analgesics	Other Ingredients [b]
AF	**Arthritis Foundation Aspirin Free** McNeil Consumer	caplet	500mg				cellulose · corn starch · hydroxypropyl methylcellulose · magnesium stearate · polyethylene glycol · sodium starch glycolate · red#40
AF CA GL PR PU SO PE	**Aspirin Free Pain & Fever Relief, Children's** Hudson	chewable tablet	80mg				
AF CA GL PR PU SO	**Aspirin Free Pain Relief** Hudson	tablet	500mg				
AF CA GL PR PU	**Aspirin Free Pain Relief** Hudson	caplet	500mg				
AF CA GL PR PU	**Aspirin Free Pain Relief** Hudson	tablet	325mg				
AL AF CA PR SO PE	**Aspirin Free, Children's** Hudson	elixir	80mg/2.5ml				sorbitol · flavor
AL AF CA PR SL PE	**Aspirin Free, Infants'** Hudson	drops	80mg/0.8ml				
AF GL	**Bayer Select Aspirin-Free Headache** Bayer Consumer	caplet	500mg				caffeine, 65mg
AF CA PR	**Bromo-Seltzer** Warner Wellcome Consumer	granular effervescent	325mg/capful				sodium bicarbonate, 2.78g/capful · citric acid, 2.22g/capful
AF CA SO	**Dyspel** Dover	tablet	325mg				ephedrine sulfate, 8mg · atropine sulfate, 0.06mg
AL AF CA	**Ed-APAP Liquid** Edwards Ph'cals	liquid	80mg/2.5ml				

See Chapter 4, "Internal Analgesic and Antipyretic Products," for more information about these products.

INTERNAL ANALGESIC AND ANTIPYRETIC PRODUCTS - continued

	Product [a] Manufacturer/Supplier	Dosage Form	Acetaminophen	Aspirin	Ibuprofen	Other Analgesics	Other Ingredients [b]
** AF GL	**Excedrin Aspirin Free** Bristol-Myers Products	geltab	500mg				caffeine, 65mg · benzoic acid · corn starch · FD&C blue#1 · FD&C red#4 · FD&C yellow#6 · gelatin · glycerin · hydroxypropyl methylcellulose · magnesium stearate · microcrystalline cellulose · mineral oil · polysorbate 20 · povidone · propylene glycol · simethicone emulsion · sorbitan monolaurate · titanium dioxide
AF	**Excedrin Aspirin Free** Bristol-Myers Products	caplet	500mg				caffeine, 65mg · benzoic acid · carnauba wax · corn starch · D&C red#27 lake · D&C yellow#10 lake · FD&C blue#1 lake · hydroxypropyl methylcellulose · magnesium stearate · methylparaben · microcrystalline cellulose · mineral oil · polysorbate 20 · povidone · propylene glycol · propylparaben · simethicone emulsion · sorbitan monolaurate · stearic acid · titanium dioxide · may also contain: croscarmellose sodium · FD&C red#40 · saccharin sodium · sodium starch glycolate
PR SO	**Excedrin Extra Strength** Bristol-Myers Products	caplet · tablet	250mg	250mg			caffeine, 65mg · benzoic acid · FD&C blue#1 · hydroxypropyl methylcellulose · microcrystalline cellulose · mineral oil · polysorbate 20 · povidone · propylene glycol · saccharin sodium · simethicone emulsion · sorbitan monolaurate · stearic acid · titanium dioxide · may also contain: carnauba wax · hydroxypropyl cellulose
** GL	**Excedrin Extra Strength** Bristol-Myers Products	geltab	250mg	250mg			caffeine, 65mg · benzoic acid · D&C yellow#10 lake · disodium EDTA · FD&C blue#1 lake · FD&C red#40 lake · ferric oxide · gelatin · glycerin · hydroxypropyl cellulose · hydroxypropyl methylcellulose · maltitol solution · mineral oil · pepsin · polysorbate 20 · povidone · propylene glycol · propyl gallate · simethicone emulsion · sorbitan monolaurate · stearic acid · titanium dioxide
** AF CA GL PU SO	**Feverall Adult Strength** Upsher-Smith Labs	suppository	650mg				
AF CA GL PU SO	**Feverall Junior Strength** Upsher-Smith Labs	suppository	325mg				

See Chapter 4, "Internal Analgesic and Antipyretic Products," for more information about these products.

INTERNAL ANALGESIC AND ANTIPYRETIC PRODUCTS - continued

	Product [a] Manufacturer/Supplier	Dosage Form	Acetamin-ophen	Aspirin	Ibuprofen	Other Analgesics	Other Ingredients [b]
AF CA GL PU SO PE	**Feverall Sprinkle Caps Powder, Children's Strength** Upsher-Smith Labs	capsule	80mg				
AF CA GL PU SO PE	**Feverall Sprinkle Caps Powder, Junior Strength** Upsher-Smith Labs	capsule	160mg				
AF CA GL PU SO PE	**Feverall, Children's** Upsher-Smith Labs	suppository	120mg				
AF CA GL PU SO PE	**Feverall, Infants'** Upsher-Smith Labs	suppository	80mg				
AF	**Genapap Extra Strength** Goldline Labs	caplet · tablet	500mg				
AL AF CA PE	**Genapap, Children's** Goldline Labs	suspension	80mg/2.5ml				
AF PE	**Genapap, Children's** Goldline Labs	elixir	80mg/2.5ml				cherry flavor
AF PE	**Genapap, Children's** Goldline Labs	chewable tablet	80mg				
AF PE	**Genapap, Infants'** Goldline Labs	drops	80mg/0.8ml				fruit flavor
AF	**Genebs** Goldline Labs	tablet	325mg				
AF	**Genebs Extra Strength** Goldline Labs	tablet	500mg				
AL AF CA PE	**Liquiprin for Children** Menley & James Labs	drops	48mg/ml				dextrose · fructose · sucrose · fruit flavor · D&C red#33 · FD&C red#40 · propylparaben · methylparaben · glycerin · citric acid · polyethylene glycol · sodium citrate · sodium gluconate · sweetener
AF CA GL SO	**Midol Menstrual Regular Strength Multisymptom Formula** Bayer Consumer	caplet	325mg				pyrilamine maleate, 12.5mg

See Chapter 4, "Internal Analgesic and Antipyretic Products," for more information about these products.

INTERNAL ANALGESIC AND ANTIPYRETIC PRODUCTS - continued

	Product [a] Manufacturer/Supplier	Dosage Form	Acetaminophen	Aspirin	Ibuprofen	Other Analgesics	Other Ingredients [b]
AF	**Neopap** PolyMedica Ph'cals	suppository	125mg				
AF CA GL SO	**Panadol Junior Strength** Bayer Consumer	caplet	160mg				
AF CA GL SO	**Panadol Maximum Strength** Bayer Consumer	caplet · tablet	500mg				
AL AF CA PE	**Panadol, Children's** Bayer Consumer	liquid	32mg/ml				saccharin · sorbitol · fruit flavor
AF CA GL PE	**Panadol, Children's** Bayer Consumer	chewable tablet	80mg				fruit flavor
AL AF CA PE	**Panadol, Infants'** Bayer Consumer	drops	80mg/0.8ml				fruit flavor · saccharin
** AL AF CA DY SU PE	**PediApap** Central Ph'cals	solution	160mg				
AF CA GL PR PU	**Percogesic Coated** Procter & Gamble	tablet	325mg				phenyltoloxamine citrate, 30mg · cellulose · flavor · FD&C yellow#6 · hydroxypropyl methylcellulose · magnesium stearate · polyethylene glycol · povidone · purified water · silica gel · starch · stearic acid · sucrose
AF SO	**Rid-a-Pain Compound** Pfeiffer Ph'cals	caplet	226.8mg				salicylamide, 97.2mg · caffeine, 32.4mg
AF CA	**Stanback AF Extra-Strength** Stanback	powder	950mg				
AF	**Tapanol Extra Strength** Republic Drug	caplet · tablet	500mg				
AL AF CA PR SL PE	**Tempra 1** Bristol-Myers Products	drops	80mg/0.8ml				grape flavor · saccharin sodium
AL AF CA SL PE	**Tempra 2** Bristol-Myers Products	syrup	160mg/5ml				grape flavor · saccharin sodium

See Chapter 4, "Internal Analgesic and Antipyretic Products," for more information about these products.

INTERNAL ANALGESIC AND ANTIPYRETIC PRODUCTS - continued

	Product [a] Manufacturer/Supplier	Dosage Form	Acetaminophen	Aspirin	Ibuprofen	Other Analgesics	Other Ingredients [b]
AF CA GL PR PE	**Tempra 3** Bristol-Myers Products	chewable tablet	80mg				grape flavor · aspartame (phenylalanine, 3.3mg)
AF CA GL PR PE	**Tempra 3, Double Strength** Bristol-Myers Products	chewable tablet	160mg				grape flavor · aspartame (phenylalanine, 6.6mg)
AF CA	**Tycolene** Pfeiffer Ph'cals	tablet	325mg				
AF CA	**Tycolene Extra Strength** Pfeiffer Ph'cals	caplet	500mg				
AF CA	**Tylenol Extended Relief** McNeil Consumer	timed-release caplet	650mg (immediate release, 325mg · slow, continuous release, 325mg)				corn starch · hydroxyethyl cellulose · hydroxypropyl methylcellulose · magnesium stearate · microcrystalline cellulose · povidone · powdered cellulose · pregelatinized starch · sodium starch glycolate · titanium dioxide · triacetin
AF CA	**Tylenol Extra Strength** McNeil Consumer	tablet	500mg				magnesium stearate · cellulose · sodium starch glycolate · starch
AF CA	**Tylenol Extra Strength** McNeil Consumer	gelcap · geltab	500mg				benzyl alcohol · butylparaben · castor oil · cellulose · corn starch · edetate calcium disodium · gelatin · hydroxypropyl methylcellulose · magnesium stearate · methylparaben · propylparaben · sodium lauryl sulfate · sodium propionate · sodium starch glycolate · titanium dioxide · blue#1 · blue#2 · red#40 · yellow#10
AF CA	**Tylenol Extra Strength** McNeil Consumer	caplet	500mg				cellulose · corn starch · hydroxypropyl methylcellulose · magnesium stearate · polyethylene glycol · sodium starch glycolate · red#40
AF CA	**Tylenol Extra Strength Adult** McNeil Consumer	liquid	166.7mg/5ml				alcohol, 7% · citric acid · flavors · glycerin · polyethylene glycol · purified water · sodium benzoate · sorbitol · sucrose · blue#1 · yellow#6 · yellow#10
AF CA	**Tylenol Extra Strength Headache Plus** McNeil Consumer	caplet	500mg				calcium carbonate, 250mg · acacia · cellulose · corn starch · croscarmellose sodium · hydroxypropyl methylcellulose · magnesium stearate · maltodextrin · propylene glycol · sodium starch glycolate · titanium dioxide · triacetin · blue#1 · blue#2

See Chapter 4, "Internal Analgesic and Antipyretic Products," for more information about these products.

INTERNAL ANALGESIC AND ANTIPYRETIC PRODUCTS - continued

	Product [a] Manufacturer/Supplier	Dosage Form	Acetaminophen	Aspirin	Ibuprofen	Other Analgesics	Other Ingredients [b]
AF CA PE	**Tylenol Junior Strength Swallowable** McNeil Consumer	caplet	160mg				cellulose · corn starch · ethylcellulose · magnesium stearate · sodium lauryl sulfate · sodium starch glycolate
AF CA PE	**Tylenol Junior Strength, Fruit Flavor** McNeil Consumer	chewable tablet	160mg				aspartame · cellulose · citric acid · corn starch · ethylcellulose · flavors · magnesium stearate · mannitol · red#7
AF CA PE	**Tylenol Junior Strength, Grape Flavor** McNeil Consumer	chewable tablet	160mg				aspartame · cellulose · cellulose acetate · citric acid · corn starch · flavors · magnesium stearate · mannitol · povidone · blue#1 · red#7 · red#30
AF CA	**Tylenol Regular Strength** McNeil Consumer	caplet	325mg				cellulose · hydroxypropyl methylcellulose · magnesium stearate · polyethylene glycol · sodium starch glycolate · starch · red#40
AF CA	**Tylenol Regular Strength** McNeil Consumer	tablet	325mg				cellulose · corn starch · magnesium stearate · sodium starch glycolate
** AF CA PE	**Tylenol, Children's Bubble Gum Flavor** McNeil Consumer	chewable tablet	80mg				aspartame · cellulose · cellulose acetate · corn starch · flavors · magnesium stearate · mannitol · povidone · red#7
AL AF CA PE	**Tylenol, Children's Cherry or Grape Flavor** McNeil Consumer	elixir	80mg/2.5ml				benzoic acid · citric acid · flavors · glycerin · malic acid (Grape) · polyethylene glycol · propylene glycol · sodium benzoate · sorbitol · sucrose · purified water · red#33 (Cherry) · red#40 · blue#1(Grape)
AF CA PE	**Tylenol, Children's Fruit Flavor** McNeil Consumer	chewable tablet	80mg				aspartame · cellulose · citric acid · corn starch · ethylcellulose · flavors · magnesium stearate · mannitol · red #7
AF CA PE	**Tylenol, Children's Grape Flavor** McNeil Consumer	chewable tablet	80mg				aspartame · cellulose · cellulose acetate · citric acid · corn starch · flavors · magnesium stearate · mannitol · povidone · blue#1 · red#7 · red#30
AL AF CA PE	**Tylenol, Children's Liquid** McNeil Consumer	suspension	80mg/2.5ml				butylparaben · cellulose · citric acid · corn syrup · flavors · glycerin · propylene glycol · purified water · sodium benzoate · sorbitol · xanthan gum · FD&C red#40

See Chapter 4, "Internal Analgesic and Antipyretic Products," for more information about these products.

INTERNAL ANALGESIC AND ANTIPYRETIC PRODUCTS - continued

	Product [a] Manufacturer/Supplier	Dosage Form	Acetaminophen	Aspirin	Ibuprofen	Other Analgesics	Other Ingredients [b]
** AL AF CA PE	**Tylenol, Children's Liquid Bubble Gum Flavor** McNeil Consumer	suspension	80mg/2.5ml				butylparaben · cellulose · citric acid · corn syrup · flavors · glycerin · propylene glycol · purified water · sodium benzoate · sorbitol · xanthan gum · D&C red#33 · FD&C red#40
AL AF CA PE	**Tylenol, Infants'** McNeil Consumer	drops	80mg/0.8ml				butylparaben · citric acid · flavors · glycerin · polyethylene glycol · propylene glycol · saccharin · sodium citrate · purified water · yellow#6
AL AF CA PE	**Tylenol, Infants' Suspension** McNeil Consumer	drops	80mg/0.8ml				butylparaben · cellulose · citric acid · corn syrup · flavors · glycerin · propylene glycol · purified water · sodium benzoate · sorbitol · xanthan gum · D&C red#33 · FD&C blue#1
AF CA	**Valorin** Otis Clapp & Son	tablet	325mg				
AF CA	**Valorin Extra** Otis Clapp & Son	tablet	500mg				
AF SO	**Valorin Super** Otis Clapp & Son	tablet	500mg				caffeine, 65mg
	Aspirin						
CA	**Adprin B** Pfeiffer Ph'cals	tablet		325mg			calcium carbonate · magnesium carbonate · magnesium oxide
CA	**Adprin B Extra Strength** Pfeiffer Ph'cals	caplet		500mg			calcium carbonate · magnesium carbonate · magnesium oxide
CA PU SU	**Alka-Seltzer Extra Strength** Bayer Consumer	effervescent tablet		500mg			sodium bicarbonate, 1985mg (sodium, 588mg) · citric acid, 1000mg
CA PU SU	**Alka-Seltzer Original** Bayer Consumer	effervescent tablet		325mg			sodium bicarbonate, 1916mg (sodium, 567mg) · citric acid, 1000mg
CA PU SU	**Alka-Seltzer, Lemon-Lime** Bayer Consumer	effervescent tablet		325mg			sodium bicarbonate, 1700mg (sodium, 506mg) · citric acid, 1000mg · saccharin · flavor
	Anacin Whitehall-Robins Healthcare	tablet		400mg			caffeine, 32mg · hydroxypropyl methylcellulose · microcrystalline cellulose · polyethylene glycol · surfactant
**	**Anacin** Whitehall-Robins Healthcare	caplet		400mg			caffeine, 32mg · hydroxypropyl methylcellulose · iron oxide · microcrystalline cellulose · polyethylene glycol · starch · surfactant

See Chapter 4, "Internal Analgesic and Antipyretic Products," for more information about these products.

INTERNAL ANALGESIC AND ANTIPYRETIC PRODUCTS - continued

	Product [a] Manufacturer/Supplier	Dosage Form	Acetaminophen	Aspirin	Ibuprofen	Other Analgesics	Other Ingredients [b]
	Anacin Maximum Strength Whitehall-Robins Healthcare	tablet		500mg			caffeine, 32mg · hydroxypropyl methylcellulose · microcrystalline cellulose · polyethylene glycol · starch · surfactant
SO	**Anodynos** Buffington	tablet		410mg		salicylamide, 30mg	caffeine, 60mg
	Arthritis Foundation Safety Coated Aspirin McNeil Consumer	tablet		500mg			carnauba wax · corn starch · hydroxypropyl methylcellulose · methacrylic acid copolymer · microcrystalline cellulose · polyethylene glycol · polysorbate 80 · sodium lauryl sulfate · talc · titanium dioxide · triacetin · blue#1 · D&C red#27 · yellow#6 · yellow#10
CA GL PR SO	**Arthritis Pain Formula** Whitehall-Robins Healthcare	caplet		500mg			magnesium hydroxide, 100mg · aluminum hydroxide, 27mg · hydrogenated vegetable oil · microcrystalline cellulose · starch · surfactant
CA	**Ascriptin Arthritis Pain** Ciba Self-Medication	caplet		325mg			magnesium hydroxide, 75mg · aluminum hydroxide, 75mg · calcium carbonate · hydroxypropyl methylcellulose · magnesium stearate · microcrystalline cellulose · propylene glycol · starch · talc · titanium dioxide · other ingredients
CA	**Ascriptin Maximum Strength** Ciba Self-Medication	caplet		500mg			magnesium hydroxide, 80mg · dried aluminum hydroxide gel, 80mg · calcium carbonate · hydroxypropyl methylcellulose · magnesium stearate · microcrystalline cellulose · propylene glycol · starch · talc · titanium dioxide · other ingredients
CA	**Ascriptin Regular Strength** Ciba Self-Medication	tablet		325mg			magnesium hydroxide, 50mg · dried aluminum hydroxide gel, 50mg · calcium carbonate · hydroxypropyl methylcellulose · magnesium stearate · microcrystalline cellulose · propylene glycol · starch · talc · titanium dioxide · other ingredients
CA SO	**Aspercin** Otis Clapp & Son	tablet		324mg			
CA SO	**Aspercin Extra** Otis Clapp & Son	tablet		500mg			
CA GL PU	**Aspergum, Cherry or Orange** Schering-Plough HealthCare	gum		227mg			flavor
CA SO	**Aspermin** Buffington	tablet		324mg			

See Chapter 4, "Internal Analgesic and Antipyretic Products," for more information about these products.

INTERNAL ANALGESIC AND ANTIPYRETIC PRODUCTS - continued

	Product [a] Manufacturer/Supplier	Dosage Form	Acetaminophen	Aspirin	Ibuprofen	Other Analgesics	Other Ingredients [b]
CA SO	**Aspermin Extra** Buffington	tablet		500mg			
CA	**Aspirin** Goldline Labs	suppository		120mg			
	Aspirin Multisource	suppository		125mg; 300mg; 600mg			
	Aspirin Lite Coat Schein Ph'cal	tablet		325mg			may contain: hydroxypropyl methylcellulose · starch
AL CA	**Aspirin, Enteric Coated** Goldline Labs	tablet		81mg			
	Aspirin, Enteric Coated Paddock Labs	tablet		650mg			
CA PE	**Aspirin, Low-Dose Children's** Goldline Labs	chewable tablet		81mg			
CA GL PR PU	**Aspirin, Special Buffered** Hudson	tablet		325mg			magnesium hydroxide, 50mg · dried aluminum hydroxide gel, 50mg · calcium carbonate
CA SO	**Aspirtab** Dover	tablet		324mg			
CA SO	**Aspirtab Max** Dover	tablet		500mg			
CA SO	**Back-Quell** Otis Clapp & Son	tablet		425mg			ephedrine sulfate · atropine sulfate
CA GL SO	**Bayer 8-Hour Aspirin Extended-Release** Bayer Consumer	timed-release caplet		650mg			
CA GL SO	**Bayer Arthritis Pain Regimen Extra Strength** Bayer Consumer	caplet		500mg			
CA GL SO	**Bayer Aspirin Extra Strength** Bayer Consumer	caplet · tablet		500mg			
CA GL SO	**Bayer Aspirin Regimen Adult Low Strength** Bayer Consumer	tablet		81mg			
CA GL SO	**Bayer Aspirin Regimen Regular Strength** Bayer Consumer	caplet		325mg			
CA GL SO	**Bayer Aspirin, Genuine** Bayer Consumer	caplet · tablet		325mg			

See Chapter 4, "Internal Analgesic and Antipyretic Products," for more information about these products.

INTERNAL ANALGESIC AND ANTIPYRETIC PRODUCTS - continued

	Product [a] Manufacturer/Supplier	Dosage Form	Acetaminophen	Aspirin	Ibuprofen	Other Analgesics	Other Ingredients [b]
CA GL SO PE	**Bayer Children's Aspirin, Cherry or Orange** Bayer Consumer	chewable tablet		81mg			saccharin · flavor
CA GL	**Bayer Plus Extra Strength** Bayer Consumer	caplet		500mg			calcium carbonate · magnesium carbonate · magnesium oxide
DY PR	**BC** Block Drug	powder		650mg			salicylamide, 195mg · caffeine, 32mg
DY PR SO	**BC** Block Drug	tablet		325mg			salicylamide, 95mg · caffeine, 16mg
DY PR	**BC Arthritis Strength** Block Drug	powder		742mg			salicylamide, 222mg · caffeine, 36mg
CA SO	**Buffaprin** Buffington	tablet		325mg			magnesium oxide
CA SO	**Buffaprin Extra** Buffington	tablet		500mg			magnesium oxide
CA SO	**Buffasal** Dover	tablet		324mg			magnesium oxide
CA SO	**Buffasal Max** Dover	tablet		500mg			magnesium oxide
CA PR SO	**Bufferin Arthritis Strength, Tri-Buffered** Bristol-Myers Products	caplet		500mg			calcium carbonate, 222.3mg · magnesium oxide, 88.9mg · magnesium carbonate, 55.6mg · benzoic acid · citric acid · corn starch · FD&C blue#1 · hydroxypropyl methylcellulose · magnesium stearate · mineral oil · polysorbate 20 · povidone · propylene glycol · simethicone emulsion · sodium phosphate · sorbitan monolaurate · titanium dioxide · may also contain: carnauba wax · zinc stearate
CA PR SO	**Bufferin Extra Strength, Tri-Buffered** Bristol-Myers Products	tablet		500mg			calcium carbonate, 222.3mg · magnesium oxide, 88.9mg · magnesium carbonate, 55.6mg · benzoic acid · citric acid · corn starch · FD&C blue#1 · hydroxypropyl methylcellulose · magnesium stearate · mineral oil · polysorbate 20 · povidone · propylene glycol · simethicone emulsion · sodium phosphate · sorbitan monolaurate · titanium dioxide · may also contain: carnauba wax · zinc stearate

See Chapter 4, "Internal Analgesic and Antipyretic Products," for more information about these products.

INTERNAL ANALGESIC AND ANTIPYRETIC PRODUCTS - continued

	Product [a] Manufacturer/Supplier	Dosage Form	Acetamin-ophen	Aspirin	Ibuprofen	Other Analgesics	Other Ingredients [b]
CA PR SO	**Bufferin, Tri-Buffered** Bristol-Myers Products	tablet		325mg			calcium carbonate, 158mg · magnesium oxide, 63mg · magnesium carbonate, 39mg · benzoic acid · citric acid · corn starch · FD&C blue#1 · hydroxypropyl methylcellulose · magnesium stearate · mineral oil · polysorbate 20 · povidone · propylene glycol · simethicone emulsion · sodium phosphate · sorbitan monolaurate · titanium dioxide · may also contain: carnauba wax · zinc stearate
	Buffets II Jones Medical	tablet	162mg	226.8mg			aluminum hydroxide, 50mg · caffeine, 32.4mg
CA SO	**Buffinol** Otis Clapp & Son	tablet		325mg			magnesium oxide
CA SO	**Buffinol Extra** Otis Clapp & Son	tablet		500mg			magnesium oxide
	Cope Mentholatum	tablet		421mg			caffeine, 32mg · magnesium hydroxide · dried aluminum hydroxide gel · corn starch · hydrogenated vegetable oil · microcrystalline cellulose · sodium lauryl sulfate · talc
	Ecotrin Adult Low Strength SmithKline Beecham	tablet		81mg			carnauba wax · D&C yellow#10 · FD&C yellow#6 · hydroxypropyl methylcellulose · methacrylic acid copolymer · microcrystalline cellulose · polyethylene glycol · silicon dioxide · starch · stearic acid · talc · titanium dioxide · triethyl citrate · propylene glycol · polysorbate 80
	Ecotrin Maximum Strength SmithKline Beecham	caplet · tablet		500mg			carnauba wax · colloidal silicon dioxide · FD&C yellow#6 · hydroxypropyl methylcellulose · maltodextrin · methacrylic acid copolymer · microcrystalline cellulose · pregelatinized starch · polyethylene glycol · simethicone · sodium hydroxide · sodium starch glycolate · stearic acid · talc · titanium dioxide · triethyl citrate
	Ecotrin Regular Strength SmithKline Beecham	tablet		325mg			carnauba wax · colloidal silicon dioxide · FD&C yellow#6 · hydroxypropyl methylcellulose · maltodextrin · methacrylic acid copolymer · microcrystalline cellulose · pregelatinized starch · polyethylene glycol · simethicone · sodium hydroxide · sodium starch glycolate · stearic acid · talc · titanium dioxide · triethyl citrate

See Chapter 4, "Internal Analgesic and Antipyretic Products," for more information about these products.

INTERNAL ANALGESIC AND ANTIPYRETIC PRODUCTS - continued

	Product [a] Manufacturer/Supplier	Dosage Form	Acetaminophen	Aspirin	Ibuprofen	Other Analgesics	Other Ingredients [b]
SO	**Emagrin** Otis Clapp & Son	tablet		410mg			salicylamide, 60mg · caffeine, 30mg
CA GL	**Empirin** Warner Wellcome Consumer	tablet		325mg			potato starch · microcrystalline cellulose
	Genprin Goldline Labs	tablet		325mg			
	Gensan Goldline Labs	tablet		400mg			caffeine, 32mg
DY PR	**Goody's Extra Strength** Goody's Ph'cals	tablet	130mg	260mg			caffeine, 16.25mg
DY PR	**Goody's Extra Strength Headache** Goody's Ph'cals	powder	260mg	520mg			caffeine, 32.5mg · lactose · potassium chloride
	Halfprin Low Strength Enteric Coated Kramer Labs	tablet		81mg; 162mg			
**	**Heartline** BDI Ph'cals	tablet		81mg			
CA	**Norwich Aspirin** Chattem	caplet		500mg			starch · hydroxypropyl methylcellulose · polyethylene glycol
CA	**Norwich Aspirin** Chattem	tablet		325mg			starch · hydroxypropyl methylcellulose · polyethylene glycol
CA SO	**Norwich Aspirin, Enteric Coated** Chattem	tablet		325mg; 500mg			dioctyl sodium sulfonate · hydroxypropylcellulose · hydroxymethylcellulose · iron oxide · microcrystalline cellulose · pharmaceutical glaze · polyethylene glycol · polyvinyl acetate phthalate · pregelatinized starch · silicone dioxide · stearic acid · talc · titanium dioxide · triethyl citrate · yellow#6 · yellow#10
	P-A-C Roberts Ph'cal	tablet		400mg			anhydrous caffeine, 32mg · cellulose · corn starch · croscarmellose sodium · sucrose · FD&C blue #2 · FD&C yellow #5 (tartrazine)
	Regiprin Enteric Coated Republic Drug	tablet		81mg			
**	**Rid-a-Pain with Codeine** Pfeiffer Ph'cals	tablet	97.2mg	226.8mg			caffeine, 32.4mg · salicylamide, 32.4mg · codeine phosphate, 1mg
	St. Joseph Low Dose Adult Aspirin Schering-Plough HealthCare	chewable tablet		81mg			fruit flavor
	Stanback, Original Formula Stanback	powder		650mg		salicylamide, 200mg	caffeine, 32mg

See Chapter 4, "Internal Analgesic and Antipyretic Products," for more information about these products.

INTERNAL ANALGESIC AND ANTIPYRETIC PRODUCTS - continued

	Product [a] Manufacturer/Supplier	Dosage Form	Acetaminophen	Aspirin	Ibuprofen	Other Analgesics	Other Ingredients [b]
DY GL PR PU SO SU	**Supac** Mission Pharmacal	tablet	160mg	230mg			calcium gluconate, 60mg · caffeine, 33mg
GL SO	**Vanquish** Bayer Consumer	caplet	194mg	227mg			magnesium hydroxide, 50mg · caffeine, 33mg · dried aluminum hydroxide gel, 25mg
	Ibuprofen						
CA SU	**Addaprin** Dover	tablet			200mg		
AF CA GL PU SO	**Advil** Whitehall-Robins Healthcare	caplet · tablet			200mg		acetylated monoglyceride · beeswax and/or carnauba wax · croscarmellose sodium · iron oxides · lecithin · methylparaben · microcrystalline cellulose · pharmaceutical glaze · povidone · propylparaben · silicon dioxide · simethicone · sodium benzoate · sodium lauryl sulfate · starch · stearic acid · sucrose · titanium dioxide
** AF	**Advil** Whitehall-Robins Healthcare	gel caplet			200mg		croscarmellose sodium · FD&C red#40 · FD&C yellow#6 · gelatin · glycerin · hydroxypropyl methylcellulose · iron oxides · lecithin · pharmaceutical glaze · propyl gallate · silicon dioxide · simethicone · sodium lauryl sulfate · starch · stearic acid · titanium dioxide · triacetin
AF	**Arthritis Foundation Ibuprofen** McNeil Consumer	tablet			200mg		carnauba wax · microcrystalline cellulose · croscarmellose sodium · hydroxypropyl methylcellulose · polyethylene glycol · polysorbate 80 · povidone · silicon dioxide · sodium starch glycolate · pregelatinized starch · stearic acid · titanium dioxide
AF CA GL SO	**Bayer Select Ibuprofen Pain Relief** Bayer Consumer	caplet			200mg		
AF	**Genpril** Goldline Labs	tablet			200mg		
AF	**Haltran** Roberts Ph'cal	tablet			200mg		carnauba wax · corn starch · hydroxypropyl methylcellulose · propylene glycol · silicon dioxide · pregelatinized starch · stearic acid · titanium dioxide

See Chapter 4, "Internal Analgesic and Antipyretic Products," for more information about these products.

INTERNAL ANALGESIC AND ANTIPYRETIC PRODUCTS - continued

	Product [a] Manufacturer/Supplier	Dosage Form	Acetaminophen	Aspirin	Ibuprofen	Other Analgesics	Other Ingredients [b]
AF CA GL SO	**Midol IB Cramp Relief Formula** Bayer Consumer	tablet			200mg		
AF CA DY GL PR PU SO SU	**Motrin IB** Pharmacia & Upjohn	caplet · tablet			200mg		carnauba wax · corn starch · hydroxypropyl methylcellulose · propylene glycol · silicon dioxide · pregelatinized starch · stearic acid · titanium dioxide
AF CA GL PU SU	**Motrin IB** Pharmacia & Upjohn	gelcap			200mg		benzyl alcohol · butylparaben · butyl alcohol · castor oil · colloidal silicon dioxide · edetate calcium disodium · FD&C yellow #6 · gelatin · hydroxypropyl methylcellulose · iron oxide black · magnesium stearate · methylparaben · microcrystalline cellulose · povidone · pregelatinized starch · propylene glycol · propylparaben · SDA 3 A alcohol · sodium lauryl sulfate · sodium propionate · sodium starch glycolate · starch · titanium dioxide
** AF PE	**Motrin, Children's** McNeil Consumer	suspension			100mg/5ml		citric acid · corn starch · artificial flavors · glycerin · polysorbate 80 · purified water · sodium benzoate · sucrose · xanthan gum · FD&C red#40 · D&C yellow#10
AF CA GL PR SO	**Nuprin** Bristol-Myers Products	caplet · tablet			200mg		carnauba wax · corn starch · D&C yellow#10 · FD&C yellow#6 · hydroxypropyl methylcellulose · propylene glycol · silicon dioxide · stearic acid · titanium dioxide
AF CA	**Ultraprin** Otis Clapp & Son	tablet			200mg		
AF CA	**Valprin** Buffington	tablet			200mg		
	Other Analgesics						
** AF	**Actron** Bayer Consumer	caplet · tablet				ketoprofen, 12.5mg	corn starch · croscarmellose sodium · hydroxypropyl methylcellulose · lactose · magnesium stearate · microcrystalline cellulose · polyethylene glycol · titanium dioxide
AF CA GL PR PU	**Aleve** Procter & Gamble	caplet · tablet				naproxen sodium, 220mg · (naproxen, 200mg · sodium, 20mg)	magnesium stearate · microcrystalline cellulose · povidone · purified water · talc · Opadry YS-1-4215

See Chapter 4, "Internal Analgesic and Antipyretic Products," for more information about these products.

INTERNAL ANALGESIC AND ANTIPYRETIC PRODUCTS - continued

	Product [a] Manufacturer/Supplier	Dosage Form	Acetaminophen	Aspirin	Ibuprofen	Other Analgesics	Other Ingredients [b]
	Arthropan Purdue Frederick	liquid				choline salicylate, 174mg/ml (equivalent to aspirin, 130mg)	
** AF	**Azo-Dine [c]** Republic Drug	tablet				phenazopyridine HCl, 97.2mg	
AF	**Azo-Standard [c]** PolyMedica Ph'cals	tablet				phenazopyridine HCl, 95mg	
AF CA PR SO	**Backache from the Makers of Nuprin** Bristol-Myers Products	caplet				magnesium salicylate tetrahydrate, 580mg (equivalent to anhydrous, 467mg)	carnauba wax · hydrogenated vegetable oil · hydroxypropyl methylcellulose · magnesium stearate · microcrystalline cellulose · polyethylene glycol · polysorbate 80 · titanium dioxide
AF CA	**Baridium [c]** Pfeiffer Ph'cals	tablet				phenazopyridine HCl, 95mg	
**	**Cystex** Numark Labs	tablet				sodium salicylate, 162.5mg	methenamine, 162mg · benzoic acid, 32mg
AF CA GL PR PU SO	**Doan's Extra Strength** Ciba Self-Medication	tablet				magnesium salicylate tetrahydrate, 580mg	magnesium stearate · microcrystalline cellulose · Opadry white · polyethylene glycol · stearic acid
AF CA GL PR PU SO	**Doan's Regular Strength** Ciba Self-Medication	tablet				magnesium salicylate tetrahydrate, 377mg	FD&C yellow#6 · magnesium stearate · microcrystalline cellulose · polyethylene glycol · stearic acid · Opadry light green
**	**Magnesium Salicylate** Multisource	caplet				magnesium salicylate, 467mg	
AF DY GL SO SU	**Mobigesic** B. F. Ascher	tablet				magnesium salicylate, 325mg	phenyltoloxamine citrate, 30mg
AF CA GL PR SO	**Momentum** Whitehall-Robins Healthcare	caplet				magnesium salicylate tetrahydrate 580mg (equivalent to magnesium salicylate anhydrous, 467mg)	hydrogenated vegetable oil · hydroxypropyl methylcellulose · microcrystalline cellulose · polyethylene glycol · polysorbate 80 · titanium dioxide

See Chapter 4, "Internal Analgesic and Antipyretic Products," for more information about these products.

INTERNAL ANALGESIC AND ANTIPYRETIC PRODUCTS - continued

	Product [a] Manufacturer/Supplier	Dosage Form	Acetaminophen	Aspirin	Ibuprofen	Other Analgesics	Other Ingredients [b]
** AF CA	**Orudis KT** Whitehall-Robins Healthcare	caplet · tablet				ketoprofen, 12.5mg	cellulose · D&C yellow#10 lake · FD&C blue#1 lake · iron oxide · pharmaceutical glaze · povidone · silica · sodium benzoate · sodium lauryl sulfate · starch · stearic acid · sugar · titanium dioxide · wax · FD&C yellow#5 lake (tartrazine)
AF CA GL PR PU	**Prodium [c]** Breckenridge Ph'cal	tablet				phenazopyridine HCl, 95mg	dextrose · FD&C red#40 aluminum lake · FD&C blue#2 aluminum lake · hydroxypropyl cellulose · polysorbate · povidone · sodium starch glycolate · starch · titanium dioxide · carnauba wax · ethylcellulose · Opaspray maroon
AF	**Re-Azo [c]** Reese Chemical	tablet				phenazopyridine HCl, 97.5mg	

** New listing
[a] For products that contain an analgesic and a sleep aid, see the Sleep Aid Products table. For products that are indicated for diuresis but may also contain an analgesic, see the Menstrual Products table.
[b] Caffeine may be effective as an adjuvant analgesic.
[c] Urinary tract analgesic

See Chapter 4, "Internal Analgesic and Antipyretic Products," for more information about these products.

EXTERNAL ANALGESIC PRODUCTS

Product Manufacturer/Supplier	Dosage Form	Counterirritant	Other Ingredients
Absorbine Jr. W. F. Young	liniment	menthol, 1.27%	acetone · chloroxylenol
Absorbine Jr. Extra Strength W. F. Young	liquid	menthol, 4%	acetone · chloroxylenol
Absorbine Jr. Power Gel W. F. Young	gel	menthol, 4%	SD alcohol 40B
Arthricare Double Ice Pain Relieving Rub Del Ph'cals	gel	menthol, 4% · camphor, 3.1%	
Arthricare Odor Free Pain Relieving Rub Del Ph'cals	cream	menthol, 1.25% · methyl nicotinate, 0.25% · capsicum oleoresin	
Arthricare Triple Medicated Pain Relieving Rub Del Ph'cals	cream	methyl salicylate, 30% · menthol, 1.25% · methyl nicotinate, 0.25%	
Arthritis Hot Thompson Medical	cream	methyl salicylate, 15% · menthol, 10%	methylparaben · glyceryl monostearate · lanolin · trolamine · citric acid · propylene glycol · stearic acid · water
Arthritis Rub Extra Strength G & W Labs	ointment	methyl salicylate, 30% · menthol, 8%	
Aspercreme Thompson Medical	lotion		trolamine salicylate, 10% · glyceryl monostearate · stearic acid · lanolin · cetyl alcohol · isopropyl palmitate · propylparaben · methylparaben · propylene glycol · sodium lauryl sulfate · potassium phosphate · water · aloe
Aspercreme Thompson Medical	cream		trolamine salicylate, 10% · cetyl alcohol · stearic acid · mineral oil · propylparaben · water · methylparaben · glycerin · potassium phosphate monobasic · aloe
Banalg Muscle Pain Reliever Forest Ph'cals	lotion	methyl salicylate, 4.9% · camphor, 2% · menthol, 1%	greaseless base
Ben-Gay Arthritis Formula Non-Greasy Pain Relieving Pfizer Consumer	cream	methyl salicylate, 30% · menthol, 8%	greaseless nonstaining emulsion base
Ben-Gay Greaseless Formula Pain Relieving Pfizer Consumer	cream	methyl salicylate, 15% · menthol, 10%	greaseless nonstaining emulsion base
Ben-Gay Original Formula Pain Relieving Pfizer Consumer	ointment	methyl salicylate, 18.3% · menthol, 16%	oleaginous base
Ben-Gay Ultra Strength Pain Relieving Pfizer Consumer	cream	methyl salicylate, 30% · menthol, 10% · camphor, 4%	greaseless nonstaining emulsion base
Ben-Gay Vanishing Scent Non-Greasy Pain Relieving Pfizer Consumer	gel	menthol, 2.5%	hydroalcoholic gel base

See Chapter 5, "External Analgesic Products," for more information about these products.

EXTERNAL ANALGESIC PRODUCTS - continued

Product Manufacturer/Supplier	**Dosage Form**	**Counterirritant**	**Other Ingredients**
Betuline Ferndale Labs	lotion	methyl salicylate · camphor · menthol	peppermint oil · water soluble base
Campho-phenique Pain Relieving Antiseptic Bayer Consumer	gel · liquid	camphor, 10.8% · phenol, 4.7%	eucalyptus oil
Capzasin-P Thompson Medical	cream	capsaicin, 0.025%	benzyl alcohol · cetyl alcohol · glyceryl monostearate · isopropyl myristate · polyoxyl 40 stearate · water · sorbitol · white petrolatum
Cool Heat Republic Drug	gel	menthol, 2%	
Deep-Down BIRA	cream	methyl salicylate, 15% · menthol, 5% · camphor, 0.5%	SD alcohol, 40.5%
Dencorub Alvin Last	cream	methyl salicylate, 15% · camphor, 3.1% · menthol, 1.25%	water · stearic acid · beeswax · paraffin · glycol stearate · petrolatum · glycerin · mineral oil · triethanolamine · lanolin · eucalyptus oil · isobornyl acetate
Dencorub Alvin Last	liquid	capsaicin, 0.025% (from capsicum oleoresin)	water · quince seed · benzoic acid · disodium EDTA · algin · mullein extract · myrrh extract · valerian
Epiderm Balm Pedinol Pharmacal	ointment	methyl salicylate · menthol	propylene glycol · isopropyl alcohol
Eucalyptamint Arthritis Pain Reliever Ciba Self-Medication	ointment	menthol, 16%	lanolin · eucalyptus oil
Eucalyptamint Muscle Pain Relief Ciba Self-Medication	cream	menthol, 8%	carbomer 980 · eucalyptus oil · fragrance · propylene glycol · SD alcohol 3A · triethanolamine · Tween 80 · water
Exocaine Medicated Rub Del Ph'cals	cream	methyl salicylate, 25%	
Exocaine Odor Free Del Ph'cals	cream		trolamine salicylate, 10%
Exocaine Plus Rub Del Ph'cals	cream	methyl salicylate, 30%	
** **First Aid Medicated Powder** Johnson & Johnson Consumer	powder	menthol · eucalyptol · methyl salicylate	zinc oxide · corn starch · dipropylene glycol · thymol
Flex-All Chattem	gel	menthol, 7% · methyl salicylate	alcohol · allantoin · aloe vera gel · boric acid · carbomer 940 · diazolidinyl urea · eucalyptus oil · glycerin · iodine · methylparaben · peppermint oil · polysorbate 60 · potassium iodide · propylene glycol · propylparaben · thyme oil · triethanolamine · water
Flex-All 454 Maximum Strength Chattem	gel	menthol, 16% · methyl salicylate	allantoin · aloe vera gel · carbomer 940 · diisopropyl adipate · eucalyptus oil · glycerin · peppermint oil · SD alcohol 38-B · steareth-2 · steareth-21 · triethanolamine · thyme oil · water
Gold Bond Medicated Anti-Itch Chattem	cream	menthol · methyl salicylate	lidocaine · cetearyl alcohol · DMDM hydantoin · eucalyptol · glyceryl stearate · methylparaben · petrolatum · propylene glycol · simethicone · sorbic acid · sorbitol · thymol · tocopherol · water · zinc oxide

See Chapter 5, "External Analgesic Products," for more information about these products.

EXTERNAL ANALGESIC PRODUCTS - continued

	Product Manufacturer/Supplier	Dosage Form	Counterirritant	Other Ingredients
	Gold Bond Medicated, Regular or Extra Strength Chattem	powder	menthol · methyl salicylate	zinc oxide · boric acid · eucalyptol · salicylic acid · talc · thymol · zinc stearate
	Gordogesic Gordon Labs	cream	methyl salicylate, 10%	propylene glycol · cetyl alcohol · mineral oil · stearic acid · white wax · triethanolamine · sodium lauryl sulfate · methylparaben · propylparaben
	Heet Whitehall-Robins Healthcare	liniment	methyl salicylate, 15% · camphor, 3.6% · capsaicin, 0.025% (as capsicum oleoresin)	alcohol, 70% · acetone
**	**Icy Hot** Chattem	cream	methyl salicylate, 30% · menthol, 10%	
**	**Icy Hot Chill Stick** Chattem	stick	methyl salicylate, 30% · menthol, 10%	
	Icy Hot Extra Strength Long-Lasting Balm Pain Reliever Chattem	ointment	methyl salicylate, 29% · menthol, 7.6%	paraffin · white petrolatum
**	**Menthacin** Mentholatum	cream	capsaicin, 0.025% · menthol, 0.4%	caprylic/capric triglyceride · carbomer 1342 · carbomer 940 · cetyl alcohol · diazolidinyl urea · glyceryl stearate · sodium lauryl sulfate · maleated soybean oil · methylparaben · polysorbate 60 · propyleneglycol · propylparaben · sorbitan stearate · trolamine · water
	Mentholatum Mentholatum	ointment	camphor, 9% · natural menthol, 1.3%	fragrance · petrolatum · titanium dioxide
	Mentholatum Deep Heating Mentholatum	lotion	methyl salicylate, 20% · menthol, 6%	carbomer 941 · lanolin oil · mineral oil · polysorbate 60 · sorbitan stearate · trolamine · water
	Mentholatum Deep Heating Arthritis Formula Mentholatum	cream	methyl salicylate, 30% · menthol, 8%	glyceryl stearate · sodium lauryl sulfate · isoceteth-20 · poloxamer 407 · quaternium-15 · sorbitan stearate · water
	Mentholatum Deep Heating Rub Mentholatum	cream	methyl salicylate, 12.7% · menthol, 5.8%	chloroxylenol · fragrance · glyceryl stearate · sodium lauryl sulfate · lanolin · water
	Methagual Gordon Labs	ointment	methyl salicylate, 8% · guaiacol, 2%	petrolatum · white wax · methylparaben · propylparaben
	Minit-Rub Bristol-Myers Products	cream	methyl salicylate, 15% · menthol, 3.5% · camphor, 2.3%	calcium benzoate · lanolin · polysorbate 20 · sodium alginate · sorbitol · water · may also contain: methylchloroisothiazoline/methylisothiazoline · DMDM hydantoin
	Mobisyl B. F. Ascher	cream		trolamine salicylate, 10%
	Muscle Rub G & W Labs	ointment	methyl salicylate, 18.3% · menthol, 16%	
	Myoflex Ciba Self-Medication	cream		trolamine salicylate, 10% · greaseless base · cetyl alcohol · disodium EDTA · fragrance · propylene glycol · sodium lauryl sulfate · stearyl alcohol · water · white wax

See Chapter 5, "External Analgesic Products," for more information about these products.

EXTERNAL ANALGESIC PRODUCTS - continued

	Product Manufacturer/Supplier	Dosage Form	Counterirritant	Other Ingredients
	Noxzema Original Procter & Gamble	cream	camphor · menthol · phenol	water · stearic acid · linseed oil · soybean oil · fragrance · ammonium hydroxide · gelatin · clove oil · eucalyptus oil · calcium hydroxide
	Noxzema Original Procter & Gamble	lotion	camphor · menthol · phenol	water · stearic acid · soybean oil · propylene glycol · fragrance · linseed oil · gelatin · calcium hydroxide · cetyl alcohol · clove oil · eucalyptus oil · carbomer · triethanolamine
	Numol S.S.S. Company	liquid	methyl salicylate, 9.7%· camphor, 9.6% · menthol, 3.1% · mustard oil	turpentine · eucalyptus oil · thymol · peppermint oil · pine needle oil · cedar leaf oil · thyme oil · mineral oil
**	**Pain Doctor** E. Fougera	cream	methyl salicylate, 25% · menthol, 10% · capsaicin, 0.025% (from capsicum oleoresin)	water · stearic acid · glyceryl stearate SE · steareth 2 · triethanolamine · carbomer 934 · propylene glycol · diazolidinyl urea · methylparaben · propylparaben
	Pain Gel Plus Mentholatum	lotion	menthol, 4%	aloe vera gel · carbomer 934 · dye · fragrance · isopropyl alcohol · methylparaben · propylparaben · squalene · triethanolamine · vitamin E acetate · water
	Pain Patch Mentholatum	pad	menthol, 154mg	
	Pain Relief Goldline Labs	gel	menthol, 7%	aloe vera gel base
**	**PainBreak** Stevens Skin	cream	menthol, 5% · methyl salicylate	deionized water · glyceryl stearate · stearic acid · jojoba oil · glycerin · cetyl alcohol · apricot kernel oil · sweet almond oil · castor oil · cetyl palmitate · cetearyl octanoate · panthenol · diazolidinyl urea · methylparaben · propylparaben · magnesium aluminum silicate · squalene · methyl gluceth 20 · tocopherol acetate · avocado oil · aloe vera gel · TEA salicylate
	Rid-a-Pain Pfeiffer Ph'cals	cream	capsaicin, 0.025%	
	Rid-a-Pain Pfeiffer Ph'cals	ointment	menthol, 15%	lanolin · eucalyptus oil
**	**Rid-a-Pain HP** Pfeiffer Ph'cals	cream	capsaicin, 0.075%	
	Sarna Stiefel Labs	lotion	camphor, 0.5% · menthol, 0.5%	
	Sloan's C. B. Fleet	liniment	turpentine oil, 47% · capsaicin, 0.025% (from oleoresin capsicum)	
	Soltice Quick Rub Chattem	cream	menthol, 5.1% · camphor, 5.1%	greaseless base
	Sports Spray Extra Strength Mentholatum	aerosol spray	methyl salicylate, 35% · menthol, 10% · camphor, 5%	alcohol, 58% · isobutane
	Sportscreme Thompson Medical	cream		trolamine salicylate, 10% · cetyl alcohol · FD&C blue#1 · FD&C yellow#5 · fragrance · glycerin · methylparaben · mineral oil · potassium phosphate monobasic · propylparaben · stearic acid · water
	Sportscreme Thompson Medical	lotion		trolamine salicylate, 10% · cetyl alcohol · fragrance · glyceryl monostearate · isopropyl palmitate · lanolin anhydrous · methylparaben · potassium phosphate monobasic · propylene glycol · propylparaben · sodium lauryl sulfate · stearic acid · water

See Chapter 5, "External Analgesic Products," for more information about these products.

EXTERNAL ANALGESIC PRODUCTS - continued

	Product Manufacturer/Supplier	Dosage Form	Counterirritant	Other Ingredients
	Thera-Gesic Mission Pharmacal	cream	methyl salicylate, 15% · menthol	water · dimethylpolysiloxane · glycerin · carbopol · triethanolamine · sodium lauryl sulfate · methylparaben · propylparaben
	Therapeutic Blue Ice Pfeiffer Ph'cals	gel	menthol, 2.5%	thymol · BHT
	Therapeutic Mineral Ice Bristol-Myers Products	gel	menthol, 2%	isopropyl alcohol · carbomer · ammonium hydroxide · thymol · magnesium sulfate · sodium hydroxide · cupric sulfate · color · water
	Therapeutic Mineral Ice Exercise Formula Bristol-Myers Products	gel	menthol, 4%	isopropyl alcohol · carbomer · ammonium hydroxide · fragrance · thymol · magnesium sulfate · sodium hydroxide · cupric sulfate · color · water
	Unguentine Mentholatum	ointment	phenol, 1%	eucalyptus oil · oleostearine · petrolatum · thymos oil · zinc oxide
	Unguentine Plus Mentholatum	cream	phenol, 0.5%	lidocaine HCl, 2% · fragrance · glyceryl stearate · isoceteth-20 · isopropyl palmitate · methylparaben · mineral oil · poloxamer 407 · propylparaben · quaternium-15 · sorbitan stearate · tetrasodium EDTA · water
SL	**Vicks VapoRub** Procter & Gamble	cream	camphor, 5.2% · menthol, 2.8% · spirits of turpentine	eucalyptus oil, 1.2% · carbomer 954 · cedarleaf oil · cetyl alcohol · cetyl palmitate · cyclomethicone copolyol · dimethicone copolyol · dimethicone · EDTA · glycerin · imidazolidinyl urea · isopropyl palmitate · methylparaben · nutmeg oil · PEG-100 stearate · propylparaben · purified water · sodium hydroxide · stearic acid · stearyl alcohol · thymol · titanium dioxide
SL	**Vicks VapoRub** Procter & Gamble	ointment	camphor, 4.8% · menthol, 2.6%	eucalyptus oil, 1.2% · cedarleaf oil · nutmeg oil · special petrolatum · spirits of turpentine · thymol
SL	**Vicks VapoSteam** Procter & Gamble	liquid	camphor, 6.2% · menthol, 3.2%	alcohol, 74% · eucalyptus oil, 1.5% · cedarleaf oil · nutmeg oil · poloxamer 124 · polyoxyethylene dodecanol · silicone
	Wonder Ice Pedinol Pharmacal	gel	menthol	
	Zostrix GenDerm	cream	capsaicin, 0.025%	benzyl alcohol · cetyl alcohol · glyceryl monostearate · isopropyl myristate · polyoxyethylene stearate blend · sorbitol solution · petrolatum · water
**	**Zostrix Sports** GenDerm	cream	capsaicin, 0.075%	benzyl alcohol · cetyl alcohol · glyceryl monostearate · isopropyl myristate · PEG-100 stearate · purified water · sorbitol solution · white petrolatum
	Zostrix-HP GenDerm	cream	capsaicin, 0.075%	benzyl alcohol · cetyl alcohol · glyceryl monostearate · isopropyl myristate · polyoxyethylene stearate blend · sorbitol solution · petrolatum · water

** New listing

See Chapter 5, "External Analgesic Products," for more information about these products.

VAGINAL ANTIFUNGAL PRODUCTS

	Product Manufacturer/Supplier	Dosage Form	Antifungal	Antiseptic	Other Ingredients
**	**Femizole-7** Lake Consumer	cream	clotrimazole, 1%		benzyl alcohol · cetearyl alcohol · cetyl esters wax · 2-octyldodecanol · polysorbate 60 · purified water · sodium phosphate monobasic · sorbitan monostearate
**	**Femstat 3** Procter & Gamble	cream	butoconazole nitrate, 2%		cetyl alcohol · glyceryl stearate · PEG-100 stearate · methylparaben · propylparaben · mineral oil · polysorbate 60 · propylene glycol · sorbitan monostearate · stearyl alcohol · purified water
	Gyne-Lotrimin Schering-Plough HealthCare	cream	clotrimazole, 1%		cetyl esters wax · octyl dodecanol · polysorbate 60 · water · sorbitan monostearate · benzyl alcohol · cetearyl alcohol
	Gyne-Lotrimin Inserts Schering-Plough HealthCare	tablet	clotrimazole, 100mg	povidone	corn starch · lactose · magnesium stearate
	Monistat 7 Advanced Care	suppository	miconazole nitrate, 100mg		hydrogenated vegetable oil base
	Monistat 7 Advanced Care	cream	miconazole nitrate, 2%	benzoic acid	BHA · mineral oil · peglicol 5 oleate · pegoxyol 7 stearate · purified water
**	**Monistat 7 Prefilled Applicators** Advanced Care	cream	miconazole nitrate, 2%	benzoic acid	BHA · mineral oil · peglicol 5 oleate · pegoxyol 7 stearate · purified water
	Mycelex-7 Bayer Consumer	cream	clotrimazole, 1%		cetyl esters wax · octyldodecanol · polysorbate 60 · water · sorbitan monostearate · benzyl alcohol · cetostearyl alcohol
	Mycelex-7 Inserts Bayer Consumer	tablet	clotrimazole, 100mg	povidone	corn starch · lactose · magnesium stearate
**	**Yeast-X** C. B. Fleet	cream	miconazole nitrate, 2%		

** New listing

See Chapter 6, "Vaginal and Menstrual Products," for more information about these products.

FEMININE HYGIENE PRODUCTS

	Product Manufacturer/Supplier	Dosage Form	Antimicrobial	Antipruritic/ Anesthetic/ Counterirritant	Hydrocortisone	Other Ingredients
	Betadine Medicated Purdue Frederick	suppository	povidone-iodine, 10%			
	Betadine Medicated Douche Purdue Frederick	liquid	povidone-iodine, 10%			
	Betadine Premixed Medicated Disposable Douche Purdue Frederick	liquid	povidone-iodine, 0.3%			
**	**Feminique Douche, Baby Powder or Spring Fresh Scent** Quality Health	liquid	octoxynol-9			deionized water · lactic acid · sodium lactate · diazolidinyl urea · methylparaben · disodium EDTA · fragrance
**	**Feminique Douche, Extra Cleansing** Quality Health	liquid	octoxynol-9			deionized water · vinegar
**	**Feminique Douche, Natural Vinegar & Water** Quality Health	liquid				water · vinegar · sorbic acid
**	**Feminique Feminine Cloth Towelettes** Quality Health	wipe	octoxynol-9			water · propylene glycol · sodium benzoate · sodium lactate · fragrance · lactic acid · quaternium-15 · sodium lauryl sulfate
	Gyne-cort Combe	cream			0.5%	
	Gyne-cort Extra Strength 10 Combe	cream			1%	
	Massengill Disp. Douche, Mtn. Breeze or Spring Rain Scent SmithKline Beecham	liquid	cetylpyridinium chloride · octoxynol-9			disodium EDTA · SD alcohol 40 · diazolidinyl urea · lactic acid · fragrance · colors · propylparaben · methylparaben · propylene glycol · water · sodium lactate
	Massengill Disp. Douche, Vinegar & Water Extra Cleansing SmithKline Beecham	liquid	cetylpyridinium chloride · octoxynol-9			diazolidinyl urea · disodium EDTA · vinegar · purified water · sodium citrate · citric acid
	Massengill Disposable Douche SmithKline Beecham	liquid	povidone-iodine, 0.3%			water

See Chapter 6, "Vaginal and Menstrual Products," for more information about these products.

FEMININE HYGIENE PRODUCTS - continued

	Product Manufacturer/Supplier	Dosage Form	Antimicrobial	Antipruritic/ Anesthetic/ Counterirritant	Hydrocortisone	Other Ingredients
	Massengill Disposable Douche, Baking Soda SmithKline Beecham	liquid	sodium bicarbonate			
	Massengill Disposable Douche, Vinegar & Water Extra Mild SmithKline Beecham	liquid				vinegar · purified water · sodium citrate · citric acid
	Massengill Douche, Country Flowers or Fresh Baby Pwdr. Scent SmithKline Beecham	liquid	cetylpyridinium chloride · octoxynol-9			purified water · SD alcohol 40 · diazolidinyl urea · sodium citrate · citric acid · disodium EDTA · fragrance · colors
	Massengill Douche, Unscented SmithKline Beecham	powder		methyl salicylate · phenol · thymol · menthol		eucalyptus oil · ammonium alum · sodium chloride · PEG-8 · D&C yellow#10 · FD&C yellow#6
	Massengill Towelette SmithKline Beecham	wipe			0.5%	diazolidinyl urea · DMDM hydantoin · isopropyl myristate · methylparaben · propylparaben · polysorbate 60 · propylene glycol · sorbitan stearate · steareth-2 · steareth-21 · water
	Massengill Towelette, Baby Powder or Unscented SmithKline Beecham	wipe	cetylpyridinium chloride · octoxynol-9			lactic acid · sodium lactate · potassium sorbate · disodium EDTA · water · fragrance
	Norforms, Fresh Flowers Scent C. B. Fleet	suppository	benzethonium chloride			PEG-18 · PEG-32 · PEG-20 stearate · fragrance · methylparaben · lactic acid
FR	**Norforms, Unscented** C. B. Fleet	suppository	benzethonium chloride			PEG-18 · PEG-32 · PEG-20 stearate · methylparaben · lactic acid
	Oxyzal Wet Dressing Gordon Labs	solution	benzalkonium chloride, 0.05% · oxyquinoline sulfate			
	PMC Disposable Douche Thomas & Thompson	liquid	boric acid, 82%	thymol, 0.3% · phenol, 0.2% · menthol		ammonium aluminum sulfate, 16% · eucalyptus oil · peppermint oil
	PMC Douche Thomas & Thompson	powder	boric acid, 82%	thymol, 0.3% · phenol, 0.2% · menthol		ammonium aluminum sulfate, 16% · eucalyptus oil · peppermint oil
	Summer's Eve Disposable Douche, Vinegar & Water C. B. Fleet	liquid	benzoic acid			vinegar · water
	Summer's Eve Douche C. B. Fleet	liquid	povidone-iodine, 0.3%			water · citric acid

See Chapter 6, "Vaginal and Menstrual Products," for more information about these products.

FEMININE HYGIENE PRODUCTS - continued

	Product Manufacturer/Supplier	Dosage Form	Antimicrobial	Antipruritic/ Anesthetic/ Counterirritant	Hydrocortisone	Other Ingredients
**	**Summer's Eve Douche, Extra-Cleansing Vinegar & Water** C. B. Fleet	liquid	benzoic acid			purified water · sodium chloride · vinegar
	Summer's Eve Douche; Musk, Touch of Spring, or White Flowers C. B. Fleet	liquid	octoxynol-9			citric acid · sodium benzoate · disodium EDTA · fragrance · water
**	**Summer's Eve Feminine Powder** C. B. Fleet	powder	octoxynol-9 · benzethonium chloride			corn starch · tricalcium phosphate · fragrance
**	**Summer's Eve Feminine Wash Cleansing Cloths** C. B. Fleet	wipe	octoxynol-9			purified water · sodium benzoate · fragrance · citric acid · disodium EDTA
	Trimo-San Milex Products	jelly	oxyquinoline sulfate, 0.025%			glycerin · carbomer · sodium citrate · citric acid · methylparaben · simethicone · lilac perfume · sodium lauryl sulfate · triethanolamine
	Tucks Warner Wellcome Consumer	pad				witch hazel, 50% · glycerin, 10% · alcohol
**	**Vaginex Douche** Quality Health	liquid	povidone-iodine, 30%			
**	**Vaginex Medicated** Quality Health	powder	8-hydroxyquinoline · 8-hydroxyquinoline sulfate			zinc oxide · corn starch · fragrance · isostearic acid · PPG-20 methyl glucose ether · talc
**	**Vaginex, Scented or Unscented** Quality Health	cream			1%	
	Vagisil Combe	cream	resorcinol, 2%	benzocaine, 5%		
**	**Yeast-X** C. B. Fleet	cream			1%	
**	**Yeast·Guard Advanced Sensitive Formula** Lake Consumer	cream	benzalkonium chloride, 0.13%	benzocaine, 5%		deionized water · glyceryl stearate · mineral oil · cetyl alcohol · PEG-100 stearate · aloe vera gel · isopropyl palmitate · isopropyl myristate · isopropyl stearate · lanolin alcohol · triethanolamine · methylparaben · propylparaben · carbomer 940 · vitamin E · fragrance · trisodium HEDTA
**	**Yeast·Guard Disposable Douche** Lake Consumer	solution	povidone-iodine, 0.3%			purified water

See Chapter 6, "Vaginal and Menstrual Products," for more information about these products.

FEMININE HYGIENE PRODUCTS - continued

	Product Manufacturer/Supplier	Dosage Form	Antimicrobial	Antipruritic/ Anesthetic/ Counterirritant	Hydrocortisone	Other Ingredients
**	**Yeast·Guard Disposable Douche Premix** Lake Consumer	liquid	octoxynol-9			purified water · lactic acid · sodium lactate · sodium benzoate · aloe vera
**	**Yeast·Guard Douche Concentrate** Lake Consumer	liquid	povidone-iodine, 10%			
**	**Yeast·Guard Maximum Strength** Lake Consumer	cream	benzalkonium chloride, 0.13%	benzocaine, 20%		deionized water · propylene glycol · cetyl alcohol · isopropyl palmitate · glyceryl stearate · sodium lauryl sulfate · aloe vera gel · methylparaben · propylparaben · vitamin E · fragrance · tetrasodium HEDTA

** New listing

See Chapter 6, "Vaginal and Menstrual Products," for more information about these products.

MENSTRUAL PRODUCTS

	Product [a] Manufacturer/Supplier	Dosage Form	Analgesic	Diuretic	Other Ingredients
AF CA GL PR PU SO	**Aqua-Ban** Thompson Medical	tablet		pamabrom, 50mg	FD&C blue#1 aluminum lake · titanium dioxide · hydroxypropyl methylcellulose · microcrystalline cellulose · propylene glycol · croscarmellose sodium · carnauba wax · lactose · magnesium stearate · polyethylene glycol · polysorbate 80 · starch
AF CA GL PR SO SU	**Backaid Pills** Alva-Amco Pharmacal	caplet	acetaminophen, 500mg	pamabrom, 25mg	
AF CA GL	**Bayer Select Aspirin-Free Menstrual** Bayer Consumer	caplet	acetaminophen, 500mg	pamabrom, 25mg	
GL PR SO	**Diurex Long Acting** Alva-Amco Pharmacal	timed-release capsule	potassium salicylate · acetaminophen	caffeine, 195mg	
** AF CA GL PR SO	**Diurex MPR** Alva-Amco Pharmacal	caplet	acetaminophen, 500mg	pamabrom, 25mg	
** AF CA GL PR SO	**Diurex PMS** Alva-Amco Pharmacal	caplet	acetaminophen, 500mg	pamabrom, 25mg	pyrilamine maleate, 15mg
AF CA GL PR SO SU	**Diurex Water Caplet** Alva-Amco Pharmacal	timed-release caplet	acetaminophen, 325mg	pamabrom, 50mg	
GL PR SO	**Diurex Water Pills** Alva-Amco Pharmacal	tablet	potassium salicylate · salicylamide	caffeine	
AF CA GL PR SO	**Diurex-2 Water Pills** Alva-Amco Pharmacal	tablet	acetaminophen, 162.5mg	pamabrom, 25mg	iron · calcium
**	**Fem-1** BDI Ph'cals	tablet	acetaminophen, 500mg	pamabrom, 25mg	
AF CA GL PR PU SU	**Lurline PMS** Fielding	tablet	acetaminophen, 500mg	pamabrom, 25mg	pyridoxine HCl, 50mg
AF	**Midol Menstrual Maximum Strength Multisymptom Formula** Bayer Consumer	gelcap	acetaminophen, 500mg	caffeine, 60mg	pyrilamine maleate, 15mg

See Chapter 6, "Vaginal and Menstrual Products," for more information about these products.

MENSTRUAL PRODUCTS - continued

	Product [a] Manufacturer/Supplier	Dosage Form	Analgesic	Diuretic	Other Ingredients
AF GL SO	**Midol Menstrual Maximum Strength Multisymptom Formula** Bayer Consumer	caplet	acetaminophen, 500mg	caffeine, 60mg	pyrilamine maleate, 15mg
** AF CA	**Midol PMS Maximum Strength Multisymptom Formula** Bayer Consumer	gelcap	acetaminophen, 500mg	pamabrom, 25mg	pyrilamine maleate, 15mg · croscarmellose sodium · D&C red#27 lake · disodium EDTA · FD&C blue#1 · FD&C red#40 lake · gelatin · glycerin · hydroxypropyl methylcellulose · iron oxide · magnesium stearate · microcrystalline cellulose · starch · stearic acid · titanium dioxide · triacetin
AF CA GL SO	**Midol PMS Multisymptom Formula** Bayer Consumer	caplet	acetaminophen, 500mg	pamabrom, 25mg	pyrilamine maleate, 15mg
AF CA GL SO	**Midol Teen Multisymptom Formula** Bayer Consumer	caplet	acetaminophen, 400mg	pamabrom, 25mg	
AF CA	**Odrinil Water Pills** Fox Pharmacal	tablet		pamabrom, 25mg	dicalcium phosphate · cellulose · stearic acid · silica · coating materials · yellow#10 · yellow#6
CA	**Pamprin Maximum Pain Relief** Chattem	caplet	acetaminophen, 250mg · magnesium salicylate, 250mg	pamabrom, 25mg	
AF CA	**Pamprin MultiSymptom Formula** Chattem	caplet · tablet	acetaminophen, 500mg	pamabrom, 25mg	pyrilamine maleate, 15mg
AF CA	**Premsyn PMS** Chattem	caplet	acetaminophen, 500mg	pamabrom, 25mg	pyrilamine maleate, 15mg

** New listing
[a] This table lists only products that contain a diuretic; some may contain an analgesic and a diuretic. For other products used in the management of dysmenorrhea, see the Internal Analgesic and Antipyretic Products table.

See Chapter 6, "Vaginal and Menstrual Products," for more information about these products.

VAGINAL LUBRICANT PRODUCTS

	Product Manufacturer/Supplier	Dosage Form	Lubricant	Preservative	Other Ingredients
	Astroglide Biofilm	gel		glycerin · propylene glycol · polyquaternium #5 · methylparaben · propylparaben	purified water
	Feminease Parnell Ph'cals	cream	mineral oil · stearic acid	glycerin · propylene glycol · benzoic acid · BHT	purified water · yerba santa · cetyl alcohol · glyceryl stearate · isopropyl myristate · PEG-40 stearate · squalene · dimethicone · diazolidinyl urea · lecithin · PEG-12 oleate · sulfated castor oil
	Gyne-Moistrin Moisturizing Schering-Plough HealthCare	gel		propylene glycol · methylparaben · propylparaben	polyglyceryl methacrylate · water
	H-R Lubricating Carter Products	jelly		propylene glycol · propylparaben · methylparaben	hydroxypropyl methylcellulose · carbomer 934P · sodium hydroxide
	K-Y Jelly Johnson & Johnson Consumer	jelly		chlorhexidine gluconate · glycerin · methylparaben	glucono delta lactone · sodium hydroxide · hydroxyethyl cellulose · purified water · sodium hydroxide
	Lubrin Inserts Kenwood Labs	suppository		glycerin	PEG-6-32 · PEG-20 · caprylic/capric triglyceride · PEG-40 stearate · polysorbate 80
** FR	**Maxilube** Mission Pharmacal	jelly	silicone oil · sodium lauryl sulfate	glycerin · methylparaben · propylparaben	water · triethanolamine · carbomer 934
	Moist Again Vaginal Moisturizing Lake Consumer	gel		glycerin · chlorhexidine gluconate · sodium benzoate · potassium sorbate · diazolidinyl urea · sorbic acid	water · carbomer · triethanolamine · aloe vera · citric acid
	Replens Warner Wellcome Consumer	gel	mineral oil · hydrogenated palm oil glyceride	sorbic acid · glycerin	carbomer 934P · polycarbophil
**	**Surgel** Ulmer	gel		propylene glycol · glycerin	sodium carboxymethylcellulose · phenyl mercuric nitrate
	Touch Personal Lubricant London Int'l U.S. Holdings	gel		propylene glycol · benzoic acid	water · hydroxyethyl cellulose · sodium hydroxide
	Women's Health Institute Lubricating Lake Consumer	gel		chlorhexidine gluconate · methylparaben · glycerin	glucono delta lactone · hydroxyethyl cellulose · sodium hydroxide · water

** New listing

See Chapter 6, "Vaginal and Menstrual Products," for more information about these products.

CONDOM PRODUCTS

	Product Manufacturer/Supplier	Material [a]	Spermicide	Comments
**	**Avanti** London Int'l U.S. Holdings	polyurethane	No	lubricated
**	**Avanti Super Thin** London Int'l U.S. Holdings	polyurethane	No	lubricated
**	**Class Act Sensitive** Carter Products	latex	No	reservoir end · lubricated · ribbed or ultra thin
	Class Act Sensitive with Spermicide Carter Products	latex	Yes	reservoir end · spermicidal lubricant · ribbed or ultra thin
**	**Fourex [a]** London Int'l U.S. Holdings	animal membrane[a]	No	pre-moistened capsule or pre-moistened foil
	Fourex with Spermicide [a] London Int'l U.S. Holdings	animal membrane [a]	nonoxynol-9, 7%	spermicidally lubricated foil
	Gold Circle Coin Aladan	latex	No	reservoir end
	Gold Circle Rainbow Coin Aladan	latex	No	reservoir end · contoured shape · colored
	Mentor Carter Products	latex	No	reservoir end · adhesive seal and applicator hood · lubricated
	Mentor Plus with Spermicide Carter Products	latex	Yes	reservoir end · adhesive seal and applicator hood · packaged with silicone spermicidal lubricant
	Naturalamb [a] Carter Products	lamb cecum [a]	No	lubricated
	Naturalamb with Spermicide [a] Carter Products	lamb cecum [a]	Yes	spermicidal lubricant
	Ramses Extra Strength with Spermicide London Int'l U.S. Holdings	latex	nonoxynol-9, 8%	reservoir end · spermicidal lubricant
**	**Ramses Extra with Spermicide** London Int'l U.S. Holdings	latex	nonoxynol-9, 5%	reservoir end · spermicidal lubricant · regular or ribbed
	Ramses Sensitol London Int'l U.S. Holdings	latex	No	reservoir end · lubricated
**	**Ramses Ultra Thin** London Int'l U.S. Holdings	latex	No	reservoir end · lubricated · regular or ribbed
	Ramses Ultra Thin with Spermicide London Int'l U.S. Holdings	latex	nonoxynol-9, 5%	reservoir end · spermicidal lubricant · regular or ribbed
	Reality Female Condom Female Health	polyurethane	No	thin, soft, loose-fitting sheath with two flexible rings · inner ring aids in insertion and holds device in place over the cervix · outer ring remains outside the vagina after insertion · may be inserted hours before intercourse · prelubricated with silicone · packaged with extra water-based lubricant · disposable, for one-time use only

See Chapter 7, "Contraceptive Methods and Products," for more information about these products.

CONDOM PRODUCTS - continued

	Product Manufacturer/Supplier	Material [a]	Spermicide	Comments
	Saxon Gold Rainbow Aladan	latex	No	reservoir end · contoured shape · colored · lubricated
	Saxon Gold Ultra with Spermicide, Clear or Rainbow Aladan	latex	nonoxynol-9, 6.6%	reservoir end · contoured shape · clear or colored · spermicidal lubricant
	Saxon Gold Ultra Lube Aladan	latex	No	reservoir end · contoured shape · water-based lubricant
	Saxon Gold Ultra Ribbed Aladan	latex	No	reservoir end · contoured shape · lubricated
	Saxon Gold Ultra Sensitive Aladan	latex	No	reservoir end · contoured shape · lubricated
**	**Sheik Classic** London Int'l U.S. Holdings	latex	No	reservoir end · regular or lubricated
	Sheik Classic with Spermicide London Int'l U.S. Holdings	latex	nonoxynol-9, 8%	reservoir end · spermicidal lubricant
	Sheik Excita Extra with Spermicide London Int'l U.S. Holdings	latex	nonoxynol-9, 8%	reservoir end · spermicidal lubricant · ribbed
	Sheik Fiesta London Int'l U.S. Holdings	latex	No	reservoir end · assorted colors · lubricated
	Sheik Super Thin London Int'l U.S. Holdings	latex	No	reservoir end · lubricated · regular or ribbed
	Sheik Super Thin with Spermicide London Int'l U.S. Holdings	latex	nonoxynol-9, 8%	reservoir end · spermicidal lubricant · regular or ribbed
**	**Sure** Aladan	latex	No	reservoir end · lubricated
**	**Sure with Spermicide** Aladan	latex	nonoxynol-9	reservoir end · contoured shape · spermicidal lubricant
**	**Touch** London Int'l U.S. Holdings	latex	No	reservoir end · available styles are regular, ribbed, sunrise colors, and thin ultra sensitive
**	**Touch Lubricated** London Int'l U.S. Holdings	latex	No	reservoir end · lubricated
	Touch with Spermicide London Int'l U.S. Holdings	latex	nonoxynol-9, 8%	reservoir end · spermicidal lubricant
	Trojan Extra Strength Carter Products	latex	No	reservoir end · colored · lubricated
	Trojan Extra Strength with Spermicide Carter Products	latex	Yes	reservoir end · spermicidal lubricant
	Trojan Magnum Carter Products	latex	No	reservoir end · larger size · lubricated

See Chapter 7, "Contraceptive Methods and Products," for more information about these products.

CONDOM PRODUCTS - continued

	Product Manufacturer/Supplier	Material [a]	Spermicide	Comments
	Trojan Magnum with Spermicide Carter Products	latex	Yes	reservoir end · larger size · spermicidal lubricant
	Trojan Naturalube Carter Products	latex	No	reservoir end · contoured shape · lubricated · ribbed/textured
	Trojan Plus Carter Products	latex	No	reservoir end · contoured shape · colored · lubricated
	Trojan Plus 2 with Spermicide Carter Products	latex	Yes	reservoir end · contoured shape · spermicidal lubricant
	Trojan Ribbed Carter Products	latex	No	reservoir end · colored · lubricated · ribbed/textured
	Trojan Ribbed with Spermicide Carter Products	latex	Yes	reservoir end · spermicidal lubricant · ribbed/textured
**	**Trojan Ultra Texture** Carter Products	latex	No	reservoir end · lubricated · textured
**	**Trojan Ultra Texture with Spermicide** Carter Products	latex	Yes	reservoir end · spermicidal lubricant · textured
	Trojan Very Sensitive Carter Products	latex	No	reservoir end · contoured shape · lubricated
	Trojan Very Sensitive with Spermicide Carter Products	latex	Yes	reservoir end · contoured shape · spermicidal lubricant
	Trojan Very Thin Carter Products	latex	No	receptacle end · lubricated
	Trojan Very Thin with Spermicide Carter Products	latex	Yes	receptacle end · spermicidal lubricant
	Trojan-Enz Carter Products	latex	No	reservoir end · regular or lubricated
	Trojan-Enz Large Carter Products	latex	No	reservoir end · larger size · lubricated
	Trojan-Enz Large with Spermicide Carter Products	latex	Yes	reservoir end · larger size · spermicidal lubricant
	Trojan-Enz with Spermicide Carter Products	latex	Yes	reservoir end · spermicidal lubricant
	Trojans Carter Products	latex	No	

** New listing

[a] Animal membrane condoms are more porous than latex ones and may allow transmission of the AIDS virus. Animal membrane condoms are not to be used for the prevention of sexually transmitted diseases.

See Chapter 7, "Contraceptive Methods and Products," for more information about these products.

SPERMICIDE PRODUCTS

	Product Manufacturer/Supplier	Dosage Form	Spermicide	Other Ingredients
	Advantage 24 [a] Lake Consumer	gel	nonoxynol-9, 3.5%	purified water · glycerin · mineral oil · polycarbophil · hydrogenated palm oil glyceride · carbomer 934P · methylparaben · sorbic acid · sodium hydroxide
	Conceptrol Advanced Care	gel	nonoxynol-9, 4%	cellulose gum · lactic acid · methylparaben · povidone · propylene glycol · purified water · sorbic acid · sorbitol solution
	Conceptrol Inserts Advanced Care	suppository	nonoxynol-9, 8.34%	lauroamphodiacetate · sodium trideceth sulfate · polyethylene glycol 1000 · polyethylene glycol 1450 · povidone
	Conceptrol Prefilled Disposable Advanced Care	gel	nonoxynol-9, 4%	cellulose gum · lactic acid · methylparaben · povidone · propylene glycol · purified water · sorbic acid · sorbitol solution
	Delfen Advanced Care	foam	nonoxynol-9, 12.5%	benzoic acid · cetyl alcohol · diethylaminoethyl stearamide · glacial acetic acid · methylparaben · perfume · polyvinyl alcohol · propylene glycol · purified water · sodium carboxymethylcellulose · sorbic acid · stearic acid
	Emko Schering-Plough HealthCare	foam	nonoxynol-9, 12%	benzethonium chloride · propellants · glyceryl stearate
	Encare Thompson Medical	suppository	nonoxynol-9, 100mg	polyethylene glycol · tartaric acid · sodium citrate · sodium bicarbonate
	Gynol II [a] Advanced Care	jelly	nonoxynol-9, 2%	lactic acid · methylparaben · povidone · propylene glycol · purified water · sodium carboxymethylcellulose · sorbic acid · sorbitol solution
	Gynol II ES [a] Advanced Care	jelly	nonoxynol-9, 3%	lactic acid · methylparaben · povidone · propylene glycol · purified water · sodium carboxymethylcellulose · sorbic acid · sorbitol solution
	K-Y Plus [a] Johnson & Johnson Consumer	jelly	nonoxynol-9, 2.2%	cremophor · hydroxyethyl cellulose · methylparaben · propylene glycol · purified water · sorbic acid
	Koromex Quality Health	foam	nonoxynol-9, 12.5%	acetic acid · cetyl alcohol · fragrance · isobutane · isopropyl alcohol · laureth-4 · PEG-50 stearate · propylene glycol · sodium acetate water
	Koromex [a] Quality Health	jelly	nonoxynol-9, 3%	
	Koromex Crystal Clear [a] Quality Health	gel	nonoxynol-9, 3%	
**	**Koromex Inserts** Quality Health	suppository	nonoxynol-9, 125mg (5%)	lactic acid · polyethylene glycol
	Ortho-Creme Advanced Care	cream	nonoxynol-9, 2%	benzoic acid · castor oil · cetyl alcohol · fragrance · glacial acetic acid · methylparaben · potassium hydroxide · propylene glycol · propylparaben · purified water · cellulose gum · sodium lauryl sulfate · sorbic acid · stearic acid · trolamine

See Chapter 7, "Contraceptive Methods and Products," for more information about these products.

SPERMICIDE PRODUCTS - continued

	Product Manufacturer/Supplier	Dosage Form	Spermicide	Other Ingredients
	Ortho-Gynol [a] Advanced Care	jelly	octoxynol-9, 1%	boric acid · castor oil · fragrance · glacial acetic acid · methylparaben · potassium hydroxide · propylene glycol · purified water · sorbic acid · sodium carboxymethylcellulose
**	**Ramses Personal Spermicidal Lubricant** London Int'l U.S. Holdings	gel	nonoxynol-9, 3%	
	Semicid Inserts Whitehall-Robins Healthcare	suppository	nonoxynol-9, 100mg	benzethonium chloride · citric acid · D&C red#21 lake · D&C red#33 lake · methylparaben · polyethylene glycol · water
	Shur-Seal [a] Milex Products	jelly	nonoxynol-9, 2%	water · propylene glycol · methylcellulose · methylparaben · simethicone · boric acid · citric acid
	VCF [a] Apothecus Ph'cal	gel	nonoxynol-9, 3%	propylene glycol · cellulose gum · sorbitol · polyvinylpyrrolidone · lactic acid · methylparaben · EDTA · water
	VCF Vaginal Contraceptive Film Apothecus Ph'cal	film square	nonoxynol-9, 28%	glycerin · polyvinyl alcohol

** New listing
[a] For use with a diaphragm

See Chapter 7, "Contraceptive Methods and Products," for more information about these products.

MISCELLANEOUS NASAL PRODUCTS

	Product Manufacturer/Supplier	Dosage Form	Primary Ingredients	Preservative	Other Ingredients
	Ayr B. F. Ascher	drops · spray	sodium chloride, 0.65%	benzalkonium chloride · thimerosal	
**	**Ayr Saline** B. F. Ascher	gel	sodium chloride, 0.5%	glycerin · propylene glycol · methylparaben · propylparaben	diazolidinyl urea · carbomer · tocopherol acetate · glyceryl polymethacrylate · aloe vera gel
SL	**Breathe Free** Thompson Medical	spray	sodium chloride, 0.65%	benzalkonium chloride	monobasic sodium · dibasic sodium
SL	**HuMIST Saline** Scherer Labs	spray	sodium chloride, 0.65%	chlorobutanol, 0.35% · disodium EDTA	sodium phosphate dibasic anhydrous · sodium phosphate monobasic
PE	**Little Noses Saline** Vetco	drops · spray	sodium chloride, 0.65%	benzalkonium chloride · thimerosal	disodium phosphate · sodium phosphate
	Mycinaire Saline Mist Pfeiffer Ph'cals	spray	sodium chloride	phenylmercuric acetate, 0.002% · benzalkonium chloride	disodium phosphate · sodium phosphate
SL	**Nasal Moist** Blairex Labs	solution	sodium chloride, 0.65%	benzyl alcohol	
SL	**Nasal Moist** Blairex Labs	pump spray	sodium chloride, 0.65%	benzyl alcohol	
	NaSal Saline Moisturizer Bayer Consumer	drops	sodium chloride, 0.65%	thimerosal, 0.001% · benzalkonium chloride	
	NaSal Saline Moisturizer Bayer Consumer	spray	sodium chloride, 0.65%	thimerosal, 0.001% · benzalkonium chloride	
PR	**Nichols Nasal Douche** Alvin Last	powder	sodium chloride		sodium bicarbonate · sodium borate · menthol · eucalyptol
**	**Nose Better** Lee Ph'cals	spray	sodium chloride, 0.35%	glycerin, 1% · benzalkonium chloride	water · potassium phosphate · fragrance · disodium EDTA · hydroxypropyl methylcellulose · sodium hydroxide
SL	**Ocean** Fleming	spray	sodium chloride, 0.65%	benzyl alcohol · benzalkonium chloride	
SL	**Pretz** Parnell Ph'cals	drops · solution · spray		glycerin, 3% · phenylmercuric nitrate	citric acid · sodium citrate · sodium chloride · yerba santa
	Salinex Muro Ph'cal	drops · spray	sodium chloride, 0.4%	benzalkonium chloride, 0.01% · propylene glycol	disodium edetate · hydroxypropyl methylcellulose · polyethylene glycol · purified water · sodium phosphate
	Sea Mist Schein Ph'cal	spray	sodium chloride	benzyl alcohol · benzalkonium chloride	sodium bicarbonate

** New listing

See Chapter 8, "Cold, Cough and Allergy Products," for more information about these products.

COLD, COUGH, AND ALLERGY PRODUCTS

	Product Manufacturer/Supplier	Dosage Form	Decongestant	Antihistamine
AF	**12-Hour Cold** Goldline Labs	tablet		dexbrompheniramine maleate, 6mg
AF	**A.R.M.** Menley & James Labs	caplet	phenylpropanolamine HCl, 25mg	chlorpheniramine maleate, 4mg
AF GL	**Actifed** Warner Wellcome Consumer	tablet	pseudoephedrine HCl, 60mg	triprolidine HCl, 2.5mg
AF	**Actifed Allergy Daytime/Nighttime** Warner Wellcome Consumer	Daytime, caplet Nighttime, caplet	Daytime: pseudoephedrine HCl, 30mg Nighttime: pseudoephedrine HCl, 30mg	Nighttime: diphenhydramine HCl, 25mg
AF	**Actifed Cold & Sinus** Warner Wellcome Consumer	caplet · tablet	pseudoephedrine HCl, 30mg	triprolidine HCl, 1.25mg
AF	**Actifed Sinus Daytime/Nighttime** Warner Wellcome Consumer	Daytime, caplet Nighttime, caplet	Daytime: pseudoephedrine HCl, 30mg Nighttime: pseudoephedrine HCl, 30mg	Nighttime: diphenhydramine HCl, 25mg
AF GL SO	**Advil Cold & Sinus** Whitehall-Robins Healthcare	caplet · tablet	pseudoephedrine HCl, 30mg	
	Alka-Seltzer Plus Cold & Cough Medicine Bayer Consumer	effervescent tablet	phenylpropanolamine bitartrate, 24.08mg	chlorpheniramine maleate, 2mg
	Alka-Seltzer Plus Cold & Cough Medicine Liqui-Gels Bayer Consumer	softgel	pseudoephedrine HCl, 30mg	chlorpheniramine maleate, 2mg
PU	**Alka-Seltzer Plus Cold Medicine** Bayer Consumer	effervescent tablet	phenylpropanolamine bitartrate, 24mg	chlorpheniramine maleate, 2mg
	Alka-Seltzer Plus Cold Medicine Liqui-Gels Bayer Consumer	softgel	pseudoephedrine HCl, 30mg	chlorpheniramine maleate, 2mg
**	**Alka-Seltzer Plus Flu & Body Aches** Bayer Consumer	effervescent tablet	phenylpropanolamine bitartrate, 20mg	chlorpheniramine maleate, 2mg
**	**Alka-Seltzer Plus Flu & Body Aches Liqui-Gels** Bayer Consumer	softgel	pseudoephedrine HCl, 30mg	
PU	**Alka-Seltzer Plus Maximum Strength Sinus Medicine** Bayer Consumer	effervescent tablet	phenylpropanolamine bitartrate, 24.08mg	brompheniramine maleate, 2mg
PU	**Alka-Seltzer Plus Night-Time Cold Medicine** Bayer Consumer	effervescent tablet	phenylpropanolamine bitartrate, 20mg	brompheniramine maleate, 2mg
	Alka-Seltzer Plus Night-Time Cold Medicine Liqui-Gels Bayer Consumer	softgel	pseudoephedrine HCl, 30mg	doxylamine succinate, 6.25mg
	Alka-Seltzer Plus Sinus Medicine Bayer Consumer	effervescent tablet		
**	**Aller-med** Republic Drug	caplet		diphenhydramine HCl, 25mg

See Chapter 8, "Cold, Cough and Allergy Products," for more information about these products.

Analgesic	Expectorant	Antitussive	Other Ingredients
pseudoephedrine sulfate, 120mg			
			D&C yellow#10 · FD&C yellow#6 · lactose · starch · magnesium stearate · gelatin · carnauba wax · hydroxypropyl methylcellulose · polyethylene glycol · sodium starch glycolate
			lactose · sucrose · magnesium stearate · potato starch · titanium dioxide · flavor · hydroxypropyl methylcellulose · polyethylene glycol · povidone · corn starch
			carnauba wax · lactose · polyethylene glycol · titanium dioxide · crospovidone · hydroxypropyl methylcellulose · Nighttime only: FD&C blue#1 lake · polysorbate 80 · magnesium stearate · microcrystalline cellulose
acetaminophen, 500mg			FD&C blue#1aluminum lake · D&C yellow#10 aluminum lake · polysorbate 80 · pregelatinized starch · titanium dioxide · carnauba wax · crospovidone · hydroxypropyl methylcellulose · magnesium stearate · microcrystalline cellulose · polyethylene glycol · povidone · stearic acid
Daytime: acetaminophen, 500mg Nighttime: acetaminophen, 500mg			carnauba wax · crospovidone · hydroxypropyl methylcellulose · magnesium stearate · microcrystalline cellulose · polyethylene glycol · povidone · pregelatinized corn starch · stearic acid · titanium dioxide · Nighttime only: FD&C blue#1 aluminum lake · polysorbate 80 · sodium starch glycolate
ibuprofen, 200mg			carnauba or equivalent wax · croscarmellose sodium · iron oxides · methylparaben · microcrystalline cellulose · propylparaben · silicon dioxide · sodium benzoate · sodium lauryl sulfate · starch · stearic acid · sucrose · titanium dioxide
aspirin, 500mg		dextromethorphan hydrobromide, 10mg	aspartame · citric acid · flavor · sodium bicarbonate (sodium, 506mg)
acetaminophen, 250mg		dextromethorphan hydrobromide, 10mg	
aspirin, 325mg			sodium, 506mg
acetaminophen, 250mg			
acetaminophen, 325mg		dextromethorphan hydrobromide, 10mg	aspartame · calcium carbonate · citric acid · croscarmellose sodium · D&C yellow#10 · flavor · maltodextrin · mannitol · polyvinylpyrrolidone · sodium bicarbonate · saccharin sodium · sorbitol · starch · stearic acid · tableting aids
acetaminophen, 250mg		dextromethorphan hydrobromide, 10mg	FD&C red#40 · gelatin · glycerin · polyethylene glycol · povidone · propylene glycol · purified water · sorbitol · titanium dioxide
aspirin, 500mg			sodium, 506mg
aspirin, 500mg		dextromethorphan hydrobromide, 10mg	sodium, 506mg
acetaminophen, 250mg		dextromethorphan hydrobromide, 10mg	

COLD, COUGH, AND ALLERGY PRODUCTS - continued

	Product Manufacturer/Supplier	Dosage Form	Decongestant	Antihistamine
AF GL PU	**Allerest Maximum Strength** Ciba Self-Medication	tablet	pseudoephedrine HCl, 30mg	chlorpheniramine maleate, 2mg
AF GL PU SO	**Allerest No Drowsiness** Ciba Self-Medication	tablet	pseudoephedrine HCl, 30mg	
AF GL PU	**Allerest Sinus Pain Formula** Ciba Self-Medication	tablet	pseudoephedrine HCl, 30mg	chlorpheniramine maleate, 2mg
AF GL PU	**Allergy Relief** Hudson	tablet		chlorpheniramine maleate, 4mg
AF	**AllerMax** Pfeiffer Ph'cals	caplet		diphenhydramine HCl, 50mg
	AllerMax Pfeiffer Ph'cals	syrup		diphenhydramine HCl, 12.5mg/5ml
LA SL	**Anti-Tuss** Century Ph'cals	syrup		
DY GL LA SL	**Anti-Tuss DM** Century Ph'cals	syrup		
AF	**Antihist-1** Goldline Labs	tablet		clemastine fumarate, 1.34mg (equivalent to clemastine, 1mg)
AL DY PE	**Babee Cof** Pfeiffer Ph'cals	syrup		
AF GL SO	**Bayer Select Aspirin-Free Sinus Pain Relief** Bayer Consumer	caplet	pseudoephedrine HCl, 30mg	
DY	**BC Allergy·Sinus·Cold** Block Drug	powder	phenylpropanolamine HCl, 25mg	chlorpheniramine maleate, 4mg
DY	**BC Sinus·Cold** Block Drug	powder	phenylpropanolamine HCl, 25mg	
AF PU SO	**Benadryl Allergy** Warner Wellcome Consumer	capsule		diphenhydramine HCl, 25mg
AF PU	**Benadryl Allergy** Warner Wellcome Consumer	tablet		diphenhydramine HCl, 25mg
AL SL	**Benadryl Allergy** Warner Wellcome Consumer	liquid		diphenhydramine HCl, 12.5mg/5ml
** PE	**Benadryl Allergy** Warner Wellcome Consumer	chewable tablet		diphenhydramine HCl, 12.5mg
AL SL	**Benadryl Allergy Decongestant** Warner Wellcome Consumer	liquid	pseudoephedrine HCl, 30mg/5ml	diphenhydramine HCl, 12.5mg/5ml
** AF	**Benadryl Allergy Decongestant** Warner Wellcome Consumer	tablet	pseudoephedrine HCl, 60mg	diphenhydramine HCl, 25mg

See Chapter 8, "Cold, Cough and Allergy Products," for more information about these products.

Analgesic	Expectorant	Antitussive	Other Ingredients
			corn starch · blue#1 · hydroxypropyl methylcellulose · lactose · microcrystalline cellulose · polyethylene glycol · polysorbate 80 · stearic acid · titanium dioxide
acetaminophen, 325mg			corn starch · hydroxypropyl methylcellulose · microcrystalline cellulose · polyethylene glycol · polysorbate 80 · stearic acid · titanium dioxide
acetaminophen, 500mg			corn starch · hydroxypropyl methylcellulose · microcrystalline cellulose · polyethylene glycol · polysorbate 80 · polyvinylpyrrolidone · stearic acid · titanium dioxide
		menthol	sucrose · raspberry flavor
	guaifenesin, 100mg/5ml		alcohol, 3.5%
	guaifenesin, 100mg/5ml	dextromethorphan hydrobromide, 15mg/5ml	
		dextromethorphan hydrobromide, 7.5mg/5ml	sucrose · tartaric acid · cherry flavor
acetaminophen, 500mg			
aspirin, 650mg			
aspirin, 650mg			
			lactose · magnesium stearate · FD&C red#3 · FD&C red#40 · FD&C blue#1 · gelatin · glyceryl monooleate · titanium dioxide
			candellila wax · croscarmellose sodium · dibasic calcium phosphate dihydrate · D&C red#27 aluminum lake · hydroxypropyl methylcellulose · microcrystalline cellulose · polyethylene glycol · polysorbate 80 · stearic acid · titanium dioxide · zinc stearate · pregelatinized starch
			FD&C red#40 · D&C red#33 · glycerin · sodium citrate · flavors · sodium benzoate · citric acid · poloxamer 407 · polysorbate 20 · sugar · water · sodium chloride
			aspartame · dextrates · D&C red#27 aluminum lake · FD&C blue#1 aluminum lake · flavors · magnesium stearate · magnesium trisilicate · tartaric acid
			saccharin sodium · sodium citrate · sodium benzoate · sorbitol · glycerin · flavors · FD&C red #40 · FD&C blue #1 · citric acid · poloxamer 407 · polysorbate 20 · sodium chloride
			croscarmellose sodium · dibasic calcium phosphate dihydrate · FD&C blue#1 aluminum lake · hydroxypropyl methylcellulose · microcrystalline cellulose · polyethylene glycol · polysorbate 80 · pregelatinized starch · stearic acid · titanium dioxide · zinc stearate

COLD, COUGH, AND ALLERGY PRODUCTS - continued

	Product Manufacturer/Supplier	Dosage Form	Decongestant	Antihistamine
AL DY	**Benadryl Allergy Dye-Free** Warner Wellcome Consumer	liquid		diphenhydramine HCl, 6.25mg/5ml
** DY	**Benadryl Allergy Dye-Free Liqui-gels** Warner Wellcome Consumer	softgel		diphenhydramine HCl, 25mg
AF	**Benadryl Allergy/Cold** Warner Wellcome Consumer	tablet	pseudoephedrine HCl, 30mg	diphenhydramine HCl, 12.5mg
** AF	**Benadryl Allergy/Sinus/Headache Formula** Warner Wellcome Consumer	caplet	pseudoephedrine HCl, 30mg	diphenhydramine HCl, 12.5mg
AL SU	**Benylin Adult Cough Formula** Warner Wellcome Consumer	liquid		
AL	**Benylin Cough Suppressant Expectorant** Warner Wellcome Consumer	liquid		
AL SU	**Benylin Multi-Symptom Formula** Warner Wellcome Consumer	liquid	pseudoephedrine HCl, 15mg/5ml	
AL PE	**Benylin Pediatric Cough Formula** Warner Wellcome Consumer	liquid		
	Bromatapp Extended Release Copley Pharm'cal	tablet	phenylpropanolamine HCl	brompheniramine maleate
AL LA	**Bromfed** Muro Ph'cal	syrup	pseudoephedrine HCl, 30mg/5ml	brompheniramine maleate, 2mg/5ml
	Bromotap Goldline Labs	elixir	phenylpropanolamine HCl, 12.5mg/5ml	brompheniramine maleate, 2mg/5ml
AL GL LA SL PE	**Cenafed** Century Ph'cals	syrup	pseudoephedrine HCl, 30mg/5ml	
AF GL PU	**Cenafed** Century Ph'cals	tablet	pseudoephedrine HCl, 30mg	
AF DY GL PU	**Cenafed** Century Ph'cals	tablet	pseudoephedrine HCl, 60mg	
AF DY GL PU	**Cenafed Plus** Century Ph'cals	tablet	pseudoephedrine HCl, 60mg	triprolidine HCl, 2.5mg
**	**Cepacol Maximum Strength, Mint** J. B. Williams	lozenge		
**	**Cepacol Sore Throat, Cherry** J. B. Williams	lozenge		

See Chapter 8, "Cold, Cough and Allergy Products," for more information about these products.

Analgesic	Expectorant	Antitussive	Other Ingredients
			glycerin · sodium citrate · saccharin sodium · sodium benzoate · flavor · citric acid · sodium carboxymethyl cellulose · sorbitol solution · water
			gelatin · glycerin · polyethylene glycol · sorbitol
acetaminophen, 500mg			candellila wax · croscarmellose sodium · hydroxypropyl cellulose · hydroxypropyl methylcellulose · magnesium stearate · microcrystalline cellulose · polyethylene glycol · pregelatinized starch · propylene glycol · sodium starch glycolate · starch · stearic acid · titanium dioxide · zinc stearate · edible ink
acetaminophen, 500mg			candelilla wax · starch · croscarmellose sodium · D&C yellow#10 aluminum lake · FD&C yellow#6 aluminum lake · hydroxypropyl cellulose · hydroxypropyl methylcellulose · microcrystalline cellulose · polyethylene glycol · polysorbate 80 · stearic acid · titanium dioxide · zinc stearate · FD&C blue#1 · pregelatinized starch · sodium starch glycolate · edible ink
		dextromethorphan hydrobromide, 15mg/5ml	glycerin · saccharin sodium · sodium benzoate · sodium citrate · citric acid · D&C red#33 · FD&C red#40 · flavors · poloxamer 407 · polysorbate 20 · sodium carboxymethyl cellulose · sorbitol solution · caramel · water
	guaifenesin, 100mg/5ml	dextromethorphan hydrobromide, 5mg/5ml	sodium benzoate · sodium citrate · saccharin sodium · caramel · citric acid · D&C red#33 · disodium edetate · FD&C red#40 · flavor · poloxamer 407 · polyethylene glycol · propyl gallate · propylene glycol · sodium chloride · sorbitol solution · purified water
	guaifenesin, 100mg/5ml	dextromethorphan hydrobromide, 5mg/5ml	saccharin sodium · sodium benzoate · sodium citrate · caramel · citric acid · D&C red#33 · edetate disodium · FD&C red#40 · flavor · poloxamer 407 · polyethylene glycol 1450 · propyl gallate · propylene glycol · sodium chloride · sorbitol solution
		dextromethorphan hydrobromide, 7.5mg/5ml	glycerin · flavors · saccharin sodium · sodium benzoate · sodium citrate · citric acid · FD&C blue#1 · FD&C red#40 · poloxamer 407 · polysorbate 20 · sodium carboxymethyl cellulose · sorbitol solution · water
			citric acid · FD&C yellow#6 · flavor · glycerin · methylparaben · sodium benzoate · sodium citrate · saccharin sodium · sorbitol · sucrose · purified water
			alcohol, 2.3% · saccharin · sorbitol · grape flavor
		menthol, 2mg	benzocaine, 10mg · cetylpyridinium chloride · D&C yellow#10 · FD&C yellow#6 · flavor · glucose · sucrose
		menthol, 3.6mg	cetylpyridinium chloride · D&C red#33 · FD&C red#40 · flavor · glucose · sucrose

COLD, COUGH, AND ALLERGY PRODUCTS - continued

	Product Manufacturer/Supplier	Dosage Form	Decongestant	Antihistamine
**	**Cepacol Sore Throat, Mint** J. B. Williams	lozenge		
	Cepacol, Cherry or Honey-Lemon J. B. Williams	lozenge		
	Cepacol, Menthol-Eucalyptus J. B. Williams	lozenge		
	Cerose-DM Wyeth-Ayerst Labs	liquid	phenylephrine HCl, 10mg/5ml	chlorpheniramine maleate, 4mg/5ml
	Cheracol D Roberts Ph'cal	liquid		
	Cheracol Plus Roberts Ph'cal	syrup	phenylpropanolamine HCl, 25mg	chlorpheniramine, 4mg
	Chlor-Trimeton 12-Hour Allergy Schering-Plough HealthCare	tablet		chlorpheniramine maleate, 12mg
	Chlor-Trimeton 12-Hour Allergy Decongestant Schering-Plough HealthCare	tablet	pseudoephedrine sulfate, 120mg	chlorpheniramine maleate, 8mg
	Chlor-Trimeton 4-Hour Allergy Schering-Plough HealthCare	tablet		chlorpheniramine maleate, 4mg
	Chlor-Trimeton 4-Hour Allergy Decongestant Schering-Plough HealthCare	tablet	pseudoephedrine sulfate, 60mg	chlorpheniramine maleate, 4mg
	Chlor-Trimeton 8-Hour Allergy Schering-Plough HealthCare	tablet		chlorpheniramine maleate, 8mg
AL	**Chlor-Trimeton Allergy** Schering-Plough HealthCare	syrup		chlorpheniramine maleate, 2mg/5ml
AF	**Chlor-Trimeton Allergy, Sinus, Headache** Schering-Plough HealthCare	caplet	phenylpropanolamine HCl, 12.5mg	chlorpheniramine maleate, 2mg
	Chlor-Trimeton Non-Drowsy 4-Hour Schering-Plough HealthCare	tablet	pseudoephedrine sulfate, 60mg	
AL DY SU	**Clear Cough DM** Vetco	liquid		
** AL DY SU	**Clear Cough Night Time** Vetco	liquid		doxylamine succinate, 2.08mg/5ml
AL	**Clear Tussin 30** Goldline Labs	liquid		
AL GL SO	**Codimal** Central Ph'cals	capsule	pseudoephedrine HCl, 30mg	chlorpheniramine maleate, 2mg
** AF GL LA SO	**Codimal** Central Ph'cals	tablet	pseudoephedrine HCl, 30mg	chlorpheniramine maleate, 2mg

See Chapter 8, "Cold, Cough and Allergy Products," for more information about these products.

Analgesic	Expectorant	Antitussive	Other Ingredients
		menthol, 2mg	cetylpyridinium chloride · D&C yellow#10 · FD&C yellow#6 · flavor · glucose · sucrose
		menthol, 3.6mg	cetylpyridinium chloride · dyes · glucose · sucrose
		menthol, 5mg · eucalyptol	cetylpyridinium chloride · glucose · sucrose
		dextromethorphan hydrobromide, 15mg/5ml	alcohol, 2.4% · flavors · citric acid · disodium edetate · FD&C yellow#6 · glycerin · saccharin sodium · sodium benzoate · sodium citrate · sodium propionate · water
	guaifenesin, 100mg	dextromethorphan hydrobromide, 10mg	alcohol, 4.75% · benzoic acid · fructose · glycerin · propylene glycol · sodium chloride · sucrose
		dextromethorphan hydrobromide, 20mg	alcohol, 8% · glycerin · methylparaben · propylene glycol · propylparaben · sodium chloride · sorbitol solution
acetaminophen, 500mg			
	guaifenesin, 100mg/5ml	dextromethorphan hydrobromide, 15mg/5ml	purified water · benzoic acid · citric acid · glycerin · sorbitol · flavor
acetaminophen, 166.67mg/5ml		dextromethorphan hydrobromide, 5mg/5ml	ascorbic acid · benzoic acid · citric acid · gelatin · glycerin · potassium citrate · propylene glycol · purified water · sorbitol · polysorbate 80 · berry flavor
	guaifenesin, 100mg/5ml	dextromethorphan hydrobromide, 15mg/5ml	
acetaminophen, 325mg			
acetaminophen, 325mg			

COLD, COUGH, AND ALLERGY PRODUCTS - continued

	Product Manufacturer/Supplier	Dosage Form	Decongestant	Antihistamine
AL DY GL LA SU	**Codimal DM** Central Ph'cals	syrup	phenylephrine HCl, 5mg/5ml	pyrilamine maleate, 8.3mg/5ml
AL GL LA	**Codimal PH** Central Ph'cals	syrup	phenylephrine HCl, 5mg/5ml	pyrilamine maleate, 8.3mg/5ml
AF	**Cold & Allergy Maximum Strength 4-Hour Liquid Gelcaps** Goldline Labs	gelcap	phenylpropanolamine HCl, 25mg	brompheniramine maleate, 4mg
AF	**Cold and Allergy Extended-Release** Goldline Labs	timed-release tablet	phenylpropanolamine HCl, 75mg	brompheniramine maleate, 12mg
AF SO	**Coldonyl** Dover	tablet	phenylephrine HCl, 5mg	
AF GL LA	**Comtrex Allergy-Sinus** Bristol-Myers Products	caplet · tablet	pseudoephedrine HCl, 30mg	chlorpheniramine maleate, 2mg
AF GL LA SO	**Comtrex Maximum Strength** Bristol-Myers Products	caplet · tablet	pseudoephedrine HCl, 30mg	chlorpheniramine maleate, 2mg
LA PR	**Comtrex Maximum Strength** Bristol-Myers Products	liquid	pseudoephedrine HCl, 60mg/30ml	chlorpheniramine maleate, 4mg/30ml
AF GL LA SO	**Comtrex Maximum Strength** Bristol-Myers Products	liqui-gel	phenylpropanolamine HCl, 12.5mg	chlorpheniramine maleate, 2mg
AF LA	**Comtrex Maximum Strength Day & Night** Bristol-Myers Products	Day, caplet Night, liquid	Day: pseudoephedrine HCl, 30mg Night: pseudoephedrine HCl, 60mg/30ml	Night: chlorpheniramine maleate, 4mg/30ml
AF GL LA	**Comtrex Maximum Strength Day & Night** Bristol-Myers Products	Day, caplet Night, tablet	Day: pseudoephedrine HCl, 30mg Night: pseudoephedrine HCl, 30mg	Night: chlorpheniramine maleate, 2mg
AF SO	**Comtrex Maximum Strength Non-Drowsy** Bristol-Myers Products	caplet	pseudoephedrine HCl, 30mg	
AF GL LA SO	**Comtrex Maximum Strength Non-Drowsy** Bristol-Myers Products	liqui-gel	phenylpropanolamine HCl, 12.5mg	

See Chapter 8, "Cold, Cough and Allergy Products," for more information about these products.

Analgesic	Expectorant	Antitussive	Other Ingredients
		dextromethorphan hydrobromide, 10mg/5ml	
		codeine phosphate, 10mg/5ml[a]	
acetaminophen, 325mg			
acetaminophen, 500mg			benzoic acid · carnauba wax · corn starch · D&C yellow#10 lake · FD&C blue#1 lake · FD&C red#40 lake · hydroxypropyl methylcellulose · mineral oil · polysorbate 20 · povidone · propylene glycol · simethicone emulsion · sodium citrate · sorbitan monolaurate · stearic acid · titanium dioxide · may also contain: crospovidone · D&C yellow#10 · erythorbic acid · FD&C blue#1 · magnesium stearate · methylparaben · microcrystalline cellulose · polysorbate 80 · propylparaben · silicon dioxide · wood cellulose
acetaminophen, 500mg		dextromethorphan hydrobromide, 15mg	benzoic acid · carnauba wax · corn starch · D&C yellow#10 aluminum lake · FD&C red#40 aluminum lake · hydroxypropyl methylcellulose · magnesium stearate · methylparaben · mineral oil · polysorbate 20 · povidone · propylene glycol · propylparaben · simethicone emulsion · sorbitan monolaurate · stearic acid · titanium dioxide
acetaminophen, 1000mg/30ml		dextromethorphan hydrobromide, 30mg/30ml	alcohol, 10% · sucrose · benzoic acid · D&C yellow#10 · FD&C blue#1 · FD&C red#40 · flavors · glycerin · polyethylene glycol · povidone · saccharin sodium · sodium citrate · water
acetaminophen, 500mg		dextromethorphan hydrobromide, 15mg	D&C yellow#10 · FD&C red#40 · gelatin · glycerin · polyethylene glycol · povidone · propylene glycol · silicon dioxide · sorbitol · titanium dioxide · water
Day: acetaminophen, 500mg Night: acetaminophen, 1000mg/30ml		Day: dextromethorphan hydrobromide, 15mg Night: dextromethorphan hydrobromide, 30mg/30ml	Day: benzoic acid · corn starch · D&C yellow#10 lake · D&C red#40 lake · hydroxypropyl methylcellulose · magnesium stearate · methylparaben · polysorbate 20 · povidone · propylene glycol · propylparaben · simethicone emulsion · sorbitan monolaurate · stearic acid · titanium dioxide · may also contain: carnauba wax · D&C yellow#10 · FD&C red#40 Night: alcohol, 10% · sucrose · benzoic acid · D&C yellow#10 · FD&C blue#1 · FD&C red#40 · flavors · glycerin · polyethylene glycol · povidone · saccharin sodium · sodium citrate · water
Day: acetaminophen, 500mg Night: acetaminophen, 500mg		Day: dextromethorphan hydrobromide, 15mg Night: dextromethorphan hydrobromide, 15mg	benzoic acid · corn starch · D&C yellow#10 lake · D&C red#40 lake · FD&C blue#1 lake (Night) · hydroxypropyl methylcellulose · magnesium stearate · methylparaben · mineral oil (Night) · polysorbate 20 · povidone · propylene glycol · propylparaben · simethicone emulsion · sorbitan monolaurate · stearic acid · titanium dioxide · may also contain: carnauba wax · sodium citrate · D&C yellow#10 · FD&C red#40
acetaminophen, 500mg		dextromethorphan hydrobromide, 15mg	benzoic acid · corn starch · D&C yellow#10 lake · FD&C red#40 lake · hydroxypropyl methylcellulose · magnesium stearate · methylparaben · polysorbate 20 · povidone · propylene glycol · propylparaben · simethicone emulsion · sorbitan monolaurate · stearic acid · titanium dioxide · may also contain: carnauba wax · D&C yellow#10 · FD&C red#40
acetaminophen, 500mg		dextromethorphan hydrobromide, 15mg	FD&C yellow#6 · gelatin · glycerin · polyethylene glycol · povidone · propylene glycol · silicon dioxide · sorbitol · titanium dioxide · water

COLD, COUGH, AND ALLERGY PRODUCTS - continued

	Product Manufacturer/Supplier	Dosage Form	Decongestant	Antihistamine
AF	**Congestac** Menley & James Labs	caplet	pseudoephedrine HCl, 60mg	
	Congestion Relief Schein Ph'cal	tablet	pseudoephedrine HCl, 60mg	
	Contac 12-Hour Allergy SmithKline Beecham	tablet		clemastine fumarate, 1.34mg (equivalent to clemastine, 1mg)
	Contac 12-Hour Cold SmithKline Beecham	timed-release capsule	phenylpropanolamine HCl, 75mg	chlorpheniramine maleate, 8mg
	Contac 12-Hour Maximum Strength SmithKline Beecham	caplet	phenylpropanolamine HCl, 75mg	chlorpheniramine maleate, 12mg
	Contac Day & Night Allergy/Sinus SmithKline Beecham	Day, caplet Night, caplet	Day: pseudoephedrine HCl, 60mg Night: pseudoephedrine HCl, 60mg	Night: diphenhydramine hydrochloride, 50mg
	Contac Day & Night Cold/Flu SmithKline Beecham	Day, caplet Night, caplet	Day: pseudoephedrine HCl, 60mg Night: pseudoephedrine HCl, 60mg	Day: dextromethorphan hydrobromide, 30mg Night: diphenhydramine HCl, 50mg
	Contac Non-Drowsy SmithKline Beecham	caplet	pseudoephedrine HCl, 30mg	dextromethorphan hydrobromide, 15mg
	Contac Severe Cold & Flu Maximum Strength SmithKline Beecham	caplet	phenylpropanolamine HCl, 12.5mg	chlorpheniramine maleate, 2mg
AF	**Coricidin Cold & Flu** Schering-Plough HealthCare	tablet		chlorpheniramine maleate, 2mg
**	**Coricidin Cough & Cold** Schering-Plough HealthCare	tablet		chlorpheniramine maleate, 4mg
AF	**Coricidin D** Schering-Plough HealthCare	tablet	phenylpropanolamine HCl, 12.5mg	chlorpheniramine maleate, 2mg
DY	**Cough-X** B. F. Ascher	lozenge		
** AL GL LA SL	**Creomulsion Complete** Summit	syrup	pseudoephedrine HCl, 20mg/5ml	chlorpheniramine maleate, 1.33mg/5ml
** AL DY GL LA SL	**Creomulsion Cough Medicine** Summit	syrup		
** AL GL LA SL PE	**Creomulsion for Children** Summit	syrup		

See Chapter 8, "Cold, Cough and Allergy Products," for more information about these products.

Analgesic	Expectorant	Antitussive	Other Ingredients
	guaifenesin, 400mg		microcrystalline cellulose · croscarmellose sodium · starch · povidone · hydroxypropyl methylcellulose · magnesium stearate · polyethylene glycol · silicon dioxide
			colloidal silicon dioxide · lactose anhydrous · magnesium stearate · microcrystalline cellulose
			colloidal silicon dioxide · corn starch · lactose · povidone · pregelatinized starch · stearic acid
			benzyl alcohol · butylparaben · colors · edetate calcium disodium · gelatin · methylparaben · pharmaceutical glaze · polysorbate 80 · propylparaben · sodium lauryl sulfate · sodium propionate · starch · sucrose
			acetylated monoglycerides · carnauba wax · colloidal silicon dioxide · ethylcellulose · hydroxypropyl methylcellulose · lactose · stearic acid · titanium dioxide
Day: acetaminophen, 650mg Night: acetaminophen, 650mg			carnauba wax · colors · hydroxypropyl methylcellulose · magnesium stearate · microcrystalline cellulose · polyethylene glycol · polysorbate 80 · silicon dioxide · starch · stearic acid · titanium dioxide
Day: acetaminophen, 650mg Night: acetaminophen, 650mg			carnauba wax · color · hydroxypropyl methylcellulose · magnesium stearate · microcrystalline cellulose · polyethylene glycol · polysorbate 80 · silicon dioxide · starch · stearic acid · titanium dioxide · white wax
acetaminophen, 325mg			microcrystalline cellulose · starch · hydroxypropyl methylcellulose · stearic acid · colloidal silicon dioxide · polyethylene glycol · polysorbate 80 · magnesium stearate · carnauba wax · titanium dioxide
acetaminophen, 500mg		dextromethorphan hydrobromide, 15mg	FD&C blue#1 · cellulose · hydroxypropyl methylcellulose · propylene glycol · polysorbate 80 · povidone · sodium starch glycolate · starch · stearic acid · titanium dioxide
acetaminophen, 325mg			
		dextromethorphan hydrobromide, 30mg	
acetaminophen, 325mg			
		dextromethorphan hydrobromide, 5mg	benzocaine, 2mg
		dextromethorphan hydrobromide, 6mg/5ml	caramel · citric acid · corn syrup · FD&C red#40 · flavor · potassium sorbate · sodium benzoate · water
		dextromethorphan hydrobromide, 6.67mg/5ml	beechwood creosote · ipecac · menthol · caramel · citric acid · potassium sorbate · sodium benzoate · corn syrup · sucrose · water
		dextromethorphan hydrobromide, 5mg/5ml	menthol · caramel · citric acid · corn syrup · FD&C red#40 · flavor · potassium sorbate · sodium benzoate · sucrose · water

COLD, COUGH, AND ALLERGY PRODUCTS - continued

	Product Manufacturer/Supplier	Dosage Form	Decongestant	Antihistamine
** AL GL LA SL PE	**Creomulsion Pediatric** Summit	syrup	pseudoephedrine HCl, 1mg/5ml	chlorpheniramine maleate, 0.67mg/5ml
AL LA SL PE	**Dallergy-D** Laser	syrup	phenylephrine HCl, 5mg/5ml	chlorpheniramine maleate, 2mg/5ml
**	**DayGel** Republic Drug	liquid-cap	pseudoephedrine HCl, 30mg	
	Decongestant Cough Formula D Goldline Labs	liquid	pseudoephedrine HCl, 20mg/5ml	
AL LA	**Delsym Extended Release** Fisons	suspension		
	Demazin Schering-Plough HealthCare	timed-release tablet	phenylpropanolamine HCl, 25mg	chlorpheniramine maleate, 4mg
AL	**Demazin** Schering-Plough HealthCare	syrup	phenylpropanolamine HCl, 12.5mg/5ml	chlorpheniramine maleate, 2mg/5ml
** AL DY SU	**Diabe-tuss DM** Paddock Labs	syrup		
AL DY SU	**Diabetic Tussin Allergy Relief** Health Care Products	syrup		chlorpheniramine maleate, 2mg
** DY SO SU	**Diabetic Tussin Cough Drops, Cherry** Health Care Products	tablet		
** DY SO SU	**Diabetic Tussin Cough Drops, Menthol-Eucalyptus** Health Care Products	tablet		
AL DY SU	**Diabetic Tussin DM** Health Care Products	syrup		
** AL DY SU	**Diabetic Tussin DM Maximum Strength** Health Care Products	syrup		
AL DY SU	**Diabetic Tussin EX** Health Care Products	syrup		
AL DY SU PE	**Diabetic Tussin, Children's** Health Care Products	syrup		

See Chapter 8, "Cold, Cough and Allergy Products," for more information about these products.

Analgesic	Expectorant	Antitussive	Other Ingredients
		dextromethorphan hydrobromide, 5mg/5ml	citric acid · corn syrup · FD&C yellow#6 · flavor · potassium sorbate · sodium benzoate · sucrose · water
			raspberry/vanilla flavor · sugar
acetaminophen, 250mg	guaifenesin, 100mg	dextromethorphan hydrobromide, 10mg	
		dextromethorphan hydrobromide, 10mg/5ml	alcohol, 10%
		dextromethorphan polistirex (equivalent to 30mg/5ml dextromethorphan hydrobromide)	citric acid · ethylcellulose · FD&C yellow#6 · flavor · high fructose corn syrup · methylparaben · polyethylene glycol 3350 · polysorbate 80 · propylene glycol · propylparaben · purified water · sucrose · tragacanth · vegetable oil · xanthan gum
		dextromethorphan, 15mg/5ml	sorbitol
			hydroxypropyl methylcellulose · calcium saccharin · methylparaben · artificial flavors · purified water · may contain citric acid
		menthol, 5mg · eucalyptus oil	acesulfame potassium · flavor · isomalt
		menthol, 6mg · eucalyptus oil	acesulfame potassium · flavor · isomalt
	guaifenesin, 100mg/5ml	dextromethorphan hydrobromide, 10mg/5ml	hydroxypropyl methylcellulose · calcium saccharin · methylparaben · potassium sorbate · povidone · artificial flavors · menthol · purified water · may contain citric acid
	guaifenesin, 200mg/5ml	dextromethorphan hydrobromide, 10mg/5ml	acesulfame K · hydroxypropyl methylcellulose · aspartame · methylparaben · potassium sorbate · artificial flavors · menthol · purified water · may contain citric acid
	guaifenesin, 100mg/5ml	menthol	hydroxypropyl methylcellulose · calcium saccharin · methylparaben · potassium sorbate · povidone · artificial flavors · purified water · may contain citric acid
	guaifenesin, 100mg/5ml	dextromethorphan hydrobromide, 10mg/5ml · menthol	hydroxypropyl methylcellulose · calcium saccharin · methylparaben · potassium sorbate · povidone · artificial flavors · purified water · may contain citric acid

COLD, COUGH, AND ALLERGY PRODUCTS - continued

	Product Manufacturer/Supplier	Dosage Form	Decongestant	Antihistamine
	Dimacol Whitehall-Robins Healthcare	caplet	pseudoephedrine HCl, 30mg	
	Dimetane Allergy Extentabs Whitehall-Robins Healthcare	timed-release tablet		brompheniramine maleate, 12mg
AL	**Dimetapp** Whitehall-Robins Healthcare	elixir	phenylpropanolamine HCl, 12.5mg/5ml	brompheniramine maleate, 2mg/5ml
	Dimetapp 12-Hour Maximum Strength Extentabs Whitehall-Robins Healthcare	timed-release tablet	phenylpropanolamine HCl, 75mg	brompheniramine maleate, 12mg
	Dimetapp 4-Hour Maximum Strength Whitehall-Robins Healthcare	tablet	phenylpropanolamine HCl, 25mg	brompheniramine maleate, 4mg
	Dimetapp 4-Hour Maximum Strength Liqui-Gels Whitehall-Robins Healthcare	softgel	phenylpropanolamine HCl, 25mg	brompheniramine maleate, 4mg
	Dimetapp Allergy Whitehall-Robins Healthcare	tablet		brompheniramine maleate, 4mg
	Dimetapp Allergy Liqui-Gels Whitehall-Robins Healthcare	softgel		brompheniramine maleate, 4mg
**	**Dimetapp Allergy Sinus** Whitehall-Robins Healthcare	caplet	phenylpropanolamine HCl, 12.5mg	brompheniramine maleate, 2mg
** AL DY SU PE	**Dimetapp Allergy, Children's** Whitehall-Robins Healthcare	elixir		brompheniramine maleate, 2mg/5ml
	Dimetapp Cold & Allergy Whitehall-Robins Healthcare	chewable tablet	phenylpropanolamine HCl, 6.25mg	brompheniramine maleate, 1mg
	Dimetapp Cold & Cough Maximum Strength Liqui-Gels Whitehall-Robins Healthcare	softgel	phenylpropanolamine HCl, 25mg	brompheniramine maleate, 4mg
** AL PE	**Dimetapp Cold & Fever, Children's** Whitehall-Robins Healthcare	suspension	pseudoephedrine HCl, 15mg/5ml	brompheniramine maleate, 1mg/5ml
	Dimetapp Decongestant Non-Drowsy Liqui-Gels Whitehall-Robins Healthcare	softgel	pseudoephedrine HCl, 30mg	
AL PE	**Dimetapp Decongestant, Pediatric** Whitehall-Robins Healthcare	drops	pseudoephedrine HCl, 7.5mg/0.8ml	

See Chapter 8, "Cold, Cough and Allergy Products," for more information about these products.

Analgesic	Expectorant	Antitussive	Other Ingredients
	guaifenesin, 100mg	dextromethorphan hydrobromide, 10mg	D&C yellow#10 aluminum lake · FD&C yellow#6 aluminum lake · flavor · hydroxypropyl methylcellulose · magnesium stearate · methacrylic acid copolymer · methylparaben · microcrystalline cellulose · polysorbate 20 · potassium sorbate · povidone · propylene glycol · propylparaben · saccharin sodium · silicon dioxide · titanium dioxide · triethyl citrate · xanthan gum
			acacia · acetylated monoglycerides · calcium carbonate · calcium sulfate · carnauba wax · cellulose acetate phthalate · corn starch · diethyl phthalate · edible ink · FD&C blue#2 aluminum lake · FD&C red#3 · gelatin · guar gum · magnesium stearate · pharmaceutical glaze · polysorbates · stearic acid · sucrose · titanium dioxide · wheat flour · white wax · may contain: FD&C red#40 aluminum lake · FD&C yellow#6 aluminum lake
			citric acid · FD&C blue#1 · FD&C red#40 · grape flavor · glycerin · saccharin sodium · sodium benzoate · sorbitol · water
			acacia · acetylated monoglycerides · calcium sulfate · carnauba wax · castor wax or oil · citric acid · edible inks · FD&C blue#1 · FD&C blue#2 aluminum lake · gelatin · magnesium stearate · magnesium trisilicate · pharmaceutical glaze · polysorbates · povidone · silicon dioxide · stearyl alcohol · sucrose · titanium dioxide · wheat flour · white wax · may contain: FD&C red#40 aluminum lake · FD&C yellow#6 aluminum lake
			corn starch · FD&C blue#1 aluminum lake · magnesium stearate · microcrystalline cellulose
			D&C red#33 · FD&C blue#1 · gelatin · glycerin · mannitol · pharmaceutical glaze · polyethylene glycol · povidone · propylene glycol · sorbitan · sorbitol · titanium dioxide · water
			corn starch · D&C yellow#10 aluminum lake · dibasic calcium phosphate · FD&C yellow#6 aluminum lake · lactose · magnesium stearate · polyethylene glycol
			FD&C green#3 · gelatin · glycerin · mannitol · pharmaceutical glaze · polyethylene glycol · povidone · propylene glycol · sorbitan · sorbitol · titanium dioxide · water
acetaminophen, 500mg			corn starch · hydroxypropyl cellulose · hydroxypropyl methylcellulose · magnesium stearate · methylparaben · microcrystalline cellulose · polysorbate 20 · povidone · propylparaben · propylene glycol · stearic acid · titanium dioxide
			citric acid · grape flavor · glycerin · sodium benzoate · sorbitol · water
			aspartame · citric acid · crospovidone · D&C red#30 aluminum lake · D&C red#7 calcium lake · FD&C blue#1 aluminum lake · grape flavor · glycine · magnesium stearate · mannitol · microcrystalline cellulose · pregelatinized starch · silicon dioxide · sorbitol · stearic acid
		dextromethorphan hydrobromide, 20mg	FD&C red #40 · gelatin · glycerin · mannitol · pharmaceutical glaze · polyethylene glycol · povidone · propylene glycol · sorbitan · sorbitol · titanium dioxide · water
acetaminophen, 160mg/5ml			carboxymethylcellulose sodium · citric acid · D&C red#33 · disodium edetate · FD&C blue#1 · flavors · glycerin · high fructose corn syrup · maltol · methylparaben · microcrystalline cellulose · polysorbate 80 · potassium sorbate · propylene glycol · propylparaben · sorbitol · sucrose · water · xanthan gum
			FD&C blue#1 · gelatin · glycerin · mannitol · pharmaceutical glaze · polyethylene glycol · povidone · propylene glycol · sorbitan · sorbitol · titanium dioxide · water
			caramel · citric acid · FD&C blue#1 · D&C red #33 · grape flavor · glycerin · high fructose corn syrup · maltol · menthol · polyethylene glycol · propylene glycol · sodium benzoate · sorbitol · sucrose · water

COLD, COUGH, AND ALLERGY PRODUCTS - continued

	Product Manufacturer/Supplier	Dosage Form	Decongestant	Antihistamine
AL	**Dimetapp DM** Whitehall-Robins Healthcare	elixir	phenylpropanolamine HCl, 12.5mg/5ml	brompheniramine maleate, 2mg/5ml
PE	**Diphenadryl** Schein Ph'cal	elixir		diphenhydramine HCl, 12.5mg/5ml
**	**Diphenylin Cough** Schein Ph'cal	syrup		diphenhydramine 12.5mg/5ml
	Disophrol Chronotabs Sustained Action Schering-Plough HealthCare	timed-release tablet	pseudoephedrine sulfate, 120mg	dexbrompheniramine maleate, 6mg
	DM Cold & Cough Goldline Labs	elixir	phenylpropanolamine HCl, 12.5mg/5ml	brompheniramine maleate, 2mg/5ml
AL LA SL PE	**Dorcol Children's Cough** Sandoz Consumer	syrup	pseudoephedrine HCl, 15mg/5ml	
**	**Dristan Cold & Cough Liqui-Gels** Whitehall-Robins Healthcare	softgel	pseudoephedrine HCl, 30mg	
	Dristan Cold Maximum Strength No Drowsiness Whitehall-Robins Healthcare	gel caplet	pseudoephedrine HCl, 30mg	
AF GL	**Dristan Cold Maximum Strength No Drowsiness** Whitehall-Robins Healthcare	caplet	pseudoephedrine HCl, 30mg	
AF GL SO	**Dristan Cold Multi-Symptom** Whitehall-Robins Healthcare	tablet	phenylephrine HCl, 5mg	chlorpheniramine maleate, 2mg
AF GL	**Dristan Cold Multi-Symptom Maximum Strength** Whitehall-Robins Healthcare	gel caplet	pseudoephedrine HCl, 30mg	brompheniramine maleate, 2mg
AF GL SO	**Dristan Sinus** Whitehall-Robins Healthcare	caplet	pseudoephedrine HCl, 30mg	
AF	**Drixoral Allergy Sinus Extended Release** Schering-Plough HealthCare	timed-release tablet	pseudoephedrine sulfate, 60mg	dexbrompheniramine maleate, 3mg
	Drixoral Cold & Allergy Sustained Action Schering-Plough HealthCare	timed-release tablet	pseudoephedrine sulfate, 120mg	dexbrompheniramine maleate, 6mg
AF	**Drixoral Cold & Flu** Schering-Plough HealthCare	timed-release tablet	pseudoephedrine sulfate, 60mg	dexbrompheniramine maleate, 3mg
	Drixoral Cough & Congestion Liquid Caps Schering-Plough HealthCare	capsule	pseudoephedrine HCl, 60mg	
AF	**Drixoral Cough & Sore Throat Liquid Caps** Schering-Plough HealthCare	capsule		

See Chapter 8, "Cold, Cough and Allergy Products," for more information about these products.

Analgesic	Expectorant	Antitussive	Other Ingredients
		dextromethorphan hydrobromide, 10mg/5ml	citric acid · FD&C blue#1 · FD&C red#40 · red grape flavor · glycerin · propylene glycol · saccharin sodium · sodium benzoate · sorbitol · water
			alcohol, 14% · D&C red#33 · FD&C red#40 · flavor · methylparaben · sugar · purified water
		menthol	alcohol 5% · ammonium chloride · citric acid · D&C red#33 · D&C yellow#10 · flavor · FD&C blue#1 · FD&C red#40 · methylparaben · propylene glycol · propylparaben · purified water · sodium citrate · sucrose
		dextromethorphan hydrobromide, 10mg/5ml	alcohol, 2.3%
	guaifenesin, 50mg/5ml	dextromethorphan hydrobromide, 5mg/5ml	benzoic acid · flavors · purified water · sodium hydroxide · sucrose · red#40 · tartaric acid · blue#1 · edetate disodium · glycerin · propylene glycol
acetaminophen, 250mg	guaifenesin, 100mg	dextromethorphan hydrobromide, 10mg	D&C yellow#10 · FD&C red#40 · gelatin · glycerin · mannitol · polyethylene glycol · povidone · propylene glycol · sorbitan · sorbitol · water
acetaminophen, 500mg			calcium stearate · croscarmellose sodium · D&C red#27 lake · D&C yellow#10 lake · EDTA · FD&C blue#1 lake · FD&C red#40 lake · gelatin · glycerin · hydrogenated vegetable oil · hydroxypropyl methylcellulose · iron oxide · lecithin · microcrystalline cellulose · pharmaceutical glaze · polyethylene glycol · povidone · simethicone · starch · stearic acid · titanium dioxide
acetaminophen, 500mg			calcium stearate · croscarmellose sodium · D&C red#7 lake · D&C yellow#10 lake · FD&C yellow#6 lake · hydrogenated vegetable oil · hydroxypropyl methylcellulose · microcrystalline cellulose · pharmaceutical glaze · polyethylene glycol · povidone · starch · stearic acid · titanium dioxide
acetaminophen, 325mg			calcium stearate · croscarmellose sodium · D&C yellow#10 lake · FD&C yellow#10 lake · hydroxypropyl methylcellulose · microcrystalline cellulose · polyethylene glycol · povidone · starch · stearic acid · may also contain: D&C red#7 lake · pharmaceutical glaze · titanium dioxide
acetaminophen, 500mg			calcium stearate · croscarmellose sodium · D&C red#30 · EDTA D&C red#40 lake · gelatin · glycerin · hydrogenated vegetable oil · hydroxypropyl methylcellulose · iron oxide · lecithin · microcrystalline cellulose · pharmaceutical glaze · polyethylene glycol · povidone · simethicone · starch · stearic acid · titanium dioxide · triacetin
ibuprofen, 200mg			carnauba or equivalent wax · croscarmellose sodium · iron oxide · methylparaben · microcrystalline cellulose · propylparaben · silicon dioxide · sodium benzoate · sodium lauryl sulfate · starch · stearic acid · sucrose · titanium dioxide
acetaminophen, 500mg			
acetaminophen, 500mg			
		dextromethorphan hydrobromide, 30mg	
acetaminophen, 325mg		dextromethorphan hydrobromide, 15mg	

COLD, COUGH, AND ALLERGY PRODUCTS - continued

	Product Manufacturer/Supplier	Dosage Form	Decongestant	Antihistamine
	Drixoral Cough Liquid Caps Schering-Plough HealthCare	capsule		
	Drixoral Non-Drowsy Extended Release Schering-Plough HealthCare	timed-release tablet	pseudoephedrine sulfate, 120mg	
**	**Duadacin** Kenwood Labs	capsule	phenylpropanolamine HCl, 12.5mg	chlorpheniramine maleate, 2mg
**	**Dynafed Jr.** BDI Ph'cals	tablet	pseudoephedrine HCl, 30mg	
	Dynafed Plus BDI Ph'cals	tablet	pseudoephedrine HCl, 30mg	
**	**Dynafed Pseudo** BDI Ph'cals	tablet	pseudoephedrine HCl, 60mg	
**	**Efidac 24 Chlorpheniramine** Ciba Self-Medication	timed-release tablet		chlorpheniramine maleate, 16mg
AF GL PU	**Efidac/24** Ciba Self-Medication	timed-release tablet	pseudoephedrine HCl, 240mg	
AF SO	**Emagrin Forte** Otis Clapp & Son	tablet	phenylephrine HCl, 5mg	
AF GL LA SO	**Excedrin Sinus** Bristol-Myers Products	caplet	pseudoephedrine HCl, 30mg	
GL	**Fedahist** Schwarz Pharma	tablet	pseudoephedrine HCl, 60mg	chlorpheniramine maleate, 4mg
SO	**Fendol** Buffington	tablet	phenylephrine HCl, 5mg	
GL LA SU	**Fisherman's Friend, Extra Strong, Sugar Free** Bristol-Myers Products	lozenge		
GL LA	**Fisherman's Friend, Licorice Strong** Bristol-Myers Products	lozenge		
GL LA	**Fisherman's Friend, Original Extra Strong** Bristol-Myers Products	lozenge		
GL LA SU	**Fisherman's Friend, Refreshing Mint, Sugar Free** Bristol-Myers Products	lozenge		
AF	**Flu, Cold, and Cough Medicine** Goldline Labs	individual packet	pseudoephedrine HCl, 60mg	chlorpheniramine maleate, 4mg
AF	**Flu-Relief** Pfeiffer Ph'cals	tablet	pseudoephedrine HCl, 30mg	chlorpheniramine maleate, 2mg
	Genac Goldline Labs	tablet	pseudoephedrine HCl, 60mg	triprolidine HCl, 2.5mg
	Genahist Goldline Labs	elixir		diphenhydramine HCl, 12.5mg/5ml

See Chapter 8, "Cold, Cough and Allergy Products," for more information about these products.

Analgesic	Expectorant	Antitussive	Other Ingredients
		dextromethorphan hydrobromide, 30mg	
acetaminophen, 325mg			
acetaminophen, 325mg			
acetaminophen, 500mg			
			cellulose · cellulose acetate · FD&C blue#1 · hydroxypropyl methylcellulose · hydroxypropyl cellulose · polysorbate 80 · povidone · sodium chloride · titanium dioxide · magnesium stearate · polyethylene glycol
acetaminophen, 260mg	guaifenesin, 101mg		caffeine, 32mg
acetaminophen, 500mg			benzoic acid · carnauba wax · corn starch · D&C yellow#10 lake · FD&C red#40 lake · hydroxypropyl methylcellulose · mineral oil · polysorbate 20 · povidone · propylene glycol · simethicone emulsion · sorbitan monolaurate · stearic acid · titanium dioxide
			lactose · colloidal silicon dioxide · magnesium stearate · microcrystalline cellulose · stearic acid · talc
acetaminophen, 354mg · salicylamide, 65mg	guaifenesin, 101mg		caffeine, 32mg
		menthol, 10mg · eucalyptus oil	sorbitol · natural licorice · magnesium stearate · capsicum
		menthol, 6mg	sugar · licorice · edible gums · anise oil
		menthol, 10mg · eucalyptus oil	sugar · licorice · edible gums · capsicum
		menthol, 3mg · peppermint oil	sorbitol · magnesium stearate · aspartame · phenylalanine
acetaminophen, 500mg		dextromethorphan hydrobromide, 20mg	yellow#6
acetaminophen, 325mg			
			alcohol, 14%

COLD, COUGH, AND ALLERGY PRODUCTS - continued

	Product Manufacturer/Supplier	Dosage Form	Decongestant	Antihistamine
AF	**Genahist** Goldline Labs	capsule		diphenhydramine HCl, 25mg
	Genamin Goldline Labs	syrup	phenylpropanolamine HCl, 12.5mg/5ml	chlorpheniramine maleate, 2mg/5ml
AF	**Genapap Maximum Strength Sinus** Goldline Labs	caplet	pseudoephedrine HCl, 30mg	
	Genaphed Goldline Labs	tablet	pseudoephedrine HCl, 30mg	
	Genatap Goldline Labs	elixir	phenylpropanolamine HCl, 12.5mg/5ml	brompheniramine maleate, 2mg/5ml
	Genatuss Goldline Labs	syrup		
	Genatuss DM Goldline Labs	syrup		
	Gencold Goldline Labs	capsule	phenylpropanolamine HCl, 75mg	chlorpheniramine maleate, 8mg
AF	**Gendecon** Goldline Labs	tablet	phenylephrine HCl, 5mg	chlorpheniramine maleate, 2mg
	Genite Goldline Labs	liquid	pseudoephedrine HCl, 10mg/5ml	doxylamine succinate, 1.25mg/5ml
AF GL LA	**GG-Cen** Central Ph'cals	capsule		
AL LA	**Guaifed** Muro Ph'cal	syrup	pseudoephedrine HCl, 30mg/5ml	
	GuiaCough Schein Ph'cal	syrup		
	GuiaCough CF Schein Ph'cal	syrup	phenylpropanolamine HCl, 12.5mg/5ml	
	GuiaCough PE Schein Ph'cal	syrup	pseudoephedrine HCl, 30mg/5ml	
AL	**Guiatuss CF** Goldline Labs	liquid	phenylpropanolamine HCl, 12.5mg/5ml	
AF	**Guiatuss Cold & Cough** Goldline Labs	gelcap	pseudoephedrine HCl, 30mg	
** SU PE	**Halls Juniors Sugar Free Cough Drops, Grape or Orange** Warner-Lambert	lozenge		
	Halls Mentho-Lyptus Cough Supp. Drops, Cherry or Mentho-L. Warner-Lambert	lozenge		

See Chapter 8, "Cold, Cough and Allergy Products," for more information about these products.

Analgesic	Expectorant	Antitussive	Other Ingredients
acetaminophen, 500mg			
			alcohol, 2.3% · saccharin · sorbitol · grape flavor
	guaifenesin, 100mg/5ml		alcohol, 3.5%
	guaifenesin, 100mg/5ml	dextromethorphan hydrobromide, 15mg/5ml	alcohol, 1.4% · sucrose · saccharin · glucose
acetaminophen, 325mg			
acetaminophen, 167mg/5ml		dextromethorphan hydrobromide, 5mg/5ml	alcohol, 25% · tartrazine
	guaifenesin, 200mg		
	guaifenesin, 200mg/5ml	menthol	benzoic acid · cherry flavor · citric acid · edetate disodium · FD&C red#40 · FD&C blue#1 · glycerin · polyethylene glycol · povidone · purified water · saccharin sodium · sodium citrate · sorbitol · sucrose · vanillin
	guaifenesin, 100mg/5ml	menthol	alcohol, 3.5% · citric acid · corn syrup · D&C red#33 · FD&C blue#1 · FD&C red#40 · FD&C yellow#6 · flavor · methylparaben · propylparaben · propylene glycol · purified water · saccharin sodium · sodium benzoate · sodium chloride
	guaifenesin, 100mg/5ml	dextromethorphan hydrobromide, 10mg/5ml · menthol	alcohol, 4.75% · citric acid · FD&C red#40 · flavor · methylparaben · propylene glycol · purified water · saccharin sodium · sodium benzoate · sorbitol · sucrose
	guaifenesin, 100mg/5ml		alcohol, 1.4% · citric acid · corn syrup · FD&C red#40 · flavor · methylparaben · propylene glycol · purified water · saccharin sodium · sodium benzoate
	guaifenesin, 100mg/5ml	dextromethorphan hydrobromide, 10mg/5ml	
	guaifenesin, 200mg	dextromethorphan hydrobromide, 10mg	
		menthol, 2.5 mg · eucalyptus oil	acesulfame · potassium · isomalt · natural flavor · blue#1 (Grape) · red#40 (Grape) · yellow#6 (Orange)
		menthol, 6.1mg · eucalyptus oil	carmine color · corn syrup · flavor · sucrose

COLD, COUGH, AND ALLERGY PRODUCTS - continued

	Product Manufacturer/Supplier	Dosage Form	Decongestant	Antihistamine
	Halls Mentho-Lyptus Cough Supp. Drops, Honey-Lemon Warner-Lambert	lozenge		
	Halls Mentho-Lyptus Cough Supp. Drops, Spearmint Warner-Lambert	lozenge		
	Halls Mentho-Lyptus Ex. Strength Cough Supp. Drops, Ice Blue Warner-Lambert	lozenge		
SU	**Halls Mentho-Lyptus Sugar Free Cough Supp. Drops, Bl. Cherry** Warner-Lambert	lozenge		
SU	**Halls Mentho-Lyptus Sugar Free Cough Supp. Drops, Citrus** Warner-Lambert	lozenge		
SU	**Halls Mentho-Lyptus Sugar Free Cough Supp. Drops, Menthol** Warner-Lambert	lozenge		
	Halls Plus Max. Strength; Cherry, Honey-Lemon, Mentho-Lyptus Warner-Lambert	lozenge		
AF GL PU	**Hay Fever & Allergy Relief** Hudson	tablet	phenylpropanolamine HCl, 18.7mg	chlorpheniramine maleate, 2mg
AL DY GL LA SU SL	**Hayfebrol** Scot-Tussin Pharmacal	liquid	pseudoephedrine HCl, 30mg/5ml	chlorpheniramine maleate, 2mg/5ml
** DY GL LA PU SO SU	**Herbal-Menthol** Shaklee	lozenge		
AF GL PU	**Histatab Plus** Century Ph'cals	tablet	phenylephrine HCl, 5mg	chlorpheniramine maleate, 2mg
	Hold Menley & James Labs	lozenge		
	Hydramine Cough Goldline Labs	syrup		diphenhydramine HCl, 12.5mg/5ml
AF GL PU SO	**Hytuss** Hyrex Ph'cals	tablet		
AF GL PU SO	**Hytuss 2X** Hyrex Ph'cals	capsule		

See Chapter 8, "Cold, Cough and Allergy Products," for more information about these products.

Analgesic	Expectorant	Antitussive	Other Ingredients
		menthol, 8.4mg · eucalyptus oil	flavor · corn syrup · sucrose · yellow#6 · yellow#10
		menthol, 5mg · eucalyptus oil	flavor · blue#1 · corn syrup · sucrose · yellow#10
		menthol, 12mg · eucalyptus oil	flavor · blue#1 · corn syrup · sucrose
		menthol, 5mg · eucalyptus oil	acesulfame potassium · blue#1 · flavor · isomalt · red#40
		menthol, 5mg · eucalyptus oil	acesulfame potassium · flavor · isomalt · yellow#5 · citric acid
		menthol, 6mg · eucalyptus oil	acesulfame potassium · flavor · isomalt · citric acid · blue#1 · red#40
		menthol, 10mg · eucalyptus oil	blue#2 (Cherry) · acesulfame (Lemon) · potassium (Lemon) · corn syrup · flavor (Cherry, Lemon) · citric acid (Mentho-Lyptus) · glycerin · high fructose corn syrup · red#40 (Cherry) · honey (Lemon) · sucrose · yellow#6 (Lemon) · yellow#10 (Lemon)
		menthol	methylparaben · propylparaben · cherry-mint flavor · glycerin · hydroxymethylcellulose · potassium benzoate · citric acid · propylene glycol · sorbitol
		menthol, 6mg (from peppermint) · eucalyptus oil · peppermint oil	brown rice syrup · corn syrup · honey · horehound extract · marshmallow root extract · thyme extract
		dextromethorphan hydrobromide, 5mg	corn syrup · sucrose · vegetable oil · flavors · FD&C blue#1 · FD&C red#40 · FD&C yellow#5 · FD&C yellow#10
			alcohol, 5%
	guaifenesin, 100mg		
	guaifenesin, 200mg		

COLD, COUGH, AND ALLERGY PRODUCTS - continued

	Product Manufacturer/Supplier	Dosage Form	Decongestant	Antihistamine
** AL	**Ipsatol** Kenwood Labs	syrup	phenylpropanolamine HCl, 9mg/5ml	
	Isodettes Goody's Ph'cals	lozenge		
	Kodet-SE Pfeiffer Ph'cals	tablet	pseudoephedrine HCl, 30mg	
	Koldets Cough Drops Pfeiffer Ph'cals	lozenge		
AF	**Kolephrin** Pfeiffer Ph'cals	caplet	pseudoephedrine HCl, 30mg	chlorpheniramine maleate, 2mg
AF	**Kolephrin DM** Pfeiffer Ph'cals	caplet	pseudoephedrine HCl, 30mg	chlorpheniramine maleate, 2mg
AL	**Kolephrin GG/DM** Pfeiffer Ph'cals	syrup		
AL	**Kophane Cough and Cold Medication** Pfeiffer Ph'cals	syrup	phenylpropanolamine HCl, 12.5mg/5ml	chlorpheniramine maleate, 2.0mg/5ml
** SU	**Luden's Maximum Strength Sugar Free, Cherry** Hershey	lozenge		
**	**Luden's Maximum Strength, Cherry** Hershey	lozenge		
**	**Luden's Maximum Strength, Menthol Eucalyptus** Hershey	lozenge		
	Mentholatum Mentholatum	ointment		
PE	**Mentholatum Cherry Chest Rub for Kids** Mentholatum	ointment		
	Mini Thin Pseudo BDI Ph'cals	tablet	pseudoephedrine HCl, 60mg	
	Multi-Symptom Cough Formula M Goldline Labs	liquid	pseudoephedrine HCl, 15mg/5ml	chlorpheniramine maleate, 1mg/5ml
	N'Ice 'N Clear, Cherry Eucalyptus SmithKline Beecham	lozenge		
	N'Ice 'N Clear, Menthol Eucalyptus SmithKline Beecham	lozenge		
	N'Ice Sore Throat & Cough, Assorted or Citrus SmithKline Beecham	lozenge		
AL LA SL	**Naldecon DX, Adult** Apothecon	liquid	phenylpropanolamine HCl, 12.5mg/5ml	

See Chapter 8, "Cold, Cough and Allergy Products," for more information about these products.

Analgesic	Expectorant	Antitussive	Other Ingredients
	guaifenesin, 100mg/5ml	dextromethorphan hydrobromide, 10mg/5ml	
		menthol, 10mg	benzocaine, 6mg · corn syrup · flavor · FD&C red#40 · FD&C blue#1 · sucrose · propylene glycol · sodium bicarbonate · water
		menthol, 6.1mg · eucalyptus oil	citric acid
acetaminophen, 325mg			
acetaminophen, 325mg		dextromethorphan hydrobromide, 10mg	
	guaifenesin, 150mg/5ml	dextromethorphan hydrobromide, 10mg/5ml	sucrose · cherry flavor
		dextromethorphan hydrobromide, 10mg/5ml · menthol	sodium citrate · sucrose · cherry-vanilla flavor
		menthol, 10mg · eucalyptus oil	isomalt · hydrogenated starch hydrolysate · citric acid · malic acid · flavoring · acesulfame potassium · artificial color
		menthol, 10mg · eucalyptus oil	sugar · corn syrup · citric acid · malic acid · flavoring · artificial color
		menthol, 10mg · eucalyptus oil	sugar · corn syrup
		camphor, 9% · natural menthol, 1.3%	fragrance · petrolatum · titanium dioxide
		camphor, 4.7% · natural menthol, 2.6% · eucalyptus oil, 1.2%	fragrance · petrolatum · steareth-2 · titanium dioxide
acetaminophen, 125mg/5ml		dextromethorphan hydrobromide, 7.5mg/5ml	
		menthol, 7mg	flavors · D&C red#33 · sorbitol · tartaric acid · FD&C yellow#6
		menthol, 5mg	citric acid · flavors · sorbitol
		menthol, 5mg	citric acid · D&C yellow#10 · D&C red#33 (Asst.) · FD&C blue#2 (Asst.) · FD&C yellow#6 (Asst.) · flavors · maltitol solution (Asst.) · saccharin sodium · sodium citrate · sorbitol · tartaric acid (Asst.)
	guaifenesin, 200mg/5ml	dextromethorphan hydrobromide, 10mg/5ml	

COLD, COUGH, AND ALLERGY PRODUCTS - continued

	Product Manufacturer/Supplier	Dosage Form	Decongestant	Antihistamine
AL LA SL PE	**Naldecon DX, Children's** Apothecon	syrup	phenylpropanolamine HCl, 6.25mg/5ml	
AL LA PE	**Naldecon DX, Pediatric** Apothecon	drops	phenylpropanolamine HCl, 6.25mg/ml	
AL LA SL PE	**Naldecon EX, Children's** Apothecon	syrup	phenylpropanolamine HCl, 6.25mg/5ml	
AL LA SL PE	**Naldecon EX, Pediatric** Apothecon	drops	phenylpropanolamine HCl, 6.25mg/ml	
AL LA SL GE	**Naldecon Senior DX** Apothecon	liquid		
AL LA SL GE	**Naldecon Senior EX** Apothecon	liquid		
AF GL PU SO	**Napril** Randob Labs	tablet	pseudoephedrine HCl, 60mg	chlorpheniramine maleate, 4mg
** AF DY GL LA PU SU	**Nasal-D** Shaklee	tablet	pseudoephedrine HCl, 60mg (from ephedra)	
AF GL PU SO	**ND-Gesic** Hyrex Ph'cals	tablet	phenylephrine HCl, 5mg	pyrilamine maleate, 12.5mg · chlorpheniramine maleate, 2mg
AL	**Night Time Cold Medicine** Goldline Labs	liquid	pseudoephedrine HCl, 60mg/oz	doxylamine succinate, 7.5mg/oz
AF	**Night Time Cold Medicine Softgels** Goldline Labs	gelcap	pseudoephedrine HCl, 30mg	doxylamine succinate, 6.25mg
**	**NiteGel** Republic Drug	liquid-cap	pseudoephedrine HCl, 30mg	doxylamine succinate, 6.25mg
AF DY GL LA PU SO	**Nolahist** Carnrick Labs	tablet		phenindamine tartrate, 25mg
	Novahistine SmithKline Beecham	elixir	phenylephrine HCl, 5mg/5ml	chlorpheniramine maleate, 2mg/5ml
	Novahistine DH SmithKline Beecham	liquid	pseudoephedrine HCl, 30mg/5ml	chlorpheniramine maleate, 2mg/5ml

See Chapter 8, "Cold, Cough and Allergy Products," for more information about these products.

Analgesic	Expectorant	Antitussive	Other Ingredients
	guaifenesin, 100mg/5ml	dextromethorphan hydrobromide, 5mg/5ml	
	guaifenesin, 50mg/ml	dextromethorphan hydrobromide, 5mg/ml	
	guaifenesin, 100mg/5ml		
	guaifenesin, 50mg/ml		
	guaifenesin, 200mg/5ml	dextromethorphan hydrobromide, 10mg/5ml	citric acid · D&C yellow#10 · FD&C yellow#6 · natural and artificial flavors · propylene glycol · Prosweet MM24 · saccharin sodium · sodium benzoate · sodium citrate · sorbitol solution · purified water
	guaifenesin, 200mg/5ml		citric acid · FD&C blue#1 · FD&C red#40 · natural and artificial flavors · polyethylene glycol · saccharin sodium · sodium benzoate · sodium citrate · sorbitol solution · purified water
			lactose · cornstarch · stearic acid · magnesium stearate
			calcium stearate · croscarmellose sodium · dicalcium phosphate · eucalyptus leaf extract · eucalyptus oil · glycerin · hydroxypropyl methylcellulose · maltodextrin · microcrystalline cellulose · peppermint leaf extract
acetaminophen, 300mg			
acetaminophen, 1000mg/oz		dextromethorphan hydrobromide, 30mg/oz	
acetaminophen, 250mg		dextromethorphan hydrobromide, 10mg	
acetaminophen, 250mg		dextromethorphan hydrobromide, 10mg	
			alcohol, 5% · sorbitol · D&C yellow#10 · FC&C blue#1 · flavors · glycerin · sodium chloride · water
		codeine phosphate, 10mg/5ml[a]	alcohol, 5% · invert sugar · saccharin sodium · sorbitol · FD&C blue#1 · FD&C red#40 · flavors · glycerin · hydrochloric acid · sodium chloride · water

COLD, COUGH, AND ALLERGY PRODUCTS - continued

	Product Manufacturer/Supplier	Dosage Form	Decongestant	Antihistamine
	Novahistine DMX SmithKline Beecham	syrup	pseudoephedrine HCl, 30mg/5ml	
	Novahistine Expectorant SmithKline Beecham	liquid	pseudoephedrine HCl, 30mg/5ml	
AF SO	**Oranyl** Otis Clapp & Son	tablet	pseudoephedrine HCl, 30mg	
AF SO	**Oranyl Plus** Otis Clapp & Son	tablet	pseudoephedrine HCl, 30mg	
**	**Ornex Maximum Strength** Menley & James Labs	caplet	pseudoephedrine HCl, 30mg	
**	**Ornex Regular Strength** Menley & James Labs	caplet	pseudoephedrine HCl, 30mg	
	P.C. Nasal Decongestant Republic Drug	tablet	pseudoephedrine, 30mg	
AL PE	**PediaCare Cough-Cold Formula** McNeil Consumer	liquid	pseudoephedrine HCl, 15mg/5ml	chlorpheniramine maleate, 1mg/5ml
AF PE	**PediaCare Cough-Cold Formula** McNeil Consumer	chewable tablet	pseudoephedrine HCl, 15mg	chlorpheniramine maleate, 1mg
AL PE	**PediaCare Infants' Decongestant** McNeil Consumer	drops	pseudoephedrine HCl, 7.5mg/0.8ml	
** AL PE	**PediaCare Infants' Decongestant Plus Cough** McNeil Consumer	drops	pseudoephedrine HCl, 7.5mg/0.8ml	
AL PE	**PediaCare Night Rest Cough-Cold Formula** McNeil Consumer	liquid	pseudoephedrine HCl, 15mg/5ml	chlorpheniramine maleate, 1mg/5ml
AL PE	**Pediacon DX, Children's** Goldline Labs	syrup	phenylpropanolamine HCl, 6.25mg/5ml	
AL PE	**Pediacon DX, Pediatric** Goldline Labs	drops	phenylpropanolamine HCl, 6.25/1ml	
AL PE	**Pediacon EX, Pediatric** Goldline Labs	drops	phenylpropanolamine HCl, 6.25mg/1ml	
LA SL PE	**Pertussin CS** Blairex Labs	liquid		
LA SL	**Pertussin ES** Blairex Labs	liquid		
	Phenylgesic Goldline Labs	tablet		phenyltoloxamine citrate, 30mg
DY	**Pinex** Alvin Last	syrup		

See Chapter 8, "Cold, Cough and Allergy Products," for more information about these products.

Analgesic	Expectorant	Antitussive	Other Ingredients
	guaifenesin, 100mg/5ml	dextromethorphan hydrobromide, 10mg/5ml	alcohol, 10% · saccharin sodium · sorbitol · FD&C red#40 · FD&C yellow#6 · flavors · glycerin · hydrochloric acid · invert sugar · sodium chloride · water
	guaifenesin, 100mg/5ml	codeine phosphate, 10mg/5ml[a]	alcohol, 7.5% · saccharin sodium · sorbitol · invert sugar · D&C yellow#10 · FD&C blue#1 · FD&C red#40 · flavors · glycerin · hydrochloric acid · sodium chloride · sodium gluconate · water
acetaminophen, 500mg			
acetaminophen, 500mg			crospovidone · hydroxypropyl methylcellulose · magnesium stearate · microcrystalline cellulose · polyethylene glycol · polysorbate 80 · povidone · starch · titanium dioxide
acetaminophen, 325mg			crospovidone · FD&C blue#1 · hydroxypropyl methylcellulose · magnesium stearate · microcrystalline cellulose · polyethylene glycol · polysorbate 80 · povidone · starch · titanium dioxide
		dextromethorphan hydrobromide, 5mg/5ml	citric acid · corn syrup · flavors · glycerin · propylene glycol · sodium benzoate · sodium carboxymethylcellulose · sorbitol · purified water · red#40
		dextromethorphan hydrobromide, 5mg	aspartame · cellulose · citric acid · flavors · magnesium stearate · magnesium trisilicate · mannitol · corn starch · D&C red#7
			benzoic acid · citric acid · flavors · glycerin · polyethylene glycol · propylene glycol · purified water · sodium benzoate · sorbitol · sucrose · red#40
		dextromethorphan hydrobromide, 2.5mg/0.8ml	citric acid · flavors · glycerin · purified water · sodium benzoate · sorbitol
		dextromethorphan hydrobromide, 7.5mg/5ml	citric acid · corn syrup · flavors · glycerin · propylene glycol · sodium benzoate · sodium carboxymethylcellulose · sorbitol · purified water · red#40
	guaifenesin, 100mg/5ml	dextromethorphan hydrobromide, 5mg/5ml	
	guaifenesin, 50mg/1ml	dextromethorphan hydrobromide, 5mg/1ml	
	guaifenesin, 50mg/1ml		
		dextromethorphan hydrobromide, 7mg/10ml	citric acid · colors · flavor · sorbic acid · sorbitol · sucrose · water
		dextromethorphan hydrobromide, 30mg/10ml	caramel · carboxymethylcellulose sodium · citric acid · D&C red#33 · flavor · sorbic acid · sorbitol · sugar · water
acetaminophen, 325mg			
		dextromethorphan hydrobromide, 7.5mg/5ml	sucrose · purified water · glycerin · caramel · honey · flavor

COLD, COUGH, AND ALLERGY PRODUCTS - continued

	Product Manufacturer/Supplier	Dosage Form	Decongestant	Antihistamine
DY	**Pinex Concentrate** Alvin Last	syrup		
**	**Prominicol Cough** Republic Drug	syrup	phenylpropanolamine HCl, 12.5mg	chlorpheniramine maleate, 2mg
AF DY GL PU SO SU	**Propagest** Carnrick Labs	tablet	phenylpropanolamine HCl, 25mg	
**	**Protac DM** Republic Drug	liquid		
AL	**Protac SF** Republic Drug	liquid		chlorpheniramine maleate, 2mg
AF	**Pyrroxate** Roberts Ph'cal	caplet	phenylpropanolamine HCl, 25mg	chlorpheniramine maleate, 4mg
	Quelidrine Cough Abbott Labs	syrup	phenylephrine HCl, 5mg/5ml · ephedrine HCl, 5mg/5ml	chlorpheniramine maleate, 2mg/5ml
AL DY	**REM** Alvin Last	liquid		
	Ricola Cough Drops, Original Flavor Ricola	lozenge		
SU	**Ricola Sugar Free Herb Throat Drops, Alpine-Mint** Ricola	lozenge		
SU	**Ricola Sugar Free Herb Throat Drops, Cherry- or Lemon-Mint** Ricola	lozenge		
SU	**Ricola Sugar Free Herb Throat Drops, Mountain Herb** Ricola	lozenge		
	Ricola Throat Drops, Cherry-Mint Ricola	lozenge		
**	**Ricola Throat Drops, Honey-Herb** Ricola	lozenge		
	Ricola Throat Drops, Lemon-Mint or Orange-Mint Ricola	lozenge		

See Chapter 8, "Cold, Cough and Allergy Products," for more information about these products.

Analgesic	Expectorant	Antitussive	Other Ingredients
		dextromethorphan hydrobromide, 7.5mg/5ml (when diluted to 16fl.oz.)	alcohol, 16% (3% when diluted) · purified water · sucrose · glycerin · honey · flavor · caramel · sodium hydroxide
		dextromethorphan hydrobromide, 10mg	
	guaifenesin, 100mg	dextromethorphan hydrobromide, 10mg	
		dextromethorphan hydrobromide, 15mg	
acetaminophen, 500mg			benzyl alcohol · butylparaben · erythrosine sodium · gelatin · glycerin · magnesium stearate · methylparaben · propylparaben · sodium lauryl sulfate · sodium propionate · starch · talc
	ammonium chloride, 40mg/5ml · ipecac fluid extract, 0.005ml/5ml	dextromethorphan hydrobromide, 10mg/5ml	alcohol, 2% · sucrose · D&C red#33 · glycerin · liquid glucose · magnesium carbonate · methylparaben · propylparaben · tolu balsam tincture · water · artificial flavors
	citric acid · sodium citrate	dextromethorphan hydrobromide, 5mg/5ml · eucalyptol	corn syrup · sucrose · glycerin · purified water · caramel · sodium chloride · sodium benzoate · licorice · anise oil · disodium EDTA
		menthol, 3mg	sugar · glucose syrup · caramelized sugar · extracts of peppermint, lemon balm, thyme, sage, hyssop, elder, linden flowers, wild thyme, horehound, angelica root, and peppermint oil
		menthol, 4.8mg	extracts of peppermint, lemon balm, lady's mantle, linden flowers, and elder · natural flavorings · citric acid · aspartame · chlorophyll · isomalt
		menthol, 1mg	extracts of peppermint, lemon balm, lady's mantle, linden flowers, and elder · citric acid · lemon and peppermint oils (Lemon-Mint) · cherry and peppermint flavorings (Cherry-Mint) · cherry and elderberry concentrates (Cherry-Mint) · ascorbic acid · aspartame · flavorings (Lemon-Mint) · isomalt
		menthol, 1.5mg	extracts of peppermint, lemon balm, thyme, sage, hyssop, elder, linden flowers, wild thyme, horehound, and angelica root · caramel coloring · aspartame · peppermint oil · isomalt
		menthol, 1.5mg	sugar · glucose syrup · citric acid · extracts of peppermint, lemon balm, thyme, sage, hyssop, elder, linden flowers, wild thyme, horehound, and angelica root · cherry concentrate · elder concentrate · cherry flavorings · peppermint oil
		menthol, 2.4mg	honey · sugar · corn syrup · extracts of peppermint, lemon balm, thyme, sage, hyssop, elder, linden flowers, wild thyme, horehound, angelica root, and peppermint oil
		menthol, 1.25mg	sugar · glucose syrup · citric acid · extracts of lemon balm, orange-mint (Orange-Mint), peppermint, thyme, sage, hyssop, elder, linden flowers, wild thyme, horehound, and angelica root · lemon oil (Lemon-Mint) · peppermint oil · orange flavoring (Orange-Mint) · natural coloring (Lemon-Mint) · paprika extract (Orange-Mint)

COLD, COUGH, AND ALLERGY PRODUCTS - continued

	Product Manufacturer/Supplier	Dosage Form	Decongestant	Antihistamine
	Ricola Throat Drops, Menthol-Eucalyptus Ricola	lozenge		
AL	**Robitussin** Whitehall-Robins Healthcare	syrup		
AL	**Robitussin CF** Whitehall-Robins Healthcare	syrup	phenylpropanolamine HCl, 12.5mg/5ml	
	Robitussin Cold & Cough Liqui-Gels Whitehall-Robins Healthcare	softgel	pseudoephedrine HCl, 30mg	
	Robitussin Cold, Cough, & Flu Liqui-Gels Whitehall-Robins Healthcare	softgel	pseudoephedrine HCl, 30mg	
	Robitussin Cough Calmers Whitehall-Robins Healthcare	lozenge		
	Robitussin Cough Drops, Cherry or Menthol Eucalyptus Whitehall-Robins Healthcare	lozenge		
	Robitussin Cough Drops, Honey-Lemon Whitehall-Robins Healthcare	lozenge		
	Robitussin DM Whitehall-Robins Healthcare	syrup		
	Robitussin Liquid Center Cough Drops, Cherry w/ Honey-Lemon Whitehall-Robins Healthcare	lozenge		
	Robitussin Liquid Center Cough Drops, Honey-Lemon w/ Cherry Whitehall-Robins Healthcare	lozenge		
	Robitussin Liquid Center Cough Drops, Menthol Euc. w/Cherry Whitehall-Robins Healthcare	lozenge		
	Robitussin Maximum Strength Cough Whitehall-Robins Healthcare	liquid		
	Robitussin Maximum Strength Cough & Cold Whitehall-Robins Healthcare	liquid	pseudoephedrine HCl, 30mg/5ml	
AL	**Robitussin Night Relief** Whitehall-Robins Healthcare	liquid	pseudoephedrine HCl, 10mg/5ml	pyrilamine maleate, 8.33mg/5ml
**	**Robitussin Night-Time Cold Formula** Whitehall-Robins Healthcare	softgel	pseudoephedrine HCl, 30mg	doxylamine succinate, 6.25mg
AL	**Robitussin PE** Whitehall-Robins Healthcare	syrup	pseudoephedrine HCl, 30mg/5ml	
** AL PE	**Robitussin Pediatric** Whitehall-Robins Healthcare	drops	pseudoephedrine HCl, 15mg/2.5ml	

See Chapter 8, "Cold, Cough and Allergy Products," for more information about these products.

Analgesic	Expectorant	Antitussive	Other Ingredients
		menthol, 4.5mg	sugar · glucose syrup · extracts of peppermint, lemon balm, thyme, sage, hyssop, elder, linden flowers, wild thyme, horehound, angelica root, peppermint oil, and eucalyptus oil · chlorophyll
	guaifenesin, 100mg/5ml		caramel · citric acid · FD&C red#40 · flavors · glucose · glycerin · high fructose corn syrup · saccharin sodium · sodium benzoate · water
	guaifenesin, 100mg/5ml	dextromethorphan hydrobromide, 10mg/5ml	citric acid · FD&C red#40 · flavors · glycerin · propylene glycol · saccharin sodium · sodium benzoate · sorbitol · water
	guaifenesin, 200mg	dextromethorphan hydrobromide, 10mg	FD&C blue#1 · FD&C red#40 · gelatin · glycerin · mannitol · pharmaceutical glaze · polyethelene glycol · povidone · propylene glycol · sorbitan · sorbitol · titanium dioxide · water
acetaminophen, 250mg	guaifenesin, 100mg	dextromethorphan hydrobromide, 10mg	D&C yellow#10 · FD&C red#40 · gelatin · glycerin · mannitol · polyethylene glycol · povidone · propylene glycol · sorbitan · sorbitol · water
		dextromethorphan hydrobromide, 5mg	corn syrup · FD&C red #40 · cherry flavor · glycerin · gum acacia · sucrose
		menthol, 7.4mg · eucalyptus oil	corn syrup · FD&C red#40 (Cherry) · flavors (Cherry) · sucrose · titanium dioxide (Menthol Eucalyptus) · may contain starch
		menthol, 10mg · eucalyptus oil	corn syrup · D&C yellow#10 · FD&C yellow#6 · flavors · sucrose · may contain starch
	guaifenesin, 100mg/5ml	dextromethorphan hydrobromide, 10mg/5ml	citric acid · FD&C red#40 · flavors · glucose · glycerin · high fructose corn syrup · saccharin sodium · sodium benzoate · water
		menthol, 8mg · eucalyptus oil	corn syrup · FD&C red#40 · flavors · glycerin · high fructose corn syrup · honey · lemon oil · methylparaben · propylparaben · sodium benzoate · sorbitol · sucrose · titanium dioxide
		menthol, 10mg · eucalyptus oil	corn syrup · D&C yellow #10 aluminum lake · FD&C yellow #6 aluminum lake · flavors · glycerin · high fructose corn syrup · honey · lemon oil · methylparaben · povidone · propylparaben · sodium benzoate · sorbitol · sucrose · titanium dioxide · water
		menthol, 8mg · eucalyptus oil	corn syrup · flavors · glycerin · high fructose corn syrup · sorbitol · sucrose · water
		dextromethorphan hydrobromide, 15mg/5ml	alcohol, 1.4% · citric acid · FD&C red#40 · flavors · glycerin · glucose · high fructose corn syrup · saccharin sodium · sodium benzoate · water
		dextromethorphan hydrobromide, 15mg/5ml	alcohol, 1.4% · citric acid · FD&C red#40 · flavors · glycerin · glucose · high fructose corn syrup · saccharin sodium · sodium benzoate · water
acetaminophen, 108.33mg/5ml		dextromethorphan hydrobromide, 5mg/5ml	citric acid · FD&C blue#1 · FD&C red#40 · cherry flavor · glycerin · propylene glycol · saccharin sodium · sodium benzoate · sorbitol · water
acetaminophen, 325mg		dextromethorphan hydrobromide, 15mg	D&C green#5 · D&C yellow#10 · FD&C green#3 · FD&C yellow#6 · gelatin · glycerin · mannitol · pharmaceutical glaze · polyethylene glycol · povidone · propylene glycol · sodium acetate · sorbitan · sorbitol · titanium dioxide · water
	guaifenesin, 100mg/5ml		citric acid · FD&C red#40 · flavors · glucose · glycerin · high fructose corn syrup · maltol · propylene glycol · saccharin sodium · sodium benzoate · water
	guaifenesin, 100mg/2.5ml	dextromethorphan hydrobromide, 5mg/2.5ml	citric acid · FD&C red#40 · flavors · glycerin · high fructose corn syrup · menthol · polyethylene glycol · propylene glycol · saccharin sodium · sodium benzoate · sodium carboxymethylcellulose · sorbitol · water

COLD, COUGH, AND ALLERGY PRODUCTS - continued

	Product Manufacturer/Supplier	Dosage Form	Decongestant	Antihistamine
AL PE	**Robitussin Pediatric Cough** Whitehall-Robins Healthcare	liquid		
AL PE	**Robitussin Pediatric Cough & Cold** Whitehall-Robins Healthcare	liquid	pseudoephedrine HCl, 15mg/5ml	
AL PE	**Robitussin Pediatric Night Relief** Whitehall-Robins Healthcare	liquid	pseudoephedrine HCl, 15mg/5ml	chlorpheniramine maleate, 1mg/5ml
	Robitussin Severe Congestion Liqui-Gels Whitehall-Robins Healthcare	softgel	pseudoephedrine HCl, 30mg	
SU	**Robitussin Sugar Free Cough Drops, Cherry or Peppermint** Whitehall-Robins Healthcare	lozenge		
AL SU	**Safe Tussin 30** Kramer Labs	liquid		
AL DY GL LA SU SL	**Scot-Tussin Allergy Relief Formula** Scot-Tussin Pharmacal	liquid		diphenhydramine HCl, 12.5mg/5ml
AL DY GL LA SU SL	**Scot-Tussin DM** Scot-Tussin Pharmacal	liquid		chlorpheniramine maleate, 2mg/5ml
AF DY GL LA PU SO SU	**Scot-Tussin DM Cough Chasers** Scot-Tussin Pharmacal	lozenge		
AL DY GL LA SU SL	**Scot-Tussin Expectorant** Scot-Tussin Pharmacal	liquid		
AL DY GL LA SU SL	**Scot-Tussin Original** Scot-Tussin Pharmacal	liquid	phenylephrine HCl, 4.2mg/5ml	pheniramine maleate, 13.33mg/5ml
** AL DY GL LA SU SL	**Scot-Tussin Senior** Scot-Tussin Pharmacal	liquid		
AF SO	**Sinapils** Pfeiffer Ph'cals	tablet	phenylpropanolamine HCl, 12.5mg	chlorpheniramine maleate, 2mg

See Chapter 8, "Cold, Cough and Allergy Products," for more information about these products.

Analgesic	Expectorant	Antitussive	Other Ingredients
		dextromethorphan hydrobromide, 7.5mg/5ml	citric acid · FD&C red#40 · cherry flavor · glycerin · propylene glycol · saccharin sodium · sodium benzoate · sorbitol · water
		dextromethorphan hydrobromide, 7.5mg/5ml	citric acid · FD&C red#40 · cherry flavor · glycerin · propylene glycol · saccharin sodium · sodium benzoate · sorbitol · water
		dextromethorphan hydrobromide, 7.5mg/5ml	citric acid · FD&C blue#1 · FD&C red#40 · flavors · glycerin · high fructose corn syrup · propylene glycol · saccharin sodium · sodium benzoate · sorbitol · water
	guaifenesin, 200mg		FD&C green#3 · gelatin · glycerin · mannitol · pharmaceutical glaze · polyethylene glycol · povidone · propylene glycol · sorbitan · sorbitol · titanium dioxide · water
		menthol, 10mg	aspartame · canola oil · FD&C blue#1 aluminum lake · FD&C red#40 aluminum lake (Cherry) · flavors · hydrogenated glucose syrup · isomalt
	guaifenesin, 200mg/5ml	dextromethorphan hydrobromide, 30mg/5ml	citric acid · benzoic acid · glycerin · sorbitol · peppermint · menthol · water
		menthol	methylparaben · propylparaben · propylene glycol · glycerin · cherry-strawberry flavor · benzoic acid · citric acid · hydroxymethylcellulose · Magnasweet-110
		dextromethorphan hydrobromide, 15mg/5ml · menthol	glycerin · propylene glycol · citric acid · potassium benzoate · hydroxymethylcellulose · methylparaben · propylparaben · cherry-strawberry flavor · Magnasweet-110
		dextromethorphan hydrobromide, 2.5mg · peppermint oil	sorbitol
	guaifenesin, 100mg/5ml	menthol	glycerin · propylene glycol · citric acid · benzoic acid · ethyl alcohol, 3.5% · methylparaben · propylparaben · hydroxypropyl methylcellulose · aspartame · grape flavor
sodium salicylate, 83.3mg/5ml	sodium citrate, 83.3mg/5ml		caffeine citrate, 25mg/5ml · glycerin · potassium benzoate · saccharin sodium · methylparaben · propylparaben · hydroxymethylcellulose · cherry-strawberry flavor · Magnasweet-110
	guaifenesin, 200mg/5ml	dextromethorphan hydrobromide, 15mg/5ml	aspartame · citric acid · hydroxypropyl methylcellulose · benzoic acid · methylparaben · propylparaben · menthol · glycerin · propylene glycol · peppermint-stick flavor
acetaminophen, 325mg			caffeine, 32.5mg

COLD, COUGH, AND ALLERGY PRODUCTS - continued

	Product Manufacturer/Supplier	Dosage Form	Decongestant	Antihistamine
AF GL PU SO	**Sinarest Extra Strength** Ciba Self-Medication	tablet	pseudoephedrine HCl, 30mg	chlorpheniramine maleate, 2mg
AF GL PU SO	**Sinarest No Drowsiness** Ciba Self-Medication	tablet	pseudoephedrine HCl, 30mg	
AF GL PU SO	**Sinarest Sinus Medicine** Ciba Self-Medication	tablet	pseudoephedrine HCl, 30mg	chlorpheniramine maleate, 2mg
	Sine-Aid IB McNeil Consumer	caplet	pseudoephedrine HCl, 30mg	
AF	**Sine-Aid Maximum Strength** McNeil Consumer	tablet	pseudoephedrine HCl, 30mg	
AF	**Sine-Aid Maximum Strength** McNeil Consumer	gelcap	pseudoephedrine HCl, 30mg	
	Sine-Aid Maximum Strength McNeil Consumer	caplet	pseudoephedrine HCl, 30mg	
	Sine-Off Maximum Strength No Drowsiness Formula Hogil Ph'cal	caplet	pseudoephedrine HCl, 30mg	
	Sine-Off Sinus Medicine Hogil Ph'cal	caplet	pseudoephedrine HCl, 30mg	chlorpheniramine maleate, 2mg
**	**Singlet** SmithKline Beecham	caplet	pseudoephedrine HCl, 60mg	chlorpheniramine maleate, 4mg
AF LA PU SO SU	**Sinulin** Carnrick Labs	tablet	phenylpropanolamine HCl, 25mg	chlorpheniramine maleate, 4mg
AF	**Sinus** Goldline Labs	tablet	pseudoephedrine HCl, 30mg	
AF GL PU	**Sinus Relief Extra Strength** Hudson	tablet	pseudoephedrine HCl, 30mg	chlorpheniramine maleate, 2mg
AF	**Sinutab Non-Drying** Warner Wellcome Consumer	liquid-cap	pseudoephedrine HCl, 30mg	
AF	**Sinutab Sinus Allergy Medication Maximum Strength** Warner Wellcome Consumer	caplet · tablet	pseudoephedrine HCl, 30mg	chlorpheniramine maleate, 2mg
AF GL PU	**Sinutab Sinus Non-Drowsiness** Warner Wellcome Consumer	tablet	pseudoephedrine HCl, 30mg	

See Chapter 8, "Cold, Cough and Allergy Products," for more information about these products.

Analgesic	Expectorant	Antitussive	Other Ingredients
acetaminophen, 500mg			corn starch · hydroxypropyl methylcellulose · microcrystalline cellulose · polyethylene glycol · polysorbate 80 · polyvinylpyrrolidone · stearic acid · titanium dioxide
acetaminophen, 325mg			corn starch · hydroxypropyl methylcellulose · microcrystalline cellulose · polyethylene glycol · polysorbate 80 · stearic acid · titanium dioxide
acetaminophen, 325mg			corn starch · yellow#10 · yellow#6 · hydroxypropyl methylcellulose · microcrystalline cellulose · polyethylene glycol · polysorbate 80 · polyvinylpyrrolidone · stearic acid · titanium dioxide
ibuprofen, 200mg			cellulose · corn starch · glyceryl triacetate · hydroxypropyl methylcellulose · silicon dioxide · sodium lauryl sulfate · sodium starch glycolate · stearic acid · titanium dioxide · red#40 aluminum lake · yellow#10 aluminum lake
acetaminophen, 500mg			cellulose · corn starch · magnesium stearate · sodium starch glycolate
acetaminophen, 500mg			benzyl alcohol · butylparaben · castor oil · cellulose · corn starch · edetate calcium disodium · gelatin · hydroxypropyl methylcellulose · iron oxide black · magnesium stearate · methylparaben · propylparaben · sodium lauryl sulfate · sodium propionate · sodium starch glycolate · titanium dioxide · FD&C red#40
acetaminophen, 500mg			cellulose · corn starch · hydroxypropyl methylcellulose · magnesium stearate · polyethylene glycol · sodium starch glycolate · titanium dioxide · blue#1 · red#40
acetaminophen, 500mg			crospovidone · FD&C red#40 · hydroxypropyl methylcellulose · magnesium stearate · microcrystalline cellulose · polyethylene glycol · polysorbate 80 · povidone · starch · titanium dioxide
acetaminophen, 500mg			carnauba wax · hydroxypropyl methylcellulose · magnesium stearate · microcrystalline cellulose · polydextrose · polyethylene glycol · povidone · sodium starch · glycolate · starch · stearic acid · titanium dioxide · triacetin · FD&C yellow#6 · D&C yellow#10
acetaminophen, 650mg			D&C red#7 · D&C yellow#10 · FD&C blue#1 · hydroxypropyl cellulose · hydroxypropyl methylcellulose 2910 · magnesium stearate · microcrystalline cellulose · polyethylene glycol 8000 · pregelatinized starch · sodium starch glycolate · sucrose · titanium dioxide
acetaminophen, 650mg			
acetaminophen, 325mg			
acetaminophen, 500mg			
	guaifenesin, 200mg		gelatin · sorbitol · FD&C blue#1 · povidone · polyethylene glycol · propylene glycol · glycerin
acetaminophen, 500mg			pregelatinized starch · FD&C yellow#6 aluminum lake · D&C yellow#10 aluminum lake · croscarmellose sodium · crospovidone · microcrystalline cellulose · povidone · stearic acid · zinc stearate · caplet only: carnauba wax · hydroxypropyl cellulose · hydroxypropyl methylcellulose · polyethylene glycol · titanium dioxide
acetaminophen, 325mg			croscarmellose sodium · D&C red#33 · FD&C red#40 · hydroxypropyl cellulose · hydroxypropyl methylcellulose · magnesium stearate · microcrystalline cellulose · pregelatinized starch · propylene glycol · simethicone · titanium dioxide · zinc stearate

COLD, COUGH, AND ALLERGY PRODUCTS - continued

	Product Manufacturer/Supplier	Dosage Form	Decongestant	Antihistamine
AF	**Sinutab Sinus without Drowsiness Maximum Strength** Warner Wellcome Consumer	caplet · tablet	pseudoephedrine HCl, 30mg	
**	**Sinutol Maximum Strength** Republic Drug	tablet	pseudoephedrine HCl, 30mg	
	Spec-T Sore Throat Cough Suppressant Apothecon	lozenge		
	Spec-T Sore Throat Decongestant Apothecon	lozenge	phenylpropanolamine HCl, 10.5mg · phenylephrine HCl, 5mg	
AL PE	**St. Joseph Cough Suppressant for Children** Schering-Plough HealthCare	syrup		
	Sucrets 4-Hour Cough Suppressant, Cherry or Menthol SmithKline Beecham	lozenge		
AF	**Sudafed** Warner Wellcome Consumer	tablet	pseudoephedrine HCl, 60mg	
AF	**Sudafed** Warner Wellcome Consumer	tablet	pseudoephedrine HCl, 30mg	
AF SO	**Sudafed 12-Hour Extended Release** Warner Wellcome Consumer	timed-release caplet	pseudoephedrine HCl, 120mg	
** AL LA SU PE	**Sudafed Children's Cold & Cough** Warner Wellcome Consumer	liquid	pseudoephedrine HCl, 15mg/5ml	
** AL SU PE	**Sudafed Children's Nasal Decongestant** Warner Wellcome Consumer	liquid	pseudoephedrine HCl, 15mg/5ml	
AF	**Sudafed Cold & Cough** Warner Wellcome Consumer	liquid-cap	pseudoephedrine HCl, 30mg	
** AL DY SU PE	**Sudafed Pediatric Nasal Decongestant** Warner Wellcome Consumer	drops	pseudoephedrine HCl, 7.5mg/0.8ml	
AF	**Sudafed Severe Cold Formula** Warner Wellcome Consumer	caplet · tablet	pseudoephedrine HCl, 30mg	
AF	**Sudafed Sinus Non-Drowsy Maximum Strength** Warner Wellcome Consumer	caplet · tablet	pseudoephedrine HCl, 30mg	

See Chapter 8, "Cold, Cough and Allergy Products," for more information about these products.

Analgesic	Expectorant	Antitussive	Other Ingredients
acetaminophen, 500mg			pregelatinized starch · D&C yellow#10 aluminum lake · FD&C yellow#6 aluminum lake · croscarmellose sodium · crospovidone · microcrystalline cellulose · povidone · stearic acid · zinc stearate · caplet only: carnauba wax · hydroxypropyl methylcellulose · polyethylene glycol · titanium dioxide
acetaminophen, 500mg			
		dextromethorphan hydrobromide, 10mg	benzocaine, 10mg · FD&C yellow#5 (tartrazine) · FD&C yellow#6 · dextrose · flavor · glucose · glycerin · propylene glycol · sucrose
			benzocaine, 10mg · FD&C blue#1 · yellow#5 (tartrazine) · dextrose · flavor · glucose · glycerin · propylene glycol · sucrose
		dextromethorphan hydrobromide, 7.5mg/5ml	
		dextromethorphan hydrobromide, 15mg · menthol	corn syrup · FD&C blue #1 · D&C yellow #10 (Menthol) · FD&C red#40 (Cherry) · Cherry or menthol-eucalyptus flavor · magnesium trisilicate · mineral oil · sucrose
			corn starch · dibasic calcium phosphate · sucrose · talc · sodium starch glycolate · acacia · carnauba wax · hydroxypropyl methylcellulose · magnesium stearate · pharmaceutical glaze · polysorbate 60 · stearic acid · titanium dioxide · pregelatinized corn starch · edible ink
			dibasic calcium phosphate · FD&C red#40 aluminum lake · yellow#6 aluminum lake · potato starch · sodium benzoate · acacia · carnauba wax · magnesium stearate · pharmaceutical glaze · polysorbate 60 · povidone · stearic acid · talc · titanium dioxide · corn starch · sucrose · edible ink
			hydroxypropyl methylcellulose · magnesium stearate · microcrystalline cellulose · polyethylene glycol · povidone · titanium dioxide · edible ink
	guaifenesin, 100mg/5ml	dextromethorphan hydrobromide, 5mg/5ml	caramel · citric acid · D&C red#33 · edetate disodium · FD&C red#40 · flavors · poloxamer 407 · polyethylene glycol 1450 · propyl gallate · propylene glycol · saccharin sodium · sodium benzoate · sodium chloride · sodium citrate · sorbitol solution · purified water
			citric acid · edetate disodium · FD&C red#40 · FD&C blue#1 · flavors · glycerin · poloxamer 407 · polyethylene glycol 1450 · povidone k-90 · saccharin sodium · sodium benzoate · sodium citrate · sorbitol solution · purified water
acetaminophen, 250mg	guaifenesin, 100mg	dextromethorphan hydrobromide, 10mg	D&C yellow#10 · FD&C red#40 · gelatin · glycerin · polyethylene glycol · povidone · propylene glycol · purified water · sorbitol · edible ink
			carboxymethyl cellulose sodium · citric acid · flavors · glycerin · poloxamer 407 · saccharin sodium · sodium benzoate · sodium chloride · sodium citrate · sorbitol solution
acetaminophen, 500mg		dextromethorphan hydrobromide, 15mg	pregelatinized corn starch · microcrystalline cellulose · carnauba wax · crospovidone · hydroxypropyl methylcellulose · polyethylene glycol · povidone · stearic acid · titanium dioxide · magnesium stearate
acetaminophen, 500mg			povidone · pregelatinized corn starch · carnauba wax · crospovidone · FD&C yellow#6 lake · hydroxymethyl cellulose · magnesium stearate · microcrystalline cellulose · polyethylene glycol · polysorbate 80 · stearic acid · titanium dioxide

COLD, COUGH, AND ALLERGY PRODUCTS - continued

	Product Manufacturer/Supplier	Dosage Form	Decongestant	Antihistamine
**	**Sudafed Sinus Non-Drying Non-Drowsy Maximum Strength** Warner Wellcome Consumer	liquid-cap	pseudoephedrine HCl, 30mg	
SO	**Sudanyl** Dover	tablet	pseudoephedrine HCl, 30mg	
AF GL PU SO	**Tavist-1 Antihistamine** Sandoz Consumer	tablet		clemastine fumarate, 1.34mg
AF GL PU SO	**Tavist-D Antihistamine/Nasal Decongestant** Sandoz Consumer	tablet	phenylpropanolamine HCl, 75mg	clemastine fumarate, 1.34mg
	Teldrin Hogil Ph'cal	timed-release capsule	phenylpropanolamine HCl, 75mg	chlorpheniramine maleate, 8mg
**	**Tetrahist** Republic Drug	tablet	pseudoephedrine HCl, 30mg	chlorpheniramine maleate, 2mg
AF GL PU	**TheraFlu Flu and Cold Medicine** Sandoz Consumer	individual packet	pseudoephedrine HCl, 60mg	chlorpheniramine maleate, 4mg
AF GL PU	**TheraFlu Flu, Cold, & Cough Medicine** Sandoz Consumer	individual packet	pseudoephedrine HCl, 60mg	chlorpheniramine maleate, 4mg
** AF	**TheraFlu Max. Strength Flu & Cold Medicine For Sore Throat** Sandoz Consumer	individual packet	pseudoephedrine HCl, 60mg	chlorpheniramine maleate, 4mg
AF GL PU	**TheraFlu Max. Strength Flu, Cold & Cough Medicine NightTime** Sandoz Consumer	individual packet	pseudoephedrine HCl, 60mg	chlorpheniramine maleate, 4mg
AF	**Theraflu Maximum Strength Non-Drowsy** Sandoz Consumer	caplet	pseudoephedrine HCl, 30mg	
** AF DY	**TheraFlu Maximum Strength Sinus Non-Drowsy** Sandoz Consumer	caplet	pseudoephedrine HCl, 30mg	
	Tolu-Sed DM Scherer Labs	liquid		
**	**Tri-Fed** Republic Drug	tablet	pseudoephedrine HCl, 60mg	triprolidine HCl, 2.5mg
AF	**Tri-Nefrin Extra Strength** Pfeiffer Ph'cals	tablet	phenylpropanolamine HCl, 25mg	chlorpheniramine maleate, 4mg
AL DY PE	**Triaminic AM, Non-Drowsy Cough & Decongestant Formula** Sandoz Consumer	syrup	pseudoephedrine HCl, 15mg/5ml	

See Chapter 8, "Cold, Cough and Allergy Products," for more information about these products.

Analgesic	Expectorant	Antitussive	Other Ingredients
	guaifenesin, 200mg		FD&C blue#1 · gelatin · glycerin · polyethylene glycol · povidone · propylene glycol · sorbitol · edible ink
			lactose · povidone · starch · talc · stearic acid
			colloidal silicon dioxide · yellow#10 · dibasic calcium phosphate dihydrate · lactose · magnesium stearate · methylcellulose · polyethylene glycol · povidone · starch · synthetic polymers · titanium dioxide
			benzyl alcohol · butylparaben · D&C red#33 · edetate calcium disodium · FD&C red#3 · FD&C yellow#6 · gelatin · methylparaben · pharmaceutical glaze · propylparaben · sodium lauryl sulfate · sodium propionate · starch · sucrose · other ingredients · may also contain polysorbate 80
acetaminophen, 325mg		dextromethorphan hydrobromide, 15mg	
acetaminophen, 650mg			natural lemon flavors · sucrose · ascorbic acid · citric acid · sodium citrate · titanium dioxide · tribasic calcium phosphate · pregelatinized starch · yellow#6 · yellow#10
acetaminophen, 650mg		dextromethorphan hydrobromide, 20mg	natural lemon flavors · sucrose · ascorbic acid · citric acid · sodium citrate · titanium dioxide · tribasic calcium phosphate · pregelatinized starch · yellow#6 · yellow#10
acetaminophen, 1000mg			acesulfame · natural apple and cinnamon flavors · ascorbic acid · aspartame · blue#1 · citric acid · maltodextrin · red#40 · silicon dioxide · sodium citrate · sucrose · tribasic calcium phosphate · yellow#10
acetaminophen, 1000mg		dextromethorphan hydrobromide, 30mg	ascorbic acid · citric acid · natural lemon flavors · maltol · pregelatinized starch · silicon dioxide · sodium citrate · sucrose · titanium dioxide · tribasic calcium phosphate · yellow#6 · yellow#10
acetaminophen, 500mg		dextromethorphan hydrobromide, 15mg	colloidal silicon dioxide · croscarmellose sodium · gelatin · hydroxypropyl cellulose · hydroxypropyl methylcellulose · lactose · magnesium stearate · methylparaben · polydextrose · polyethylene glycol · pregelatinized starch · red#40 · titanium dioxide · triacetin · yellow#6 · yellow#10
acetaminophen, 500mg			colloidal silicon dioxide · croscarmellose sodium · hydroxypropyl methylcellulose · lactose · magnesium stearate · methylcellulose · methylparaben · polyethylene glycol · povidone · pregelatinized starch · titanium dioxide
	guaifenesin, 100mg/5ml	dextromethorphan hydrobromide, 10mg/5ml	alcohol, 10%
		dextromethorphan hydrobromide, 7.5mg/5ml	benzoic acid · citric acid · dibasic sodium phosphate · edetate disodium · flavors · propylene glycol · purified water · sorbitol · sucrose

COLD, COUGH, AND ALLERGY PRODUCTS - continued

	Product Manufacturer/Supplier	Dosage Form	Decongestant	Antihistamine
AL DY PE	**Triaminic AM, Non-Drowsy Decongestant Formula** Sandoz Consumer	syrup	pseudoephedrine HCl, 15mg/5ml	
AL LA SL PE	**Triaminic DM, Cough Relief** Sandoz Consumer	syrup	phenylpropanolamine HCl, 6.25mg/5ml	
AL LA SL PE	**Triaminic Expectorant, Chest & Head Congestion** Sandoz Consumer	liquid	phenylpropanolamine HCl, 6.25mg/5ml	
** AL DY LA SL PE	**Triaminic Infant, Oral Decongestant** Sandoz Consumer	drops	pseudoephedrine HCl, 7.5mg/0.8ml	
AL LA SL PE	**Triaminic Night Time** Sandoz Consumer	liquid	pseudoephedrine HCl, 15mg/5ml	chlorpheniramine maleate, 1mg/5ml
AL PE	**Triaminic Sore Throat, Throat Pain & Cough** Sandoz Consumer	liquid	pseudoephedrine HCl, 15mg/5ml	
AL LA SL PE	**Triaminic, Cold & Allergy** Sandoz Consumer	syrup	phenylpropanolamine HCl, 6.25mg/5ml	chlorpheniramine maleate, 1mg/5ml
AF GL PU	**Triaminicin** Sandoz Consumer	tablet	phenylpropanolamine HCl, 25mg	chlorpheniramine maleate, 4mg
AL LA SL PE	**Triaminicol Multi-Symptom Relief** Sandoz Consumer	liquid	phenylpropanolamine HCl, 6.25mg/5ml	chlorpheniramine maleate, 1mg/5ml
AL	**Tricodene Forte** Pfeiffer Ph'cals	syrup	phenylpropanolamine HCl, 12.5mg/5ml	chlorpheniramine maleate, 2mg/5ml
AL	**Tricodene NN Cough and Cold Medication** Pfeiffer Ph'cals	syrup	phenylpropanolamine HCl, 12.5mg/5ml	chlorpheniramine maleate, 2.0mg/5ml
AL	**Tricodene No. 1** Pfeiffer Ph'cals	syrup		pyrilamine maleate, 12.5mg/5ml
AL SU	**Tricodene Sugar Free** Pfeiffer Ph'cals	liquid		chlorpheniramine maleate, 2mg/5ml
AL PE	**Tricodene, Pediatric** Pfeiffer Ph'cals	syrup	phenylpropanolamine HCl, 12.5mg/5ml	
AF GL PU SO	**Tuss-DM** Hyrex Ph'cals	tablet		

See Chapter 8, "Cold, Cough and Allergy Products," for more information about these products.

Analgesic	Expectorant	Antitussive	Other Ingredients
			benzoic acid · edetate disodium · flavors · purified water · sodium hydroxide · sorbitol · sucrose
		dextromethorphan hydrobromide, 5mg/5ml	sorbitol · sucrose · benzoic acid · blue#1 · flavors · propylene glycol · purified water · red#40 · sodium chloride
	guaifenesin, 50mg/5ml		saccharin · sorbitol · sucrose · benzoic acid · edetate disodium · flavors · purified water · saccharin sodium · sodium hydroxide · yellow#6 · yellow#10
			benzoic acid · edetate disodium · flavors · purified water · sodium chloride · sorbitol solution · sucrose
		dextromethorphan hydrobromide, 7.5mg/5ml	sorbitol · sucrose · benzoic acid · blue#1 · citric acid · flavors · propylene glycol · purified water · red#33 · dibasic sodium phosphate
acetaminophen, 160mg/5ml		dextromethorphan hydrobromide, 7.5mg/5ml	benzoic acid · blue#1 · dibasic sodium phosphate · edetate disodium · flavors · glycerin · polyethylene glycol · propylene glycol · purified water · red#33 · red#40 · sucrose · tartaric acid
			sorbitol · sucrose · benzoic acid · edetate disodium · flavors · purified water · sodium hydroxide · yellow#6
acetaminophen, 650mg			colloidal silicon dioxide · croscarmellose sodium · hydroxypropyl cellulose · lactose · magnesium stearate · methylcellulose · methylparaben · polyethylene glycol · povidone · pregelatinized starch · red#40 · titanium dioxide · yellow#10
		dextromethorphan hydrobromide, 5mg/5ml	benzoic acid · flavor · propylene glycol · purified water · red#40 · sodium chloride · sorbitol · sucrose
		dextromethorphan hydrobromide, 10mg/5ml	sucrose · sodium citrate · strawberry-vanilla flavor
		dextromethorphan hydrobromide, 10mg/5ml · menthol	sodium citrate · sucrose · cherry-vanilla flavor
		codeine phosphate, 8.2mg/5ml[a] · menthol	sucrose · sodium citrate · cherry flavor
		dextromethorphan hydrobromide, 10mg/5ml · menthol	sorbitol · mannitol · saccharin · sodium citrate · cherry flavor
		dextromethorphan hydrobromide, 10mg/5ml	sucrose · sodium citrate · cherry-vanilla flavor
	guaifenesin, 200mg	dextromethorphan hydrobromide, 10mg	

COLD, COUGH, AND ALLERGY PRODUCTS - continued

	Product Manufacturer/Supplier	Dosage Form	Decongestant	Antihistamine
	Tussar-2 Rhône-Poulenc Rorer Ph'cals	syrup	pseudoephedrine HCl, 30mg/5ml	
AL	**Tussar-DM** Rhône-Poulenc Rorer Ph'cals	syrup	pseudoephedrine HCl, 30mg/5ml	chlorpheniramine maleate, 2mg/5ml
	Tussar-SF Rhône-Poulenc Rorer Ph'cals	syrup	pseudoephedrine HCl, 30mg/5ml	
AF	**Tylenol Allergy Sinus Maximum Strength** McNeil Consumer	caplet	pseudoephedrine HCl, 30mg	chlorpheniramine maleate, 2mg
AF	**Tylenol Allergy Sinus Maximum Strength** McNeil Consumer	gelcap	pseudoephedrine HCl, 30mg	chlorpheniramine maleate, 2mg
** AF	**Tylenol Allergy Sinus Maximum Strength** McNeil Consumer	geltab	pseudoephedrine HCl, 30mg	chlorpheniramine maleate, 2mg
AF	**Tylenol Allergy Sinus NightTime Maximum Strength** McNeil Consumer	caplet	pseudoephedrine HCl, 30mg	diphenhydramine HCl, 25mg
AL PE	**Tylenol Children's Cold Multi-Symptom** McNeil Consumer	liquid	pseudoephedrine HCl, 15mg/5ml	chlorpheniramine maleate, 1mg/5ml
AF PE	**Tylenol Children's Cold Multi-Symptom** McNeil Consumer	chewable tablet	pseudoephedrine HCl, 7.5mg	chlorpheniramine maleate, 0.5mg
AL PE	**Tylenol Children's Cold Plus Cough** McNeil Consumer	liquid	pseudoephedrine HCl, 15mg/5ml	chlorpheniramine maleate, 1mg/5ml
AF PE	**Tylenol Children's Cold Plus Cough** McNeil Consumer	chewable tablet	pseudoephedrine HCl, 7.5mg	chlorpheniramine maleate, 0.5mg
AF	**Tylenol Cold Medication Multi-Symptom Formula** McNeil Consumer	caplet · tablet	pseudoephedrine HCl, 30mg	chlorpheniramine maleate, 2mg
AF	**Tylenol Cold Multi-Symptom** McNeil Consumer	individual packet	pseudoephedrine HCl, 60mg/packet	chlorpheniramine maleate, 4mg/packet
AF	**Tylenol Cold No Drowsiness Formula** McNeil Consumer	caplet	pseudoephedrine HCl, 30mg	
AF	**Tylenol Cold No Drowsiness Formula** McNeil Consumer	gelcap	pseudoephedrine HCl, 30mg	
	Tylenol Cough Multi-Symptom McNeil Consumer	liquid		

See Chapter 8, "Cold, Cough and Allergy Products," for more information about these products.

Analgesic	Expectorant	Antitussive	Other Ingredients
	guaifenesin, 100mg/5ml	codeine phosphate, 10mg/5ml[a]	alcohol, 2.5% · artificial flavors · citric acid · D&C yellow#10 · FD&C blue#1 · glycerin · methylparaben · methyl salicylate · propylene glycol · saccharin sodium · sodium citrate · sorbitol · sucrose · water
		dextromethorphan hydrobromide, 15mg/5ml	artificial flavors · citric acid · FD&C red#40 · glucose · glycerin · methylparaben · sodium citrate · sucrose · water
	guaifenesin, 100mg/5ml	codeine phosphate, 10mg/5ml[a]	alcohol, 2.5% · artificial flavors · citric acid · FD&C red#40 · glycerin · methylparaben · methyl salicylate · propylene glycol · saccharin sodium · sodium citrate · sorbitol
acetaminophen, 500mg			carnauba wax · cellulose · corn starch · hydroxypropyl cellulose · hydroxypropyl methylcellulose · iron oxide black · magnesium stearate · polyethylene glycol · sodium starch glycolate · titanium dioxide · blue#1 · yellow#6 · yellow#10
acetaminophen, 500mg			benzyl alcohol · butylparaben · castor oil · corn starch · cellulose · edetate calcium disodium · gelatin · hydroxypropyl methylcellulose · magnesium stearate · methylparaben · propylparaben · sodium lauryl sulfate · sodium propionate · sodium starch glycolate · titanium dioxide · blue#1 · blue#2 · yellow#10
acetaminophen, 500mg			benzyl alcohol · butylparaben · castor oil · corn starch · cellulose · edetate calcium disodium · gelatin · hydroxypropyl methylcellulose · magnesium stearate · methylparaben · propylparaben · sodium lauryl sulfate · sodium propionate · sodium starch glycolate · titanium dioxide · blue#1 · blue#2 · yellow#10
acetaminophen, 500mg			cellulose · corn starch · hydroxypropyl methylcellulose · iron oxide black · magnesium stearate · polyethylene glycol · polysorbate 80 · sodium citrate · sodium starch glycolate · titanium dioxide · blue#1 · yellow#10
acetaminophen, 160mg/5ml			benzoic acid · citric acid · flavors · glycerin · malic acid · polyethylene glycol · propylene glycol · sodium benzoate · sorbitol · sucrose · purified water · blue#1 · red#40
acetaminophen, 80mg			aspartame · basic polymethacrylate · cellulose acetate · citric acid · flavors · hydroxypropyl methylcellulose · magnesium stearate · mannitol · microcrystalline cellulose · blue#1 · red#7
acetaminophen, 160mg/5ml		dextromethorphan hydrobromide, 5mg/5ml	citric acid · corn syrup · flavors · polyethylene glycol · propylene glycol · sodium benzoate · sodium carboxymethylcellulose · sorbitol · purified water · red#33 · red#40
acetaminophen, 80mg		dextromethorphan hydrobromide, 2.5mg	aspartame · basic polymethacrylate · cellulose acetate · colloidal silicon dioxide · flavors · hydroxypropyl methylcellulose · mannitol · microcrystalline cellulose · stearic acid · red #7
acetaminophen, 325mg		dextromethorphan hydrobromide, 15mg	cellulose · corn starch · glyceryl triacetate (caplet) · hydroxypropyl methylcellulose (caplet) · iron oxide black (caplet) · magnesium stearate · sodium starch glycolate (caplet) · titanium dioxide (caplet) · blue#1 (caplet) · yellow#6 · yellow#10
acetaminophen, 650mg/packet		dextromethorphan hydrobromide, 30mg/packet	aspartame · citric acid · corn starch · flavors · sodium citrate · sucrose · red#40 · yellow#10
acetaminophen, 325mg		dextromethorphan hydrobromide, 15mg	cellulose · corn starch · glyceryl triacetate · hydroxypropyl methylcellulose · iron oxide black · magnesium stearate · sodium starch glycolate · titanium dioxide · blue#1 · yellow#10
acetaminophen, 325mg		dextromethorphan hydrobromide, 15mg	benzyl alcohol · butylparaben · castor oil · cellulose · corn starch · edetate calcium disodium · gelatin · hydroxypropyl methylcellulose · magnesium stearate · methylparaben · propylparaben · sodium propionate · sodium lauryl sulfate · sodium starch glycolate · titanium dioxide · red #40 · yellow #10
acetaminophen, 650mg/15ml		dextromethorphan hydrobromide, 30mg/15ml	alcohol, 5% · citric acid · flavors · high fructose corn syrup · polyethylene glycol · propylene glycol · purified water · sodium benzoate · sodium carboxymethylcellulose · saccharin sodium · sorbitol · red #40

COLD, COUGH, AND ALLERGY PRODUCTS - continued

	Product Manufacturer/Supplier	Dosage Form	Decongestant	Antihistamine
	Tylenol Cough with Decongestant Multi-Symptom McNeil Consumer	liquid	pseudoephedrine, HCl, 60mg/15ml	
AF	**Tylenol Flu Maximum Strength** McNeil Consumer	gelcap	pseudoephedrine HCl, 30mg	
AF	**Tylenol Flu NightTime Maximum Strength** McNeil Consumer	gelcap	pseudoephedrine HCl, 30mg	diphenhydramine HCl, 25mg
** AF	**Tylenol Flu NightTime Maximum Strength Hot Medication** McNeil Consumer	individual packet	pseudoephedrine HCl, 60mg/packet	diphenhydramine HCl, 50mg/packet
** AL PE	**Tylenol Infants' Cold Decongestant and Fever Reducer** McNeil Consumer	drops	pseudoephedrine HCl, 7.5mg/0.8ml	
** AF	**Tylenol Severe Allergy Maximum Strength** McNeil Consumer	caplet		diphenhydramine HCl, 12.5mg
AF	**Tylenol Sinus Maximum Strength** McNeil Consumer	caplet · tablet	pseudoephedrine HCl, 30mg	
** AF	**Tylenol Sinus Maximum Strength** McNeil Consumer	gelcap · geltab	pseudoephedrine HCl, 30mg	
PR SL	**Vaporizer in a Bottle Air Wick Inhaler** Columbia Labs	nasal inhaler		
AF PU SO	**Vicks 44 LiquiCaps Cough, Cold, & Flu Relief** Procter & Gamble	softgel	pseudoephedrine HCl, 30mg	chlorpheniramine maleate, 2mg
AF PU SO	**Vicks 44 LiquiCaps Non-Drowsy Cough & Cold Relief** Procter & Gamble	softgel	pseudoephedrine HCl, 60mg	
LA SL	**Vicks 44 Soothing Cough Relief** Procter & Gamble	liquid		
AL LA SL PE	**Vicks 44d Pediatric Cough & Head Congestion Relief** Procter & Gamble	liquid	pseudoephedrine HCl, 30mg/15ml	
LA SL	**Vicks 44D Soothing Cough & Head Congestion Relief** Procter & Gamble	liquid	pseudoephedrine HCl, 20mg/5ml	

See Chapter 8, "Cold, Cough and Allergy Products," for more information about these products.

Analgesic	Expectorant	Antitussive	Other Ingredients
acetaminophen, 650mg/15ml		dextromethorphan hydrobromide, 30mg/15ml	alcohol, 5% · citric acid · flavors · high fructose corn syrup · polyethylene glycol · propylene glycol · purified water · sodium benzoate · sodium carboxymethylcellulose · saccharin sodium · sorbitol · blue#1 · red #40
acetaminophen, 500mg		dextromethorphan hydrobromide, 15mg	benzyl alcohol · butylparaben · castor oil · cellulose · corn starch · edetate calcium disodium · gelatin · hydroxypropyl methylcellulose · iron oxide black · magnesium stearate · methylparaben · propylparaben · sodium lauryl sulfate · sodium propionate · sodium starch glycolate · titanium dioxide · red#40 · blue#1
acetaminophen, 500mg			benzyl alcohol · butylparaben · castor oil · cellulose · corn starch · edetate calcium disodium · gelatin · hydroxypropyl methylcellulose · iron oxide black · magnesium stearate · methylparaben · propylparaben · sodium citrate · sodium lauryl sulfate · sodium propionate · sodium starch glycolate · titanium dioxide · D&C red#28 · FD&C blue#1
acetaminophen, 1000mg/packet			ascorbic acid · aspartame · citric acid · flavors · sodium citrate · sucrose · yellow#10 · blue#1 · red#40 · yellow#6 · may also contain silicon dioxide
acetaminophen, 80mg/0.8ml			citric acid · corn syrup · flavors · polyethylene glycol · propylene glycol · purified water · sodium benzoate · saccharin · FD&C red#40
acetaminophen, 500mg			cellulose · corn starch · hydroxypropyl cellulose · hydroxypropyl methylcellulose · iron oxide black · magnesium stearate · polyethylene glycol · sodium citrate · sodium starch glycolate · titanium dioxide · yellow#6 · yellow#10
acetaminophen, 500mg			carnauba wax (caplet) · cellulose · corn starch · hydroxypropyl methylcellulose (caplet) · magnesium stearate · polyethylene glycol (caplet) · polysorbate 80 (caplet) · sodium starch glycolate · titanium dioxide (caplet) · blue#1 · yellow#6 (tablet) · red#40 (caplet) · yellow#10
acetaminophen, 500mg			benzyl alcohol · butylparaben · castor oil · cellulose · corn starch · edetate calcium disodium · gelatin · hydroxypropyl methylcellulose · iron oxide black · magnesium stearate · methylparaben · propylparaben · sodium lauryl sulfate · sodium propionate · sodium starch glycolate · titanium dioxide · FD&C blue#1 · D&C yellow #10
		camphor, 3.6% · menthol, 0.55% · eucalyptus oil · oil of peppermint	isopropyl alcohol, 71.4% · methyl salicylate · oil of white camphor · isobornyl acetate · oil of spike lavender · propylene glycol · isoamyl acetate · resin fixative-D
acetaminophen, 250mg		dextromethorphan hydrobromide, 10mg	D&C red#33 lake · FD&C blue#1 · gelatin · glycerin · polyethylene glycol · povidone · propylene glycol · purified water
		dextromethorphan hydrobromide, 30mg	D&C red#33 · FD&C blue#1 · FD&C red#40 · gelatin · glycerin · polyethylene glycol · povidone · purified water · sorbitol
		dextromethorphan hydrobromide, 10mg/5ml	alcohol, 5% · carboxymethylcellulose sodium · citric acid · FD&C blue#1 · FD&C red#40 · flavor · high fructose corn syrup · polyethylene oxide · polyoxyl 40 stearate · propylene glycol · purified water · sodium benzoate · sodium citrate
		dextromethorphan hydrobromide, 15mg/15ml	carboxymethylcellulose sodium · cellulose · citric acid · FD&C red#40 · flavor · glycerin · polysorbate 80 · potassium sorbate · propylene glycol · purified water · sodium citrate · sorbitol · sucrose
		dextromethorphan hydrobromide, 10mg/5ml	alcohol, 5% · citric acid · FD&C blue#1 · FD&C red#40 · flavor · high fructose corn syrup · polyethylene oxide · polyoxyl 40 stearate · propylene glycol · purified water · saccharin sodium · sodium benzoate · sodium citrate · sucrose

COLD, COUGH, AND ALLERGY PRODUCTS - continued

	Product Manufacturer/Supplier	Dosage Form	Decongestant	Antihistamine
AL SL PE	**Vicks 44e Pediatric Cough & Chest Congestion Relief** Procter & Gamble	liquid		
LA SL	**Vicks 44E Soothing Cough & Chest Congestion Relief** Procter & Gamble	liquid		
AL LA SL PE	**Vicks 44m Pediatric Cough & Cold Relief** Procter & Gamble	liquid	pseudoephedrine HCl, 30mg/15ml	chlorpheniramine maleate, 2mg/15ml
LA SL	**Vicks 44M Soothing Cough, Cold, & Flu Relief** Procter & Gamble	liquid	pseudoephedrine HCl, 15mg/5ml	chlorpheniramine maleate, 1mg/5ml
	Vicks Chloraseptic Cough and Throat Drops, several flavors Procter & Gamble	lozenge		
**	**Vicks Cough Drops, Cherry** Procter & Gamble	lozenge		
**	**Vicks Cough Drops, Menthol** Procter & Gamble	lozenge		
AF GL PU	**Vicks DayQuil Allergy Relief 12-Hour** Procter & Gamble	tablet	phenylpropanolamine HCl, 75mg	brompheniramine maleate, 12mg
AL LA SL PE	**Vicks DayQuil Children's Allergy Relief** Procter & Gamble	liquid	pseudoephedrine HCl, 30mg/15ml	chlorpheniramine maleate, 2mg/15ml
AF GL PU SO	**Vicks DayQuil LiquiCaps Multi-Symptom Cold/Flu Relief** Procter & Gamble	softgel	pseudoephedrine HCl, 30mg	
AL LA SL	**Vicks DayQuil Multi-Symptom Cold/Flu Relief** Procter & Gamble	liquid	pseudoephedrine HCl, 60mg/30ml	
AF GL PU	**Vicks DayQuil Sinus Pressure & Congestion Relief** Procter & Gamble	caplet	phenylpropanolamine HCl, 25mg	
AF PU	**Vicks DayQuil Sinus Pressure & Pain Relief with Ibuprofen** Procter & Gamble	caplet	pseudoephedrine HCl, 30mg	
AL LA SL PE	**Vicks NyQuil Children's Cold/Cough Medicine** Procter & Gamble	liquid	pseudoephedrine HCl, 30mg/15ml	chlorpheniramine maleate, 2mg/15ml
AF GL PU SO	**Vicks Nyquil Hot Therapy** Procter & Gamble	individual packet	pseudoephedrine HCl, 60mg	doxylamine succinate, 12.5mg

See Chapter 8, "Cold, Cough and Allergy Products," for more information about these products.

Analgesic	Expectorant	Antitussive	Other Ingredients
	guaifenesin, 100mg/15ml	dextromethorphan hydrobromide, 10mg/15ml	carboxymethylcellulose sodium · cellulose · citric acid · FD&C red#40 · flavor · glycerin · polysorbate 80 · potassium sorbate · propylene glycol · purified water · sodium citrate · sorbitol · sucrose
	guaifenesin, 200mg/15ml	dextromethorphan hydrobromide, 20mg/15ml	alcohol, 5% · carboxymethylcellulose sodium · citric acid · FD&C blue#1 · FD&C red#40 · flavor · high fructose corn syrup · polyethylene oxide · polyoxyl 40 stearate · propylene glycol · purified water · saccharin sodium · sodium benzoate · sodium citrate · sucrose
		dextromethorphan hydrobromide, 15mg/15ml	carboxymethylcellulose sodium · cellulose · citric acid · FD&C red#40 · flavor · glycerin · polysorbate 80 · potassium sorbate · propylene glycol · purified water · sodium citrate · sorbitol · sucrose
acetaminophen, 162.5mg/5ml		dextromethorphan hydrobromide, 7.5mg/5ml	alcohol, 10% · carboxymethylcellulose sodium · citric acid · FD&C blue#1 · FD&C red#40 · flavor · high fructose corn syrup · polyethylene glycol · polyethylene oxide · propylene glycol · purified water · saccharin sodium · sodium citrate
		menthol, 10mg	corn syrup · colors · flavors · sucrose
		menthol, 1.7mg · eucalyptus oil	ascorbic acid · citric acid · corn syrup · FD&C blue#1 · FD&C red #40 · sucrose
		menthol, 3.3mg · eucalyptus oil	ascorbic acid · caramel · corn syrup · sucrose
			dimethyl polysiloxane oil · FD&C blue#1 aluminum lake · hydroxypropyl methylcellulose · lactose · magnesium stearate · polyethylene glycol · talc · titanium dioxide
			citric acid · D&C red#33 · FD&C green#3 · flavor · methylparaben · potassium sorbate · propylene glycol · purified water · sodium citrate · sorbitol · sucrose
acetaminophen, 250mg	guaifenesin, 100mg	dextromethorphan hydrobromide, 10mg	FD&C red#40 · FD&C yellow#6 · gelatin · glycerin · polyethylene glycol · povidone · propylene glycol · purified water · sorbitol special
acetaminophen, 650mg/30ml	guaifenesin, 200mg/30ml	dextromethorphan hydrobromide, 20mg/30ml	citric acid · FD&C yellow#6 · flavor · glycerin · polyethylene glycol · propylene glycol · purified water · saccharin sodium · sodium citrate · sucrose
	guaifenesin, 200mg		colloidal silicon dioxide · crospovidone · FD&C yellow#6 aluminum lake · hydroxypropyl methylcellulose · microcrystalline cellulose · polyethylene glycol · polysorbate 80 · povidone · stearic acid · titanium dioxide
ibuprofen, 200mg			carnauba or equivalent wax · croscarmellose sodium · iron oxide · methylparaben · microcrystalline cellulose · propylparaben · silicon dioxide · sodium benzoate · sodium lauryl sulfate · starch · stearic acid · sucrose · titanium dioxide
		dextromethorphan hydrobromide, 15mg/15ml	citric acid · FD&C red#40 · flavor · potassium sorbate · propylene glycol · purified water · sodium citrate · sucrose
acetaminophen, 1000mg		dextromethorphan hydrobromide, 30mg	citric acid · flavor · sucrose

COLD, COUGH, AND ALLERGY PRODUCTS - continued

	Product Manufacturer/Supplier	Dosage Form	Decongestant	Antihistamine
AF GL PU SO	**Vicks NyQuil LiquiCaps Multi-Symptom Cold/Flu Relief** Procter & Gamble	softgel	pseudoephedrine HCl, 30mg	doxylamine succinate, 6.25mg
LA SL	**Vicks NyQuil Multi-Symptom Cold/Flu Relief, Cherry** Procter & Gamble	liquid	pseudoephedrine HCl, 60mg/30ml	doxylamine succinate, 12.5mg/30ml
LA SL	**Vicks NyQuil Multi-Symptom Cold/Flu Relief, Original** Procter & Gamble	liquid	pseudoephedrine HCl, 60mg/30ml	doxylamine succinate, 12.5mg/30ml
	Vicks Original Cough Drops, Cherry Procter & Gamble	lozenge		
	Vicks Original Cough Drops, Menthol Procter & Gamble	lozenge		
SL	**Vicks VapoRub** Procter & Gamble	cream		
SL	**Vicks VapoRub** Procter & Gamble	ointment		
SL	**Vicks VapoSteam** Procter & Gamble	liquid		

** New listing
[a] Schedule V drug; nonprescription sale forbidden in some states

See Chapter 8, "Cold, Cough and Allergy Products," for more information about these products.

Analgesic	Expectorant	Antitussive	Other Ingredients
acetaminophen, 250mg		dextromethorphan hydrobromide, 10mg	D&C yellow#10 · FD&C blue#1 · gelatin · glycerin · polyethylene glycol · povidone · propylene glycol · purified water · sorbitol special
acetaminophen, 1000mg/30ml		dextromethorphan hydrobromide, 30mg/30ml	alcohol, 10% · citric acid · FD&C blue#1 · FD&C red#40 · flavor · high fructose corn syrup · polyethylene glycol · propylene glycol · purified water · saccharin sodium · sodium citrate
acetaminophen, 1000mg/30ml		dextromethorphan hydrobromide, 30mg/30ml	alcohol, 10% · citric acid · D&C yellow#10 · FD&C green#3 · FD&C yellow#6 · flavor · high fructose corn syrup · polyethylene glycol · propylene glycol · purified water · saccharin sodium · sodium citrate
		menthol, 3.1mg	citric acid · corn syrup · FD&C blue#1 · FD&C red#40 · flavor · sucrose
		menthol, 6.6mg · camphor · eucalyptus oil · thymol	caramel · corn syrup · flavor · sucrose · tolu balsam · benzyl alcohol
		camphor, 5.2% · menthol, 2.8% · eucalyptus oil, 1.2% · spirits of turpentine · thymol	carbomer 954 · cedarleaf oil · cetyl alcohol · cetyl palmitate · cyclomethicone copolyol · dimethicone · EDTA · glycerin · imidazolidinyl urea · isopropyl palmitate · methylparaben · nutmeg oil · PEG-100 stearate · propylparaben · purified water · sodium hydroxide · stearic acid · stearyl alcohol · titanium dioxide
		camphor, 4.8% · menthol, 2.6% · eucalyptus oil, 1.2% · spirits of turpentine · thymol	cedarleaf oil · nutmeg oil · special petrolatum
		camphor, 6.2% · menthol, 3.2% · eucalyptus oil, 1.5%	alcohol, 74% · cedarleaf oil · nutmeg oil · poloxamer 124 · polyoxyethylene dodecanol · silicone

TOPICAL DECONGESTANT PRODUCTS

	Product Manufacturer/Supplier	Dosage Form	Sympathomimetic	Preservative	Other Ingredients
	4-Way Fast Acting Bristol-Myers Products	nasal spray	phenylephrine HCl, 0.5% · naphazoline HCl, 0.05%	benzalkonium chloride, 0.04%	pyrilamine maleate, 0.2% · water · boric acid/sodium borate
	4-Way Long Lasting Bristol-Myers Products	nasal spray	oxymetazoline HCl, 0.05%	phenylmercuric acetate, 0.002% · benzalkonium chloride	glycine · sorbitol · water
	4-Way Mentholated Bristol-Myers Products	nasal spray	phenylephrine HCl, 0.5% · naphazoline HCl, 0.05%	benzalkonium chloride, 0.04%	pyrilamine maleate, 0.2% · camphor · eucalyptol · menthol · poloxamer 188 · polysorbate 80 · water · boric acid/sodium borate
	Afrin 12-Hour Schering-Plough HealthCare	nasal drops · nasal pump spray · nasal spray	oxymetazoline HCl, 0.05%	benzalkonium chloride · propylene glycol	disodium edetate · polyethylene glycol 1450 · povidone · sodium phosphate dibasic · sodium phosphate monobasic · water
	Afrin 12-Hour, Cherry Schering-Plough HealthCare	nasal spray	oxymetazoline HCl, 0.05%	benzalkonium chloride · benzyl alcohol · propylene glycol	disodium edetate · flavor · polyethylene glycol 1450 · sodium phosphate dibasic · sodium phosphate monobasic · water
	Afrin 12-Hour, Menthol Schering-Plough HealthCare	nasal spray	oxymetazoline HCl, 0.05%	benzalkonium chloride	camphor · eucalyptol · menthol · polysorbate 80
	Afrin Extra Moisturizing Formula Schering-Plough HealthCare	nasal spray	oxymetazoline HCl, 0.05%	benzalkonium chloride · glycerin · propylene glycol	polyethylene glycol 1450, povidone
	Afrin Sinus Schering-Plough HealthCare	nasal spray	oxymetazoline HCl, 0.05%	benzalkonium chloride · benzyl alcohol · propylene glycol	camphor · eucalyptol · menthol · polysorbate 80
	Alconefrin 12 PolyMedica Ph'cals	nasal drops	phenylephrine HCl, 0.16%		
	Alconefrin 25 PolyMedica Ph'cals	nasal drops · nasal spray	phenylephrine HCl, 0.25%		
	Alconefrin 50 PolyMedica Ph'cals	nasal drops	phenylephrine HCl, 0.5%		
	Benzedrex Menley & James Labs	nasal inhaler	propylhexedrine, 250mg		menthol · lavender oil
	Benzedrex 12 HR Menley & James Labs	nasal spray	oxymetazoline HCl, 0.05%	benzalkonium chloride · phenylmercuric acetate	glycine · sorbitol · water
	Cheracol Roberts Ph'cal	nasal pump spray	oxymetazoline HCl, 0.05%	phenylmercuric acetate, 0.02 mg/ml in an aqueous solution of benzalkonium chloride	glycine · sodium hydroxide · sorbitol · artificial cherry flavor · purified water
SL	**Dristan** Whitehall-Robins Healthcare	nasal spray	phenylephrine HCl, 0.5%	benzalkonium chloride, 0.02% · benzyl alcohol · disodium EDTA	pheniramine maleate, 0.2% · disodium phosphate · hydroxypropyl methylcellulose · phosphoric acid · sodium chloride · water
SL	**Dristan 12-Hour** Whitehall-Robins Healthcare	nasal spray	oxymetazoline HCl, 0.05%	benzalkonium chloride, 0.02% · thimerosal, 0.002%	hydroxypropyl methylcellulose · potassium phosphate · sodium chloride · sodium phosphate · water
	Duramist Plus Pfeiffer Ph'cals	nasal spray	oxymetazoline HCl, 0.05%	benzalkonium chloride, 0.01%	
	Duration Schering-Plough HealthCare	nasal spray	oxymetazoline HCl, 0.05%	benzalkonium chloride · propylene glycol	disodium edetate, polyethylene glycol 1450, povidone
	Genasal Goldline Labs	nasal solution	oxymetazoline HCl, 0.05%	phenylmercuric acetate	
** PE	**Little Noses Decongestant** Vetco	nasal drops	phenylephrine HCl, 0.125%	thimerosal, 0.001% · benzalkonium chloride	citric acid · purified water · sodium chloride · sodium citrate

See Chapter 8, "Cold, Cough and Allergy Products," for more information about these products.

TOPICAL DECONGESTANT PRODUCTS - continued

	Product Manufacturer/Supplier	Dosage Form	Sympathomimetic	Preservative	Other Ingredients
	Neo-Synephrine 12-Hour Bayer Consumer	nasal pump spray · nasal spray	oxymetazoline HCl, 0.05%	phenylmercuric acetate, 0.002% · benzalkonium chloride	
	Neo-Synephrine Extra Bayer Consumer	nasal drops · nasal spray	phenylephrine HCl, 1%	thimerosal, 0.001% · benzalkonium chloride	
**	**Neo-Synephrine Extra Moisturizing 12-Hour** Bayer Consumer	nasal spray	oxymetazoline HCl, 0.05%	phenylmercuric acetate, 0.002% · benzalkonium chloride · glycerin	glycine · purified water · sorbitol · may contain sodium chloride
	Neo-Synephrine Mild Bayer Consumer	nasal drops · nasal spray	phenylephrine HCl, 0.25%	benzalkonium chloride · thimerosal, 0.001%	
PE	**Neo-Synephrine Pediatric** Bayer Consumer	nasal drops	phenylephrine HCl, 0.125%	thimerosal, 0.001% · benzalkonium chloride	
	Neo-Synephrine Regular Bayer Consumer	nasal drops · nasal spray	phenylephrine HCl, 0.5%	thimerosal, 0.001% · benzalkonium chloride	
SL	**Otrivin** Ciba Self-Medication	nasal drops · nasal spray	xylometazoline HCl, 0.1%	benzalkonium chloride, 0.02%	disodium edetate · sodium phosphate monobasic · sodium chloride · sodium phosphate dibasic · purified water
SL PE	**Otrivin Pediatric** Ciba Self-Medication	nasal drops	xylometazoline HCl, 0.05%	benzalkonium chloride, 0.02%	disodium edetate · sodium phosphate monobasic · sodium chloride · sodium phosphate dibasic · purified water
	Oxymeta 12 Schein Ph'cal	nasal spray	oxymetazoline HCl, 0.05%	phenylmercuric acetate, 0.02mg/ml · benzalkonium chloride	purified water · glycine · sorbitol solution · sodium hydroxide
SL	**Pretz-D** Parnell Ph'cals	nasal drops	ephedrine, 0.25%	glycerin, 3% · phenylmercuric acetate	citric acid · sodium citrate · sodium chloride · yerba santa
SL	**Privine** Ciba Self-Medication	nasal drops · nasal spray	naphazoline HCl, 0.05%	benzalkonium chloride, 0.02%	disodium edetate · sodium chloride · dibasic sodium phosphate · monobasic sodium phosphate · purified water
** SL	**Privine** Ciba Self-Medication	nasal solution	naphazoline HCl, 0.05%	benzalkonium chloride	disodium edetate dihydrate · hydrochloric acid · purified water · sodium chloride · trolamine
SL	**Rhinall** Scherer Labs	nasal drops · nasal spray	phenylephrine HCl, 0.25%	chlorobutanol · benzalkonium chloride	sodium bisulfite · sodium chloride · sorbitol · Tween 80 · disodium EDTA
	Sea Mist Schein Ph'cal	nasal spray		benzyl alcohol · benzalkonium chloride	sodium chloride · sodium bicarbonate · sodium chloride
SL	**Vicks Sinex 12-Hour Ultra Fine Mist** Procter & Gamble	nasal spray	oxymetazoline HCl, 0.05%	benzalkonium chloride · chlorhexidine gluconate	camphor · menthol · eucalyptol · disodium EDTA · potassium phosphate · purified water · sodium chloride · sodium phosphate · tyloxapol
SL	**Vicks Sinex Ultra Fine Mist** Procter & Gamble	nasal spray	phenylephrine HCl, 0.5%	benzalkonium chloride · chlorhexidine gluconate	camphor · eucalyptol · menthol · citric acid · purified · disodium EDTA · water · tyloxapol
SL	**Vicks Vapor Inhaler** Procter & Gamble	nasal inhaler	levodesoxyephedrine, 50mg/inhaler		bornyl acetate · camphor · lavender oil · menthol

** New listing

See Chapter 8, "Cold, Cough and Allergy Products," for more information about these products.

SORE THROAT PRODUCTS

	Product Manufacturer/Supplier	Dosage Form	Anesthetic [a]	Antibacterial [a]	Other Ingredients
	Celestial Seasonings Soothers Herbal Throat Drops, Asst. Warner-Lambert	lozenge	menthol		pectin · cherry, elderberry, and pineapple juices (Cherry) · chamomile flower extract (Lemon) · beta carotene (Orange) · citric acid · corn syrup · honey · lemon juice (Lemon) · natural flavor · oils of angelica root and anise star · cassia bark (Orange) · ginger · lemon grass · sage · white thyme · orange juice (Orange) · sucrose · tea extract (Lemon)
	Cepacol Anesthetic J. B. Williams	lozenge	benzocaine, 10mg	cetylpyridinium chloride, 1.4%	glucose · sucrose · dyes
**	**Cepacol Maximum Strength, Mint** J. B. Williams	lozenge	benzocaine, 10mg · menthol, 2mg	cetylpyridinium chloride	D&C yellow#10 · FD&C yellow#6 · flavor · glucose · sucrose
**	**Cepacol Sore Throat, Cherry** J. B. Williams	lozenge	menthol, 3.6mg	cetylpyridinium chloride	D&C red#33 · FD&C red#40 · flavor · glucose · sucrose
**	**Cepacol Sore Throat, Mint** J. B. Williams	lozenge	menthol, 2mg	cetylpyridinium chloride	D&C yellow#10 · FD&C yellow#6 · flavor · glucose · sucrose
	Cepacol, Cherry or Honey-Lemon J. B. Williams	lozenge	menthol, 3.6mg	cetylpyridinium chloride	dyes · glucose · sucrose
	Cepacol, Menthol-Eucalyptus J. B. Williams	lozenge	menthol, 5mg · eucalyptol	cetylpyridinium chloride	glucose · sucrose
	Cepacol, Original Flavor J. B. Williams	lozenge		cetylpyridinium chloride, 1.4%	dyes · glucose · sucrose
	Cepastat Extra Strength Sore Throat SmithKline Beecham	lozenge	phenol, 29mg · eucalyptus oil · menthol		antifoam emulsion · caramel · gum crystal · sorbitol
	Cepastat Sore Throat, Cherry SmithKline Beecham	lozenge	phenol, 14.5mg · menthol		antifoam emulsion · D&C red#33 · FD&C yellow#6 · flavor · gum crystal · saccharin sodium · sorbitol
	Cheracol Sore Throat Roberts Ph'cal	spray	phenol, 1.4%	alcohol, 12.5%	glycerin · propylene glycol · sodium citrate · saccharin sodium · citric acid · sorbitol
GL LA SU	**Fisherman's Friend, Extra Strong, Sugar Free** Bristol-Myers Products	lozenge	menthol, 10mg · eucalyptus oil		sorbitol · natural licorice · magnesium stearate · capsicum
GL LA	**Fisherman's Friend, Licorice Strong** Bristol-Myers Products	lozenge	menthol, 6mg		sugar · licorice · edible gums · anise oil
GL LA	**Fisherman's Friend, Original Extra Strong** Bristol-Myers Products	lozenge	menthol, 10mg · eucalyptus oil		sugar · licorice · edible gums · capsicum

See Chapter 8, "Cold, Cough and Allergy Products," for more information about these products.

SORE THROAT PRODUCTS - continued

	Product Manufacturer/Supplier	Dosage Form	Anesthetic [a]	Antibacterial [a]	Other Ingredients
GL LA SU	**Fisherman's Friend, Refreshing Mint, Sugar Free** Bristol-Myers Products	lozenge	menthol, 3mg		sorbitol · peppermint oil · magnesium stearate · aspartame · phenylalanine
** SU PE	**Halls Juniors Sugar Free Cough Drops, Grape or Orange** Warner-Lambert	lozenge	menthol, 2.5mg · eucalyptus oil		acesulfame potassium · isomalt · natural flavor · blue#1 (Grape) · red#40 (Grape) · yellow#6 (Orange)
	Halls Mentho-Lyptus Cough Supp. Drops, Cherry or Mentho-L. Warner-Lambert	lozenge	menthol, 6.1mg · eucalyptus oil		carmine color · corn syrup · flavor · sucrose
	Halls Mentho-Lyptus Cough Supp. Drops, Honey-Lemon Warner-Lambert	lozenge	menthol, 8.4mg · eucalyptus oil ·		flavor · corn syrup · sucrose · yellow#6 · yellow#10
	Halls Mentho-Lyptus Cough Supp. Drops, Spearmint Warner-Lambert	lozenge	menthol, 5mg · eucalyptus oil		flavor · blue#1 · corn syrup · sucrose · yellow#10
	Halls Mentho-Lyptus Ex. Strength Cough Supp. Drops, Ice Blue Warner-Lambert	lozenge	menthol, 12mg · eucalyptus oil		flavor · blue#1 · corn syrup · sucrose
SU	**Halls Mentho-Lyptus Sugar Free Cough Supp. Drops, Bl. Cherry** Warner-Lambert	lozenge	menthol, 5mg · eucalyptus oil		acesulfame potassium · blue#1 · flavor · isomalt · red#40
SU	**Halls Mentho-Lyptus Sugar Free Cough Supp. Drops, Citrus** Warner-Lambert	lozenge	menthol, 5mg · eucalyptus oil		acesulfame potassium · flavor · isomalt · yellow#5 · citric acid
SU	**Halls Mentho-Lyptus Sugar Free Cough Supp. Drops, Menthol** Warner-Lambert	lozenge	menthol, 6mg · eucalyptus oil		acesulfame potassium · flavor · isomalt · citric acid · blue#1 · red#40
	Halls Plus Max. Strength; Cherry, Honey-Lemon, Mentho-Lyptus Warner-Lambert	lozenge	menthol, 10mg · eucalyptus oil		blue#2 (Cherry) · acesulfame (Lemon) · potassium (Lemon) · corn syrup · flavor (Cherry, Lemon) · citric acid (Mentho-Lyptus) · glycerin · high fructose corn syrup · red#40 (Cherry) · honey (Lemon) · sucrose · yellow#6 (Lemon) · yellow#10 (Lemon)

See Chapter 8, "Cold, Cough and Allergy Products," for more information about these products.

SORE THROAT PRODUCTS - continued

	Product Manufacturer/Supplier	Dosage Form	Anesthetic [a]	Antibacterial [a]	Other Ingredients
** DY GL LA PU SO SU	**Herbal-Menthol** Shaklee	lozenge	menthol, 6mg (from peppermint) · eucalyptus oil		brown rice syrup · corn syrup · honey · horehound extract · marshmallow root extract · peppermint oil · thyme extract
	Isodettes Goody's Ph'cals	lozenge	menthol, 10mg · benzocaine, 6mg		corn syrup · flavor · FD&C red#40 · FD&C blue#1 · sucrose · propylene glycol · sodium bicarbonate · water
	Isodettes Goody's Ph'cals	spray	phenol, 1.4% (phenol · sodium phenolate)		propylene glycol · flavor · FD&C red#40 · water · sodium hydroxide
	Koldets Cough Drops Pfeiffer Ph'cals	lozenge	menthol, 6.1mg · eucalyptus oil		citric acid
** SU	**Luden's Maximum Strength Sugar Free, Cherry** Hershey	lozenge	menthol, 10mg · eucalyptus oil		isomalt · hydrogenated starch hydrolysate · citric acid · malic acid · flavoring · acesulfame potassium · artificial color
**	**Luden's Maximum Strength, Cherry** Hershey	lozenge	menthol, 10mg · eucalyptus oil		sugar · corn syrup · citric acid · malic acid · flavoring · artificial color
**	**Luden's Maximum Strength, Menthol Eucalyptus** Hershey	lozenge	menthol, 10mg · eucalyptus oil		sugar · corn syrup
**	**Luden's Original Menthol** Hershey	lozenge	menthol		sugar · corn syrup · flavoring · caramel color
AL	**Mycinette** Pfeiffer Ph'cals	pump spray	phenol, 1.4%		alum, 0.5%
	Mycinettes Pfeiffer Ph'cals	lozenge	benzocaine, 15mg · menthol	cetylpyridinium chloride, 2.5mg	flavors · mannitol · sodium citrate · saccharin sodium · sorbitol
	N'Ice 'N Clear, Cherry Eucalyptus SmithKline Beecham	lozenge	menthol, 7mg		flavors · D&C red#33 · sorbitol · tartaric acid · FD&C yellow #6
	N'Ice 'N Clear, Menthol Eucalyptus SmithKline Beecham	lozenge	menthol, 5mg		citric acid · flavors · sorbitol
	N'Ice Sore Throat & Cough, Assorted or Citrus SmithKline Beecham	lozenge	menthol, 5mg		citric acid · D&C yellow#10 · D&C red#33 (Asst.) · FD&C blue#2 (Asst.) · FD&C yellow#6 (Asst.) · flavors · maltitol solution (Asst.) · saccharin sodium · sodium citrate · sorbitol · tartaric acid (Asst.)
	Painalay Sore Throat Gargle Medtech Labs	spray	phenol, 0.5%		
	Protac Republic Drug	lozenge	benzocaine, 10mg	cetylpyridinium chloride, 2.5mg	

See Chapter 8, "Cold, Cough and Allergy Products," for more information about these products.

SORE THROAT PRODUCTS - continued

	Product Manufacturer/Supplier	Dosage Form	Anesthetic [a]	Antibacterial [a]	Other Ingredients
	Ricola Cough Drops, Original Flavor Ricola	lozenge	menthol, 3mg		sugar · glucose syrup · caramelized sugar · extracts of peppermint, lemon balm, thyme, sage, hyssop, elder, linden flowers, wild thyme, horehound, angelica root, and peppermint oil
SU	**Ricola Sugar Free Herb Throat Drops, Alpine-Mint** Ricola	lozenge	menthol, 4.8mg		extracts of peppermint, lemon balm, lady's mantle, linden flowers, and elder · natural flavorings · citric acid · aspartame · chlorophyll · isomalt
SU	**Ricola Sugar Free Herb Throat Drops, Cherry- or Lemon-Mint** Ricola	lozenge	menthol, 1mg		extracts of peppermint, lemon balm, lady's mantle, linden flowers, and elder · citric acid · lemon and peppermint oils (Lemon-Mint) · cherry and peppermint flavorings (Cherry-Mint) · cherry and elderberry concentrates (Cherry-Mint) · ascorbic acid · aspartame · flavorings (Lemon-Mint) · isomalt
SU	**Ricola Sugar Free Herb Throat Drops, Mountain Herb** Ricola	lozenge	menthol, 1.5mg		extracts of peppermint, lemon balm, thyme, sage, hyssop, elder, linden flowers, wild thyme, horehound, and angelica root · caramel coloring · aspartame · peppermint oil · isomalt
	Ricola Throat Drops, Cherry-Mint Ricola	lozenge	menthol, 1.5mg		sugar · glucose syrup · citric acid · extracts of peppermint, lemon balm, thyme, sage, hyssop, elder, linden flowers, wild thyme, horehound, and angelica root · cherry concentrate · elder concentrate · cherry flavorings · peppermint oil
**	**Ricola Throat Drops, Honey-Herb** Ricola	lozenge	menthol, 2.4mg		honey · sugar · corn syrup · extracts of peppermint, lemon balm, thyme, sage, hyssop, elder, linden flowers, wild thyme, horehound, angelica root, and peppermint oil
	Ricola Throat Drops, Lemon-Mint or Orange-Mint Ricola	lozenge	menthol, 1.25mg		sugar · glucose syrup · citric acid · extracts of lemon balm, orange-mint (Orange-Mint), peppermint, thyme, sage, hyssop, elder, linden flowers, wild thyme, horehound, and angelica root · lemon oil (Lemon-Mint) · peppermint oil · orange flavoring (Orange-Mint) · natural coloring (Lemon-Mint) · paprika extract (Orange-Mint)
	Ricola Throat Drops, Menthol-Eucalyptus Ricola	lozenge	menthol, 4.5mg		sugar · glucose syrup · extracts of peppermint, lemon balm, thyme, sage, hyssop, elder, linden flowers, wild thyme, horehound, angelica root, peppermint oil, and eucalyptus oil · chlorophyll

See Chapter 8, "Cold, Cough and Allergy Products," for more information about these products.

SORE THROAT PRODUCTS - continued

	Product Manufacturer/Supplier	Dosage Form	Anesthetic [a]	Antibacterial [a]	Other Ingredients
	Robitussin Cough Drops, Cherry or Menthol Eucalyptus Whitehall-Robins Healthcare	lozenge	menthol, 7.4mg · eucalyptus oil		corn syrup · FD&C red#40 (Cherry) · flavors (Cherry) · sucrose · titanium dioxide (Menthol Eucalyptus) · may contain starch
	Robitussin Cough Drops, Honey-Lemon Whitehall-Robins Healthcare	lozenge	menthol, 10mg · eucalyptus oil		corn syrup · D&C yellow#10 · FD&C yellow#6 · flavors · sucrose · may contain starch
	Robitussin Liquid Center Cough Drops, Cherry w/ Honey-Lemon Whitehall-Robins Healthcare	lozenge	menthol, 8mg · eucalyptus oil		corn syrup · FD&C red#40 · flavors · glycerin · high fructose corn syrup · honey · lemon oil · methylparaben · propylparaben · sodium benzoate · sorbitol · sucrose · titanium dioxide
	Robitussin Liquid Center Cough Drops, Honey-Lemon w/ Cherry Whitehall-Robins Healthcare	lozenge	menthol, 10mg · eucalyptus oil		corn syrup · D&C yellow #10 aluminum lake · FD&C yellow #6 aluminum lake · flavors · glycerin · high fructose corn syrup · honey · lemon oil · methylparaben · povidone · propylparaben · sodium benzoate · sorbitol · sucrose · titanium dioxide · water
	Robitussin Liquid Center Cough Drops, Menthol Euc. w/Cherry Whitehall-Robins Healthcare	lozenge	menthol, 8mg · eucalyptus oil		corn syrup · flavors · glycerin · high fructose corn syrup · sorbitol · sucrose · water
SU	**Robitussin Sugar Free Cough Drops, Cherry or Peppermint** Whitehall-Robins Healthcare	lozenge	menthol, 10mg		aspartame · canola oil · FD&C blue#1 aluminum lake · FD&C red#40 aluminum lake (Cherry) · flavors · hydrogenated glucose syrup · isomalt
	Sore Throat Spray; Cherry, Menthol, or Mint Pharmaceutical Assoc.	spray	phenol, 1.4%		
	Spec-T Sore Throat Anesthetic Apothecon	lozenge	benzocaine, 10mg		agar FD&C red#40 · glucose · glycerin · sucrose · flavor
	Spec-T Sore Throat Cough Suppressant Apothecon	lozenge	benzocaine, 10mg		dextromethorphan hydrobromide, 10mg · FD&C yellow#5 (tartrazine) · FD&C yellow#6 · dextrose · flavor · glucose · glycerin · propylene glycol · sucrose
	Spec-T Sore Throat Decongestant Apothecon	lozenge	benzocaine, 10mg		phenylpropanolamine HC1, 10.5mg · phenylephrine HCl, 5mg · FD&C blue#1 · yellow#5 (tartrazine) · dextrose · flavor · glucose · glycerin · propylene glycol · sucrose
PE	**Sucrets Children's Sore Throat, Cherry** SmithKline Beecham	lozenge	dyclonine HCl, 1.2mg		citric acid · corn syrup · FD&C blue#1 · FD&C red#40 · flavor · mineral oil · silicon dioxide · sucrose

See Chapter 8, "Cold, Cough and Allergy Products," for more information about these products.

SORE THROAT PRODUCTS - continued

	Product Manufacturer/Supplier	Dosage Form	Anesthetic [a]	Antibacterial [a]	Other Ingredients
	Sucrets Maximum Strength Sore Throat, Vapor Black Cherry SmithKline Beecham	lozenge	dyclonine HCl, 3mg		corn syrup · FD&C blue#1 · FD&C red#40 · flavors · menthol · mineral oil · silicon dioxide · sucrose · tartaric acid
	Sucrets Maximum Strength Sore Throat, Wintergreen SmithKline Beecham	lozenge	dyclonine HCl, 3mg		citric acid · corn syrup · D&C yellow#10 · flavors · mineral oil · silicon dioxide · sucrose
	Sucrets Sore Throat, Assorted Flavors SmithKline Beecham	lozenge	dyclonine HCl, 2mg		citric acid · corn syrup · D&C yellow#10 · FD&C blue#1 · FD&C red#40 · flavors · mineral oil · silicon dioxide · sucrose · tartaric acid
	Sucrets Sore Throat, Original Mint SmithKline Beecham	lozenge		hexylresorcinol, 2.4mg	corn syrup · D&C yellow#10 · FD&C blue#1 · flavors · mineral oil · silicon dioxide · sucrose
	Throat Discs SmithKline Beecham	lozenge			sucrose · starch · acacia · glycyrrhiza extract · gum tragacanth · anethole · linseed · cubeb oleo resin · anise oil · peppermint oil · capsicum · mineral oil
	Throtoceptic S.S.S. Company	pump spray	phenol, 1.4%		alum, 0.5% · flavor
AL AF SO	**Vicks Chloraseptic Sore Throat, Cherry Menthol** Procter & Gamble	spray	phenol, 1.4%		colors · flavors · glycerin · purified water · saccharin sodium
	Vicks Chloraseptic Sore Throat, Cherry or Menthol Procter & Gamble	lozenge	menthol, 10mg · benzocaine, 6mg		corn syrup · FD&C yellow#10 (menthol) · FD&C blue#1 · FD&C red#40 · FD&C yellow#6 (menthol) · flavor · sucrose
**	**Vicks Cough Drops, Cherry** Procter & Gamble	lozenge	menthol, 1.7mg · eucalyptus oil		ascorbic acid · citric acid · corn syrup · FD&C blue#1 · FD&C red#40 · sucrose
**	**Vicks Cough Drops, Menthol** Procter & Gamble	lozenge	menthol, 3.3mg · eucalyptus oil		ascorbic acid · caramel · corn syrup · sucrose
	Vicks Original Cough Drops, Cherry Procter & Gamble	lozenge	menthol, 3.1mg		citric acid · corn syrup · FD&C blue#1 · FD&C red#40 · flavor · sucrose
	Vicks Original Cough Drops, Menthol Procter & Gamble	lozenge	menthol, 6.6mg · eucalyptus oil		camphor · caramel · corn syrup · flavor · sucrose · tolu balsam · thymol · benzyl alcohol

** New listing
[a] Phenol is both an anesthetic and an antibacterial agent.

See Chapter 8, "Cold, Cough and Allergy Products," for more information about these products.

ASTHMA AUXILIARY DEVICES

	Product Manufacturer/Supplier	Comments
	Peak Flow Meters	
** PE	**Assess Low Range** HealthScan	measures within range of 30-390 Liters/min · accurate to ±5% · made from virtually indestructible polycarbonate plastic · transparent, to encourage regular cleaning · one-year warranty · disposable cardboard pediatric-sized mouthpiece available · main body dimensions: 8" x 1.5" x 1.3", weight: 2.6 oz.
**	**Assess Standard Range** HealthScan	measures within range of 60-880 Liters/min · accurate to ±5% · made from virtually indestructible polycarbonate plastic · transparent, to encourage regular cleaning · one-year warranty · disposable cardboard mouthpiece available · main body dimensions: 8" x 1.5" x 1.3", weight: 2.6 oz.
** PE	**Mini-Wright Low Range** Clement Clarke	measures within range of 30-370 Liters/min · accurate to ±5% · individually custom calibrated for accuracy · made from engineering-quality plastic · disposable cardboard pediatric-sized mouthpiece/adapter available · can be disassembled for easy maintenance
**	**Mini-Wright Standard Range** Clement Clarke	measures within range of 60-800 Liters/min · accurate to ±5% · individually custom calibrated for accuracy · made from engineering-quality plastic · disposable cardboard mouthpiece available · can be disassembled for easy maintenance

** New listing

See Chapter 9, "Asthma Products," for more information about these products.

ASTHMA INHALANT PRODUCTS

	Product Manufacturer/Supplier	Dosage Form [a]	Epinephrine	Other Ingredients
AL	**Asthma Haler** Menley & James Labs	oral inhaler	0.16mg base/spray (epinephrine bitartrate, 0.3mg/spray)	cetylpyridinium chloride · propellants · sorbitan trioleate
AL	**Asthma Nefrin** Menley & James Labs	solution for nebulization	2.25% base (as racemic epinephrine HCl)	chlorobutanol, 0.5% · benzoic acid · potassium metabisulfite · sodium bisulfite · sodium chloride · propylene glycol
	Breatheasy Pascal	oral inhaler	2.2% (as epinephrine HCl)	benzyl alcohol, 1% · isotonic salts, 0.5%
AL PR SL	**Broncho Saline** Blairex Labs	solution for nebulization		sodium chloride, 0.9%
SO SL	**Bronkaid Mist and Refill** Bayer Consumer	oral inhaler	0.25mg base/spray (as nitrate and HCl salts)	alcohol, 33%
**	**Bronkaid Mist Suspension** Bayer Consumer	oral inhaler	epinephrine bitartrate, 7mg/ml	
AL PR SL	**Dey-Vial Sodium Chloride Solution** Dey Labs	solution		sodium chloride, 0.9%
	Epinephrine Mist Goldline Labs	oral inhaler	5.5mg/ml (0.22 mg/spray)	alcohol, 34%
	Micro NEFRIN Bird Products	solution for nebulization	2.25% base (as racemic epinephrine HCl)	chlorobutanol, 0.5g
SL	**Primatene Mist** Whitehall-Robins Healthcare	oral inhaler	5.5mg/ml	alcohol, 34% · ascorbic acid · fluorocarbons (propellant) · water
AL PR SL	**Sodium Chloride Inhalation Solution USP** Dey Labs	solution		sodium chloride, 0.45%; 0.9%

** New listing

[a] As this book was going to press, the FDA amended the final monograph for OTC bronchodilator drug products by removing the dosage form pressurized metered-dose inhalers (MDIs) for the ingredients epinhephrine, epinephrine bitartrate, and racepinephrine HCl (Federal Register, 1996 May 20; 61(98): 25142-7). Under this rule, which becomes effective June 19, 1996, sale of such products over-the-counter will require an approved new drug application (NDA) that contains certain information not required by the monograph. The oral inhaler products listed in this table are not affected by the ruling because they are already subjects of approved NDAs.

See Chapter 9, "Asthma Products," for more information about these products.

ASTHMA ORAL PRODUCTS

	Product Manufacturer/Supplier	Dosage Form	Ephedrine [a]	Other Ingredients
GL SO	**Bronkaid Dual Action Formula** Bayer Consumer	caplet	25mg (as sulfate)	guaifenesin, 400mg
	Dynafed Two-Way BDI Ph'cals	tablet	25mg (as HCl)	guaifenesin, 200mg · magnesium stearate · ditab
	Mini Thin Two-Way BDI Ph'cals	tablet	25mg (as HCl)	guaifenesin, 200mg · magnesium stearate · ditab
** GL PU SO	**Primatene** Whitehall-Robins Healthcare	tablet	12.5mg (as HCl)	guaifenesin, 200mg · crospovidone · D&C yellow #10 lake · FD&C yellow#6 lake · magnesium stearate · microcrystalline cellulose · povidone · silicon dioxide
	Tedrigen Goldline Labs	tablet	25mg (as HCl)	phenobarbital, 8mg

** New listing
[a] Several states have placed restrictions on the nonprescription status of ephedrine due to its abuse potential.

See Chapter 9, "Asthma Products," for more information about these products.

SLEEP AID PRODUCTS

	Product Manufacturer/Supplier	Dosage Form	Antihistamine	Other Ingredients
AF	**Anacin P.M. Aspirin Free** Whitehall-Robins Healthcare	caplet	diphenhydramine HCl, 25mg	acetaminophen, 500mg · calcium stearate · FD&C blue#1 lake · hydroxypropyl methylcellulose · magnesium stearate · microcrystalline cellulose · polyethylene glycol · povidone · starch · stearic acid · titanium dioxide · may also contain: ammonium hydroxide · iron oxide · pharmaceutical glaze · potassium hydroxide · propylene glycol
DY GL SO	**Arthriten PM** Alva-Amco Pharmacal	caplet	diphenhydramine HCl, 25mg	acetaminophen, 250mg · magnesium salicylate, 250mg · magnesium carbonate · magnesium oxide · calcium carbonate
AF	**Arthritis Foundation Nighttime** McNeil Consumer	caplet	diphenhydramine HCl, 25mg	acetaminophen, 500mg · cellulose · corn starch · hydroxypropyl methylcellulose · magnesium stearate or stearic acid · colloidal silicon dioxide · polyethylene glycol · polysorbate 80 · sodium citrate · sodium starch glycolate · titanium dioxide · blue#1 · blue#2
AF GL SO	**Backaid PM Pills** Alva-Amco Pharmacal	caplet	diphenhydramine HCl, 25mg	acetaminophen, 500mg
**	**Bayer PM Extra Strength** Bayer Consumer	caplet	diphenhydramine HCl, 25mg	aspirin, 500mg · colloidal silicon dioxide · dibasic calcium phosphate · dibutyl sebacate · ethylcellulose · FD&C blue#1 lake · FD&C blue#2 lake · hydroxypropyl methylcellulose · microcrystalline cellulose · oleic acid · propylene glycol · starch · titanium dioxide · zinc stearate
AF GL SO	**Bayer Select Aspirin-Free Night Time Pain Relief** Bayer Consumer	caplet	diphenhydramine HCl, 25mg	acetaminophen, 500mg
	Compoz Medtech Labs	gelcap	diphenhydramine HCl, 25mg	
	Compoz Medtech Labs	tablet	diphenhydramine HCl, 50mg	
** GL	**Doan's P.M. Extra Strength** Ciba Self-Medication	caplet	diphenhydramine HCl, 25mg	magnesium salicylate tetrahydrate, 580mg · carnauba wax · colloidal silicon dioxide · croscarmellose sodium · microcrystalline cellulose · magnesium stearate · Opadry blue · stearic acid · talc
	Dormarex Republic Drug	capsule	diphenhydramine HCl, 50mg	
	Dormarex 2 Republic Drug	caplet	diphenhydramine HCl, 50mg	
AF GL PU SO	**Dormin** Randob Labs	capsule	diphenhydramine HCl, 25mg	lactose · magnesium stearate · polyethylene glycol · silicon dioxide · talc
	Doxylamine Succinate Copley Pharm'cal	tablet	doxylamine succinate, 25mg	
AF GL SO	**Excedrin PM** Bristol-Myers Products	caplet · tablet	diphenhydramine citrate, 38mg	acetaminophen, 500mg · benzoic acid · carnauba wax · corn starch · D&C yellow#10 aluminum lake · FD&C blue#1 aluminum lake · hydroxypropyl methylcellulose · magnesium stearate · methylparaben · pregelatinized starch · propylparaben · simethicone emulsion · stearic acid · titanium dioxide · may also contain: D&C yellow#10 · FD&C blue#1 · polyethylene glycol · polysorbate 80 · propylene glycol

See Chapter 10, "Sleep Aid and Stimulant Products," for more information about these products.

SLEEP AID PRODUCTS - continued

	Product Manufacturer/Supplier	Dosage Form	Antihistamine	Other Ingredients
AF	**Excedrin PM LiquiGels** Bristol-Myers Products	softgel	diphenhydramine HCl, 25mg	acetaminophen, 500mg · D&C red#33 · FD&C blue#1 · FD&C green#3 · gelatin · glycerin · polyethylene glycol · povidone · propylene glycol · silicon dioxide · sorbitol · titanium dioxide · water
**	**Legatrin PM** Columbia Labs	caplet	diphenhydramine HCl, 50mg	acetaminophen, 500mg · dicalcium phosphate · croscarmellose sodium · stearic acid · microcrystalline cellulose · magnesium stearate · FD&C blue#2 aluminum lake · FD&C red#40 aluminum lake · hydroxypropyl methylcellulose · polyethylene glycol · talc · titanium dioxide
** GL SO	**Melatonex** Sunsource	timed-release tablet		pyridoxine HCl, 10mg · melatonin, 3mg · dicalcium phosphate · microcrystalline cellulose · glyceryl monstearate · magnesium stearate
**	**Melatonin** Hudson	tablet		melatonin, 200mcg · cellulose · magnesium stearate · stearic acid · silica · protein coating
AF GL SO	**Midol PM Night Time Formula** Bayer Consumer	caplet	diphenhydramine HCl, 25mg	acetaminophen, 500mg
AF	**Nervine Nighttime Sleep-Aid** Bayer Consumer	caplet	diphenhydramine HCl, 25mg	calcium phosphate dibasic · calcium sulfate · carboxymethylcellulose sodium · corn starch · magnesium stearate · microcrystalline cellulose
	Night-Time Sleep-Aid Goldline Labs	tablet	doxylamine succinate, 25mg	
**	**NiteGel** Republic Drug	liquid-cap	doxylamine succinate, 6.25mg	acetaminophen, 250mg · pseudoephedrine HCl, 30mg · dextromethorphan hydrobromide, 10mg
AF DY	**Nytol** Block Drug	caplet	diphenhydramine HCl, 25mg	cellulose · corn starch · lactose · silica · stearic acid
AF DY	**Nytol Maximum Strength** Block Drug	caplet	doxylamine succinate, 25mg	colloidal silicon dioxide · magnesium stearate · microcrystalline cellulose · stearic acid
AF GL PU	**Sleep Rite** Hudson	tablet	diphenhydramine HCl, 25mg	
AF GL SO	**Sleep-eze 3** Whitehall-Robins Healthcare	tablet	diphenhydramine HCl, 25mg	croscarmellose sodium · dicalcium phosphate · D&C yellow#10 · FD&C yellow#6 · magnesium stearate · microcrystalline cellulose · stearic acid
AF GL PU SO	**Sleepinal** Thompson Medical	softgel	diphenhydramine HCl, 50mg	D&C yellow#10 · FD&C blue#1 · gelatin · glycerin · polyethylene glycol 400 · povidone 30 · propylene glycol · sorbitol · water
AF GL PU SO	**Sleepinal** Thompson Medical	capsule	diphenhydramine HCl, 50mg	lactose · magnesium stearate · talc
	Snooze Fast BDI Ph'cals	tablet	diphenhydramine HCl, 50mg	FD&C blue#1 aluminum lake
	Sominex Maximum Strength SmithKline Beecham	caplet	diphenhydramine HCl, 50mg	carnauba wax · crospovidone · dibasic calcium phosphate · FD&C blue#1 · hydroxypropyl methylcellulose · magnesium stearate · microcrystalline cellulose · polyethylene glycol · polysorbate 80 · silicon dioxide · starch · titanium dioxide

See Chapter 10, "Sleep Aid and Stimulant Products," for more information about these products.

SLEEP AID PRODUCTS - continued

	Product Manufacturer/Supplier	Dosage Form	Antihistamine	Other Ingredients
	Sominex Original SmithKline Beecham	tablet	diphenhydramine HCl, 25mg	dibasic calcium phosphate · FD&C blue#1 · magnesium stearate · microcrystalline cellulose · silicon dioxide · starch
	Sominex Pain Relief Formula SmithKline Beecham	tablet	diphenhydramine HCl, 25mg	acetaminophen, 500mg · colloidal silicon dioxide · corn starch · crospovidone · FD&C blue#1 · stearic acid
AF DY GL SO	**Tranquil** Alva-Amco Pharmacal	tablet	diphenhydramine HCl, 25mg	lactose microcrystalline cellulose · stearic acid · magnesium stearate
AF DY GL SO	**Tranquil Plus** Alva-Amco Pharmacal	caplet	diphenhydramine HCl, 25mg	acetaminophen, 250mg · magnesium salicylate, 250mg · magnesium carbonate · magnesium oxide · calcium carbonate
	Twilite Pfeiffer Ph'cals	caplet	diphenhydramine HCl, 50mg	
AF	**Tylenol PM Extra Strength** McNeil Consumer	caplet	diphenhydramine HCl, 25mg	acetaminophen, 500mg · cellulose · corn starch · hydroxypropyl methylcellulose · magnesium stearate or stearic acid · colloidal silicon dioxide · polyethylene glycol · polysorbate 80 · sodium citrate · sodium starch glycolate · titanium dioxide · blue#1 · blue#2
AF	**Tylenol PM Extra Strength** McNeil Consumer	gelcap	diphenhydramine HCl, 25mg	acetaminophen, 500mg · benzyl alcohol · butylparaben · castor oil · cellulose · corn starch · edetate calcium disodium · gelatin · hydroxypropyl methylcellulose · magnesium stearate · propylparaben · sodium lauryl sulfate · sodium citrate · sodium propionate · sodium starch glycolate · titanium dioxide · blue#1 · red#28
** AF	**Tylenol PM Extra Strength** McNeil Consumer	geltab	diphenhydramine HCl, 25mg	acetaminophen, 500mg · benzyl alcohol · butylparaben · castor oil · cellulose · corn starch · edetate calcium disodium · gelatin · hydroxypropyl methylcellulose · magnesium stearate · propylparaben · sodium lauryl sulfate · sodium citrate · sodium propionate · sodium starch glycolate · titanium dioxide · blue #1 · red #28
AF GL PU	**Unisom Nighttime Sleep Aid** Pfizer Consumer	tablet	doxylamine succinate, 25mg	microcrystalline cellulose · dibasic calcium phosphate dihydrate · sodium starch glycolate · magnesium stearate · FD&C blue#1 aluminum lake
AF GL PU SO	**Unisom Pain Relief** Pfizer Consumer	tablet	diphenhydramine HCl, 50mg	acetaminophen, 650mg · corn starch · polyvinylpyrolidone · stearic acid · Opadry blue · Opadry clear · magnesium stearate
	Unisom Sleepgels Pfizer Consumer	softgel	diphenhydramine HCl, 50mg	polyethylene glycol 400 · water · gelatin · sorbitol special glycerin blend 50/50 · glycerin · FD&C blue#1 · pharmaceutical glaze · propylene glycol · titanium dioxide

** New listing

See Chapter 10, "Sleep Aid and Stimulant Products," for more information about these products.

STIMULANT PRODUCTS

	Product Manufacturer/Supplier	Dosage Form	Caffeine	Other Ingredients
	20/20 BDI Ph'cals	tablet	200mg	FD&C yellow#6 aluminum lake · FD&C red#10 aluminum lake · FD&C blue#1 aluminum lake · FD&C blue#2 aluminum lake
	357 Magnum II BDI Ph'cals	tablet	200mg	FD&C red#40 aluminum lake · FD&C yellow#6 aluminum lake · FD&C blue#1 aluminum lake · FD&C blue#2 aluminum lake
GL PU SO	**Caffedrine** Thompson Medical	caplet	200mg	calcium sulfate · lactose · ethylcellulose · povidone · isopropyl alcohol · stearic acid · magnesium stearate · methyl alcohol · hydroxypropyl methylcellulose · triacetin · FD&C yellow#6 aluminum lake · D&C yellow#10 aluminum lake · titanium dioxide · propylene glycol
	Dexitac Republic Drug	timed-release capsule	250mg	
	King of Hearts BDI Ph'cals	tablet	200mg	FD&C red#40 aluminum lake · FD&C red#6 aluminum lake
GL SO	**No Doz** Bristol-Myers Products	chewable tablet	100mg	aspartame · crospovidone · dicalcium phosphate · ethylcellulose · flavor · magnesium stearate · mannitol · microcrystalline cellulose
GL SO	**No Doz Maximum Strength** Bristol-Myers Products	caplet	200mg	benzoic acid · carnauba wax · corn starch · FD&C blue#1 · flavor · hydroxypropyl methylcellulose · microcrystalline cellulose · mineral oil · polysorbate 20· povidone · propylene glycol · simethicone emulsion · sorbitan monolaurate · stearic acid · sucrose · titanium dioxide · water
	Overtime BDI Ph'cals	tablet	200mg	
GL SO	**Pep-Back** Alva-Amco Pharmacal	tablet	100mg	calcium carbonate
GL SO	**Pep-Back Ultra** Alva-Amco Pharmacal	caplet	200mg	calcium carbonate
GL PU SO	**Quick-Pep** Thompson Medical	tablet	150mg	dextrose, anhydrous · microcrystalline cellulose · sodium starch glycolate · colloidal silicon dioxide · FD&C yellow#6 aluminum lake · D&C yellow#10 aluminum lake · stearic acid · magnesium stearate · FD&C red#3 · starch · sucrose · talc
	Vivarin SmithKline Beecham	caplet · tablet	200mg	dextrose · D&C yellow#10 · FD&C yellow#6 · magnesium stearate · microcrystalline cellulose · silicon dioxide · starch

** New listing

See Chapter 10, "Sleep Aid and Stimulant Products," for more information about these products.

HISTAMINE II RECEPTOR ANTAGONISTS

	Product Manufacturer/Supplier	Dosage Form	Histamine II Receptor Antagonist	Other Ingredients
**	**Axid AR** Whitehall-Robins Healthcare	tablet	nizatidine, 75mg	colloidal silicon dioxide · hydroxypropyl methylcellulose · synthetic iron oxides · magnesium stearate · microcrystalline cellulose · polyethylene glycol · pregelatinized starch · propylene glycol · corn starch · titanium dioxide
**	**Pepcid AC** Johnson & Johnson·Merck	tablet	famotidine, 10mg	hydroxypropyl cellulose · hydroxypropyl methylcellulose · red iron oxide · magnesium stearate · microcrystalline cellulose · starch · talc · titanium dioxide
** DY GL PU SO SU	**Tagamet HB** SmithKline Beecham	tablet	cimetidine, 100mg	cellulose · hydroxypropyl methylcellulose · magnesium stearate · polyethylene glycol · polysorbate 80 · povidone · sodium lauryl sulfate · sodium starch glycolate · corn starch · titanium dioxide
** SO SU	**Zantac 75** Warner Wellcome Consumer	tablet	ranitidine HCl, 84mg (equivalent to ranitidine, 75mg)	hydroxypropyl methylcellulose · magnesium stearate · microcrystalline cellulose · synthetic red iron oxide · titanium dioxide · triacetin

** New listing

See Chapter 11, "Acid-Peptic Products," for more information about these products.

ANTIFLATULENT PRODUCTS

	Product [a] Manufacturer/Supplier	Dosage Form	Simethicone	Other Ingredients
**	**Alka-Seltzer Anti-Gas** Bayer Consumer	gelcap	125mg	D&C red#33 · FD&C blue#1 · FD&C red#40 · gelatin · glycerin · peppermint oil · purified water · sorbitol · titanium dioxide
SO	**Antacid Liquid** Goldline Labs	liquid	40mg/5ml	aluminum hydroxide, 400mg/5ml (equivalent to dried gel) · magnesium hydroxide, 400mg/5ml
**	**Beano** AkPharma	tablet		alpha galactosidase enzyme (from aspergillus niger) · corn starch · mannitol · sorbitol · hydrogenated cottonseed oil
**	**Beano** AkPharma	drops		water · sorbitol · alpha galactosidase enzyme (from aspergillus niger) · salt · disodium citrate · potassium sorbate
SO	**Di-Gel** Schering-Plough HealthCare	chewable tablet	20mg	calcium carbonate, 280mg · magnesium hydroxide, 128mg · mint or lemon/orange flavor
SO	**Di-Gel** Schering-Plough HealthCare	liquid	20mg/5ml	aluminum hydroxide, 200mg/5ml · magnesium hydroxide, 200mg/5ml
GL PU SO	**Gas-X** Sandoz Consumer	chewable tablet	80mg	calcium carbonate · dextrose · maltodextrin · cherry or peppermint creme flavor · red#30
** SU	**Gas-X Extra Strength** Sandoz Consumer	softgel	125mg	blue#1 · gelatin · glycerin · peppermint oil · red#40 · sorbitol · titanium dioxide · water · yellow#10
GL PU SO	**Gas-X Extra Strength** Sandoz Consumer	chewable tablet	125mg	tribasic calcium phosphate · colloidal silicon dioxide · cherry or peppermint creme flavor · dextrose · maltodextrin · silicon dioxide · red#30 · yellow#10
PU SO	**Gelusil** Warner Wellcome Consumer	chewable tablet	25mg	aluminum hydroxide, 200mg · magnesium hydroxide, 200mg · flavors · magnesium stearate · mannitol · sorbitol · sugar
** GL SU SL	**Genasyme** Goldline Labs	drops	40mg/0.6ml	
** DY PU	**Genasyme** Goldline Labs	chewable tablet	80mg	
SO	**Kudrox** Schwarz Pharma	suspension	40mg/5ml	aluminum hydroxide, 500mg/5ml · magnesium hydroxide, 450mg/5ml
DY SO SU PE	**Little Tummys Infant Gas Relief** Vetco	drops	20mg/0.3ml	citric acid · purified water · sodium benzoate · microcrystalline cellulose · xanthan gum · natural flavor · acesulfame K
SO	**Losopan Plus** Goldline Labs	suspension	20mg/5ml	magaldrate, 540mg/5ml
PU	**Maalox Antacid Plus Anti-Gas** Ciba Self-Medication	tablet	25mg	magnesium hydroxide, 200mg · aluminum hydroxide gel, 200mg · D&C red#30 · dextrose · flavors · glycerin · magnesium stearate · mannitol · saccharin sodium · sorbitol · starch · sugar

See Chapter 11, "Acid-Peptic Products," for more information about these products.

ANTIFLATULENT PRODUCTS - continued

	Product [a] Manufacturer/Supplier	Dosage Form	Simethicone	Other Ingredients
** PU	**Maalox Antacid Plus Anti-Gas Extra Strength** Ciba Self-Medication	tablet	30mg	magnesium hydroxide, 350mg · aluminum hydroxide, 350mg · colors · dextrose · flavors · glycerin · magnesium stearate · mannitol · saccharin sodium · sorbitol · starch · sugar
PU	**Maalox Anti-Gas** Ciba Self-Medication	tablet	80mg	corn starch · D&C red#30 · D&C yellow#10 · flavor · gelatin · mannitol · sucrose · tribasic calcium · phosphate
PU	**Maalox Anti-Gas Extra Strength** Ciba Self-Medication	tablet	150mg	corn starch · D&C red#27 aluminum lake · flavor · gelatin · mannitol · sucrose · tribasic calcium · phosphate
GL SO SU SL	**Maalox Extra Strength Antacid/Anti-Gas** Ciba Self-Medication	suspension	200mg/5ml	aluminum hydroxide, 2500mg/5ml (equivalent to dried gel) · magnesium hydroxide, 2250mg/5ml · calcium saccharin · flavors · methylparaben · propylparaben · purified water · sorbitol
SO	**Mylanta** Johnson & Johnson·Merck	suspension	20mg/5ml	aluminum hydroxide, 200mg/5ml · magnesium hydroxide, 200mg/5ml
SO	**Mylanta Double Strength** Johnson & Johnson·Merck	suspension	40mg/5ml	aluminum hydroxide, 400mg/5ml · magnesium hydroxide, 400mg/5ml
	Mylanta Gas Relief Johnson & Johnson·Merck	chewable tablet	80mg	
**	**Mylanta Gas Relief** Johnson & Johnson·Merck	gelcap	62.5mg	
	Mylanta Gas Relief Maximum Strength Johnson & Johnson·Merck	chewable tablet	125mg	
PE	**Mylicon, Infant's** Johnson & Johnson·Merck	drops	40mg/0.6ml	
**	**Phazyme Gas Relief** Block Drug	tablet	95mg	acacia · carnauba wax · compressible sugar · croscarmellose sodium · FD&C red#40 lake · FD&C yellow#6 lake · hydroxypropyl methylcellulose · microcrystalline cellulose · polyoxyl 40 stearate · povidone · sodium benzoate · sucrose · talc · titanium dioxide · white wax
** DY PE	**Phazyme Gas Relief** Block Drug	drops	40mg/0.6ml	carbomer 934P · citric acid · flavor · hydroxypropyl methylcellulose · PEG-8 stearate · potassium sorbate · sodium citrate · saccharin sodium · water
**	**Phazyme Gas Relief Maximum Strength** Block Drug	chewable tablet	125mg	citric acid · D&C yellow#10 · dextrates · FD&C blue#1 · peppermint flavor · sorbitol · starch · sucrose · talc · tribasic calcium phosphate
**	**Phazyme Gas Relief Maximum Strength** Block Drug	softgel	125mg	FD&C red#40 · gelatin · glycerin · hydrogenated soybean oil · lecithin · methylparaben · polysorbate 80 · propylparaben · soybean oil · titanium dioxide · vegetable shortening · yellow wax
SO SL	**Riopan Plus** Whitehall-Robins Healthcare	suspension	40mg/5ml	magaldrate, 540mg/5ml · mint flavor · glycerin · PEG-8 stearate · potassium citrate · saccharin · sorbitan stearate · sorbitol · xanthan gum · water

See Chapter 11, "Acid-Peptic Products," for more information about these products.

ANTIFLATULENT PRODUCTS - continued

	Product [a] Manufacturer/Supplier	Dosage Form	Simethicone	Other Ingredients
GL PU SO	**Riopan Plus** Whitehall-Robins Healthcare	chewable tablet	20mg	magaldrate, 480mg · mint flavor · magnesium stearate · methylcellulose · polyethylene glycol · silicon dioxide · sorbitol · starch · sucrose · titanium dioxide
GL PU SO	**Riopan Plus Double Strength** Whitehall-Robins Healthcare	chewable tablet	20mg	magaldrate, 1080mg · mint flavor · magnesium stearate · methylcellulose · polyethylene glycol · saccharin · silicon dioxide · sorbitol · starch · sucrose · titanium dioxide
SO SL	**Riopan Plus Double Strength, Cherry or Mint** Whitehall-Robins Healthcare	suspension	40mg/5ml	magaldrate, 1080mg/5ml · flavors · glycerin · PEG-8 stearate · potassium citrate · saccharin · sorbitan stearate · sorbitol · xanthan gum · water
SO	**Simaal 2 Gel** Schein Ph'cal	liquid	40mg/5ml	aluminum hydroxide, 400mg/5ml · magnesium hydroxide, 400mg/5ml · butylparaben · carboxymethylcellulose sodium · hydroxypropyl methylcellulose · microcrystalline cellulose · potassium citrate · propylparaben · water · saccharin sodium
SO	**Simaal Gel** Schein Ph'cal	liquid	20mg/5ml	aluminum hydroxide, 200mg/5ml · magnesium hydroxide, 200mg/5ml · sorbitol · butylparaben · carboxymethylcellulose · microcrystalline cellulose · propylparaben · purified water · saccharin sodium
SO	**Tempo Drops** Thompson Medical	chewable tablet	20mg	calcium carbonate, 414mg · aluminum hydroxide, 133mg · magnesium hydroxide, 81mg · corn syrup · water · FD&C blu#1 · flavor · sorbitol · soy protein · starch · titanium dioxide
SO	**Titralac Plus** 3M Health Care	liquid	20mg/5ml	calcium carbonate, 500mg/5ml · saccharin · spearmint flavor
SO	**Titralac Plus** 3M Health Care	chewable tablet	21mg	calcium carbonate, 420mg · glycine · magnesium stearate · saccharin · spearmint oil · starch · may also contain croscarmellose sodium
GL LA PU SO	**Tums Anti-Gas/Antacid** SmithKline Beecham	chewable tablet	20mg	calcium carbonate, 500mg · adipic acid · corn syrup · colors · flavors · microcrystalline cellulose · mineral oil · sodium polyphosphate · starch · sucrose · talc · triglycerol monooleate

** New listing

[a] Combination simethicone-antacid products listed in this table are limited to those that contain at least 40mg of simethicone per dose, which is the lowest recommended adult dose (taken 4 times daily) for relief of flatulence. The Antacid and Antireflux Products table lists combination antacid-simethicone products that contain less than 40mg of simethicone per dose.

See Chapter 11, "Acid-Peptic Products," for more information about these products.

ANTACID AND ANTIREFLUX PRODUCTS

	Product Manufacturer/Supplier	Dosage Form	Calcium Carbonate	Aluminum Hydroxide	Magnesium Salts	Other Antacids	Other Ingredients
**	**Acid-X** BDI Ph'cals	tablet	250mg				acetaminophen, 500mg
SO	**Alamag** Goldline Labs	suspension		225mg/5ml	200mg/5ml (as hydroxide)		
PU	**Alka-Mints** Bayer Consumer	chewable tablet	850mg				sorbitol · flavor
**	**Alka-Seltzer** Bayer Consumer	caplet	380mg				acetaminophen, 500mg · crospovidone · docusate sodium · hydroxypropyl methylcellulose · lecithin · magnesium stearate · polyvinylpyrrolidone · sodium benzoate · sodium hexametaphosphate · sodium starch glycolate · starch · stearic acid
**	**Alka-Seltzer** Bayer Consumer	gelcap	500mg				
PU SU	**Alka-Seltzer Extra Strength** Bayer Consumer	effervescent tablet				sodium bicarbonate, 1985mg (sodium, 588mg)	citric acid, 1000mg · aspirin, 500mg
PU SU	**Alka-Seltzer Gold** Bayer Consumer	effervescent tablet				sodium bicarbonate, 958mg (sodium, 311mg)	citric acid, 832mg · potassium bicarbonate, 312mg
PU SU	**Alka-Seltzer Original** Bayer Consumer	effervescent tablet				sodium bicarbonate, 1916mg (sodium, 567mg)	citric acid, 1000mg · aspirin, 325mg
PU SU	**Alka-Seltzer, Lemon-Lime** Bayer Consumer	effervescent tablet				sodium bicarbonate, 1700mg (sodium, 506mg)	citric acid, 1000mg · aspirin, 325mg · saccharin sodium
	Alkets Roberts Ph'cal	chewable tablet	500mg				dextrose · flavors · magnesium stearate · maltodextrin
	Alkets Extra Strength Roberts Ph'cal	chewable tablet	750mg				dextrose · flavors · magnesium stearate · maltodextrin
GL LA PU SU	**Almora** Forest Ph'cals	chewable tablet			500mg (as gluconate dihydrate) · 2.8mg (as stearate)		starch 1500, 79.22mg · stearic acid hystrene 5016, 1.4mg

See Chapter 11, "Acid-Peptic Products," for more information about these products.

ANTACID AND ANTIREFLUX PRODUCTS - continued

	Product Manufacturer/Supplier	Dosage Form	Calcium Carbonate	Aluminum Hydroxide	Magnesium Salts	Other Antacids	Other Ingredients
** SO SU	**ALternaGEL** Johnson & Johnson·Merck	liquid		600mg			butylparaben · carboxymethyl cellulose sodium · flavors · hydroxypropyl methylcellulose · microcrystalline cellulose · potassium citrate · propylparaben · purified water · simethicone
	Alu-Cap 3M Ph'cals	capsule		400mg			
	Alu-Tab 3M Ph'cals	tablet		500mg			
	Aluminum Hydroxide Concentrate Roxane Labs	suspension		135mg/ml			sorbitol solution, 15% · flavor · polyethylene glycol · propylene glycol · hydroxypropyl methylcellulose · methylparaben · propylparaben · disodium edetate · sodium hypochlorite solution
SO	**Amitone** Menley & James Labs	chewable tablet	350mg				magnesium stearate · mineral oil · powdered peppermint · sodium polyphosphate · starch · stearic acid · sucrose · talc
	Amphojel Wyeth-Ayerst Labs	tablet		300mg; 600mg			flavors · cellulose · hydrogenated vegetable oil · magnesium stearate · polacrilin potassium · saccharin starch · talc
	Amphojel Wyeth-Ayerst Labs	suspension		320mg/5ml			calcium benzoate · glycerin · hydroxypropyl methylcellulose · menthol · peppermint oil · potassium butylparaben · potassium propylparaben · saccharin · simethicone · sorbitol solution · water
	Amphojel, Peppermint Wyeth-Ayerst Labs	suspension		320mg/5ml			butylparaben · calcium benzoate · glycerin · hydroxypropyl methylcellulose · methylparaben · propylparaben · saccharin · simethicone · sorbitol solution · water

See Chapter 11, "Acid-Peptic Products," for more information about these products.

ANTACID AND ANTIREFLUX PRODUCTS - continued

	Product Manufacturer/Supplier	Dosage Form	Calcium Carbonate	Aluminum Hydroxide	Magnesium Salts	Other Antacids	Other Ingredients
	Antacid Extra Strength Goldline Labs	tablet	750mg				
SO	**Antacid Liquid** Goldline Labs	liquid		400mg/5ml	400mg/5ml (as hydroxide)		simethicone, 40mg/5ml
	Antacid Liquid Goldline Labs	gelcap	311mg		232mg (as carbonate)		
** DY GL LA PU SU	**Arm & Hammer Pure Baking Soda** Church & Dwight	powder				sodium bicarbonate, 100%	
	Basaljel Wyeth-Ayerst Labs	tablet		500mg			cellulose · hydrogenated vegetable oil · magnesium stearate · polacrillin potassium · starch · talc
	Basaljel Wyeth-Ayerst Labs	suspension		400mg			flavors · butylparaben · calcium benzoate · glycerin · hydroxypropyl methylcellulose · methylparaben · mineral oil · propylparaben · saccharin · simethicone · sorbitol solution · water
	Basaljel Wyeth-Ayerst Labs	capsule		500mg			D&C yellow#10 · FD&C blue#1 · FD&C red#40 · FD&C yellow #6 · gelatin · polacrillin potassium · polyethylene glycol · talc · titanium dioxide
	Bell/ans C. S. Dent	chewable tablet				sodium bicarbonate, 520mg (sodium, 144mg)	wintergreen, ginger flavor · acacia · charcoal · corn starch · gelatin · potato starch · propylene glycol · sucrose · cream mint flavor
	Bromo-Seltzer Warner Wellcome Consumer	granular effervescent				sodium bicarbonate, 2.78mg	acetaminophen, 325mg · citric acid, 2224mg
GL LA SU	**Calcium Carbonate** Roxane Labs	tablet	500mg; 1250mg				colloidal silicon dioxide · crospovidone · magnesium stearate · povidone · titanium dioxide · cellulose · polyethylene glycol · water

See Chapter 11, "Acid-Peptic Products," for more information about these products.

ANTACID AND ANTIREFLUX PRODUCTS - continued

	Product Manufacturer/Supplier	Dosage Form	Calcium Carbonate	Aluminum Hydroxide	Magnesium Salts	Other Antacids	Other Ingredients
DY	**Calcium Carbonate** Roxane Labs	suspension	250mg/ml				sorbitol solution, 40% · spearmint flavor · glycol · methylparaben · propylparaben · water · xanthan gum · sodium hypochlorite solution
DY	**Calcium Carbonate** Roxane Labs	suspension	500mg/5ml				sorbitol · propylene glycol · methylparaben · propylparaben · flavoring · sodium hypochlorite · water · xanthan gum
SO	**Chooz** Schering-Plough HealthCare	gum	500mg				
	Citrocarbonate Roberts Ph'cal	granular effervescent				sodium bicarbonate, 2.34g	sodium citrate · citric acid anhydrous · calcium lactate pentahydrate · sodium chloride · monobasic sodium phosphate anhydrous · magnesium sulfate dried
	Dialume Rhône-Poulenc Rorer Ph'cals	tablet		500mg			calcium stearate
GL SO	**Dicarbosil** BIRA	chewable tablet	500mg				peppermint oil
GL LA PU	**Equilet** Mission Pharmacal	chewable tablet	500mg				
DY LA PU	**Gaviscon** SmithKline Beecham	chewable tablet		80mg	20mg (as trisilicate)	sodium bicarbonate, 70mg (sodium, 19mg)	alginic acid, 200mg, calcium stearate · flavor · starch (may contain corn starch) · sucrose
DY GL LA SU SL	**Gaviscon ESRF** SmithKline Beecham	suspension		50.8mg/ml	47.5mg/ml (as carbonate)		sodium alginate, 20mg/ml · benzyl alcohol · edetate disodium · flavor · glycerin · saccharin sodium · simethicone emulsion · sorbitol solution · water · xanthongum
DY LA PU	**Gaviscon Extra Strength** SmithKline Beecham	chewable tablet		160mg	105mg (as carbonate)	sodium bicarbonate	alginic acid, 200mg, calcium stearate · flavor · sucrose · May contain: sorbitol · mannitol · starch

See Chapter 11, "Acid-Peptic Products," for more information about these products.

ANTACID AND ANTIREFLUX PRODUCTS - continued

	Product Manufacturer/Supplier	Dosage Form	Calcium Carbonate	Aluminum Hydroxide	Magnesium Salts	Other Antacids	Other Ingredients
** GL LA SU SL	**Gaviscon Liquid** SmithKline Beecham	suspension		31.5mg/5ml	119.5mg/5ml (as carbonate)		benzyl alcohol · D&C yellow#10 · edetate disodium · FD&C blue#1 · flavor · glycerin · saccharin sodium · sodium alginate · sorbitol solution · water · xanthan gum
DY LA PU	**Gaviscon-2** SmithKline Beecham	chewable tablet		160mg	40mg (as trisilicate)	sodium bicarbonate, 140mg (sodium, 36.8mg)	alginic acid, 400mg, calcium stearate · flavor · starch (may contain corn starch) · sucrose
	Genalac Goldline Labs	chewable tablet	420mg				glycine base
SO	**Losopan** Goldline Labs	suspension				magaldrate, 540mg/5ml	
DY GL LA PU SU	**Maalox** Ciba Self-Medication	caplet	311mg		232mg (as carbonate)		corn starch · croscarmellose · magnesium stearate · sodium lauryl sulfate · hydroxypropyl methylcellulose · titanium dioxide
** DY GL LA SO SU SL	**Maalox** Ciba Self-Medication	suspension		225mg/5ml	200mg/5ml (as hydroxide)		calcium saccharin · methylparaben · natural flavor · propylparaben · sorbitol · purified water · other ingredients
GL LA SU SL	**Maalox Heartburn Relief** Ciba Self-Medication	suspension		140mg/5ml	175mg/5ml (carbonate)		calcium carbonate · calcium saccharin · FD&C blue#1 · FD&C yellow#5 (tartrazine) · mint flavor · magnesium alginate · methylparaben · propylparaben · potassium bicarbonate · sorbitol · purified water
DY GL LA SU SL	**Maalox Therapeutic Concentrate** Ciba Self-Medication	suspension		600mg/5ml	300mg/5ml (as hydroxide)		flavor · guar gum · methylparaben · propylparaben · sorbitol · purified water · may also contain citric acid
GL PU SO	**Mag-Ox 400** Blaine Ph'cals	tablet			400mg (as oxide)		

See Chapter 11, "Acid-Peptic Products," for more information about these products.

ANTACID AND ANTIREFLUX PRODUCTS - continued

	Product Manufacturer/Supplier	Dosage Form	Calcium Carbonate	Aluminum Hydroxide	Magnesium Salts	Other Antacids	Other Ingredients
	Magnalox Schein Ph'cal	liquid		225mg/5ml	200mg/5ml (as hydroxide)		carboxymethylcellulose sodium · citric acid · flavors · hydroxypropyl methylcellulose · methylparaben · microcrystalline cellulose · propylparaben · water · saccharin sodium · simethicone · sorbitol
DY LA SL	**Magnesia and Alumina** Roxane Labs	suspension		220mg/5ml	200mg/5ml (as hydroxide)		sorbitol solution, 15% · peppermint · glycol · propylparaben · butylparaben · magnesium aluminum silicate · sodium hypochlorite solution
	Marblen Fleming	tablet	520mg		400mg (as carbonate)		peach/apricot flavor
	Marblen Fleming	suspension	520mg/5ml		400mg/5ml (as carbonate)		peach/apricot flavor
	Milk of Magnesia Roxane Labs	suspension			400mg/5ml (as hydroxide)		
	Milk of Magnesia Pharmaceutical Assoc.	suspension			390mg/5ml (as hydroxide)		citric acid · methylparaben · propylparaben · sodium hypochlorite
	Milk of Magnesia Concentrate Roxane Labs	suspension			1200mg/5ml (as hydroxide)		
	Milk of Magnesia Concentrate Pharmaceutical Assoc.	suspension			1165mg/5ml (as hydroxide)		sorbitol solution, 29% · sugar, 8% · glycerin · lemon · benzyl alcohol (bulk formulation only) · sodium carboxymethylcellulose · sodium hexametaphosphate · sodium citrate · vanillin · sodium hypochlorite · citric acid
**	**Mylanta** Johnson & Johnson·Merck	gelcap	550mg		125mg (as hydroxide)		
**	**Mylanta Double Strength** Johnson & Johnson·Merck	chewable tablet	700mg		300mg (as hydroxide)		
** SO	**Mylanta Regular Strength** Johnson & Johnson·Merck	chewable tablet	350mg		150mg (as hydroxide)		
SO	**Mylanta Soothing** Johnson & Johnson·Merck	lozenge	600mg				
	Nephrox Fleming	suspension		320mg/5ml			mineral oil, 10% · watermelon flavor

See Chapter 11, "Acid-Peptic Products," for more information about these products.

ANTACID AND ANTIREFLUX PRODUCTS - continued

	Product Manufacturer/Supplier	Dosage Form	Calcium Carbonate	Aluminum Hydroxide	Magnesium Salts	Other Antacids	Other Ingredients
LA	**Phillips' Milk of Magnesia** Bayer Consumer	suspension			400mg/5ml (as hydroxide)		cherry, mint, or original flavor
GL	**Phillips' Milk of Magnesia** Bayer Consumer	chewable tablet			311mg (as hydroxide)		mint flavor
AL LA	**Phillips' Milk of Magnesia Concentrate** Bayer Consumer	suspension			800mg/5ml (as hydroxide)		strawberry flavor
LA SO SL	**Riopan** Whitehall-Robins Healthcare	suspension				magaldrate, 108mg/ml	mint flavor
SO	**Rolaids, Asst. Fruit Flavors** Warner-Lambert	chewable tablet	550mg				corn starch · flavoring · light mineral oil · magnesium stearate · mannitol · pregelatinized starch · silicone dioxide · sucrose · blue#1 · red#27 · red#40 · titanium dioxide · yellow#5 (tartrazine) · yellow#6
	Rolaids, Peppermint or Spearmint Flavor Warner-Lambert	chewable tablet	412mg		80mg (as hydroxide)		pregelatinized starch · mannitol · flavors · light mineral oil · magnesium stearate · microcrystalline cellulose · polyethylene glycol · silicon dioxide · sucrose
	Sodium Bicarbonate Multisource	chewable tablet				sodium bicarbonate, 325mg; 650mg	
SO	**Titralac** 3M Health Care	chewable tablet	420mg				glycine, 150mg · saccharin starch · magnesium stearate · spearmint flavor
SO	**Titralac Extra Strength** 3M Health Care	chewable tablet	750mg				glycine · magnesium stearate · saccharin · spearmint oil · starch
GL LA PU	**Tums E-X Extra Strength, Wintergreen or Asst. Fruit Flavors** SmithKline Beecham	chewable tablet	750mg				sucrose · starch · talc · mineral oil · flavors · sodium polyphosphate · May also contain: adipic acid · blue#1 lake · yellow#6 lake · yellow#10 lake · red#27 lake · red#30 lake

See Chapter 11, "Acid-Peptic Products," for more information about these products.

ANTACID AND ANTIREFLUX PRODUCTS - continued

	Product Manufacturer/Supplier	Dosage Form	Calcium Carbonate	Aluminum Hydroxide	Magnesium Salts	Other Antacids	Other Ingredients
GL LA PU	**Tums Ultra, Fruit or Mint Flavors** SmithKline Beecham	chewable tablet	1000mg				sucrose · starch · talc · mineral oil · flavors · sodium polyphosphate · May also contain: adipic acid · blue#1 lake · yellow#6 lake · yellow#10 lake · red#27 lake · red#30 lake
GL LA PU SO	**Tums, Peppermint or Asst. Fruit Flavors** SmithKline Beecham	chewable tablet	500mg				sucrose · starch · talc · mineral oil · flavor(s) · sodium polyphosphate · May also contain: adipic acid · blue#1 lake · yellow#6 lake · yellow#10 lake · red#27 lake · red#30 lake
	Tylenol Headache Plus Extra Strength McNeil Consumer	caplet	250mg				acetaminophen, 500mg · acacia · cellulose · corn starch · croscarmellose sodium · hydroxypropyl methylcellulose · magnesium stearate · maltodextrin · propylene glycol · sodium starch glycolate · titanium dioxide · triacetin · blue#1 · blue#2
GL PU SO	**Uro-Mag** Blaine Ph'cals	capsule			140mg (as oxide)		

** New listing
[a] The Antiflatulent Products table contains combination antacid-simethicone products that contain more than 40mg of simethicone per dose.

See Chapter 11, "Acid-Peptic Products," for more information about these products.

LAXATIVE PRODUCTS

	Product Manufacturer/Supplier	Dosage Form	Stimulant	Bulk	Emollient/ Lubricant	Other Laxatives	Other Ingredients
SL	**Agoral, Marshmallow or Raspberry** Warner Wellcome Consumer	emulsion	phenolphthalein, 65.67mg/5ml		mineral oil	glycerin	agar · tragacanth · acacia · benzoic acid · egg albumin · flavors · water · citric acid or sodium hydroxide · D&C red#30 aluminum lake (raspberry) · saccharin sodium · sodium benzoate
GL PU SO	**Alophen** Warner Wellcome Consumer	tablet	phenolphthalein, 60mg				acacia · calcium carbonate · candellila wax · corn starch · compressible sugar · FD&C blue#2 aluminum lake · FD&C red#40 aluminum lake · FD&C yellow#6 aluminum lake · gelatin · kaolin · microcrystalline cellulose · pregelatinized starch · polyvinylpyrrolidone · sucrose · titanium dioxide · magnesium stearate · sodium benzoate · talc
**	**Bisacodyl, Enteric Coated** Paddock Labs	tablet	bisacodyl, 10mg				
	Bisco-Lax Schein Ph'cal	suppository	bisacodyl, 10mg				hydrogenated vegetable oil
	Bisco-Lax Enteric Coated Schein Ph'cal	tablet	bisacodyl, 5mg				
	Caroid Mentholatum	tablet	cascara sagrada extract, 50mg · phenolphthalein, 32.4mg				acacia · beeswax · calcium carbonate · carnauba wax · dicalcium phosphate dihydrate · gelatin · iron oxide · lactose · microcrystalline cellulose · silica · sucrose · magnesium stearate · sodium lauryl sulfate · stearic acid
	Cascara Sagrada Multisource	various	cascara sagrada, 325mg; 450mg				
	Cascara Sagrada Aromatic Fluidextract Multisource	liquid	cascara sagrada				
DY GL LA PU SU	**Ceo-Two** Beutlich, L.P. Ph'cals	suppository					sodium bicarbonate · potassium bitartrate · polyethylene glycol

See Chapter 12, "Laxative Products," for more information about these products.

LAXATIVE PRODUCTS - continued

	Product Manufacturer/Supplier	Dosage Form	Stimulant	Bulk	Emollient/ Lubricant	Other Laxatives	Other Ingredients
	Citrucel SmithKline Beecham	powder		methylcellulose, 2g/tbsp			citric acid · FD&C yellow#6 · orange flavor · potassium citrate · riboflavin · sucrose
**	**Citrucel Sugar Free** SmithKline Beecham	powder		methylcellulose, 2g/tbsp			aspartame · dibasic calcium phosphate · FD&C yellow#6 · malic acid · maltodextrin · orange flavor · potassium citrate · riboflavin · phenylketonurics: contains phenylalanine, 52mg/dose
LA SL	**Colace** Roberts Ph'cal	syrup			docusate sodium, 20mg/5ml		
LA SL	**Colace** Roberts Ph'cal	liquid			docusate sodium, 50mg/5ml		
GL	**Colace** Roberts Ph'cal	capsule			docusate sodium, 50mg; 100mg		
**	**Correctol** Schering-Plough HealthCare	caplet · tablet	bisacodyl, 5mg				
	Correctol Extra Gentle Schering-Plough HealthCare	softgel			docusate sodium, 100mg		
**	**Correctol Herbal Tea, Honey Lemon or Cinnamon Spice** Schering-Plough HealthCare	liquid	senna (total sennosides), 30mg/teabag				natural flavors
	DC 240 Goldline Labs	capsule			docusate calcium, 240mg		
	Deficol Enteric Coated Vangard Labs	tablet	bisacodyl, 5mg				
	Dialose Johnson & Johnson·Merck	tablet			docusate sodium, 100mg		
	Dialose Plus Johnson & Johnson·Merck	tablet	yellow phenolphthalein, 65mg		docusate sodium, 100mg		
	Dioctolose Goldline Labs	capsule			docusate potassium, 100mg		
SO	**Docu-K Plus** Vangard Labs	capsule	casanthranol, 30mg		docusate potassium, 100mg		
	Docusate Calcium and Yellow Phenolphthalein Vangard Labs	capsule	yellow phenolphthalein, 65mg		docusate calcium, 60mg		
	Docusate Potassium with Casanthranol Multisource	capsule	casanthranol, 30mg		docusate potassium, 100mg		

See Chapter 12, "Laxative Products," for more information about these products.

LAXATIVE PRODUCTS - continued

	Product Manufacturer/Supplier	Dosage Form	Stimulant	Bulk	Emollient/ Lubricant	Other Laxatives	Other Ingredients
**	**Docusate Sodium** Schein Ph'cal	softgel			docusate sodium, 250mg	glycerin	FD&C red#40 · FD&C yellow#10 · gelatin · methylparaben · propylene glycol · propylparaben · sorbitol
LA SO	**Doxidan** Pharmacia & Upjohn	softgel	yellow phenolphthalein, 65mg		docusate calcium, 60mg	glycerin	alcohol, up to 1.5% · corn oil · FD&C blue#1 · FD&C red#40 · gelatin · hydrogenated vegetable oil · methylparaben · propylparaben · sorbitol · titanium dioxide · vegetable shortening · yellow wax · lecithin
LA SO SL	**Dr. Caldwell Senna** Gebauer	liquid	senna, 166.5mg/5ml				alcohol, 4.9%
SO	**Dulcolax** Ciba Self-Medication	tablet	bisacodyl, 5mg		docusate sodium	glycerin	acacia · acetylated monoglyceride · carnauba wax · cellulose acetate phthalate · corn starch · D&C red#30 aluminum lake · D&C yellow#10 aluminum lake · dibutyl phthalate · gelatin · iron oxides · kaolin · lactose · methylparaben · pharmaceutical glaze · povidone · propylparaben · sorbitan monooleate · sucrose · titanium dioxide · white wax · magnesium stearate · polyethylene glycol · sodium benzoate · talc
	Emulsoil Paddock Labs	liquid	castor oil, 95%				flavor · emulsifier
	Epsom Salt Multisource	granule				magnesium sulfate, 40mEq/5mg	
GL PU	**Espotabs** Combe	tablet	yellow phenolphthalein, 97.2mg				
	Evac-Q-Kwik Savage Labs	liquid				magnesium citrate, 25mEq/30ml	sodium, 0.095mEq/30ml · carbon dioxide · citric acid · FD&C red#4 · cherry flavor · potassium citrate · water
	Evac-Q-Kwik Savage Labs	suppository	bisacodyl, 10mg				

See Chapter 12, "Laxative Products," for more information about these products.

LAXATIVE PRODUCTS - continued

	Product Manufacturer/Supplier	Dosage Form	Stimulant	Bulk	Emollient/ Lubricant	Other Laxatives	Other Ingredients
	Evac-Q-Kwik Savage Labs	tablet	phenolphthalein, 130mg				acacia · calcium carbonate · calcium sulfate · corn starch · dibasic calcium phosphate · FD&C red#40 · lactose · polyvinylpyrolidone · shellac · titanium dioxide · water · white wax · magnesium stearate · sodium benzoate · talc
GL PU GE	**Evac-U-Gen** Walker, Corp.	chewable tablet	yellow phenolphthalein, 97.2mg				saccharin sodium (sodium, 0.004mEq) · anise oil · corn syrup solids · D&C red#7 · FD&C blue#1 · lactose · confectioner's sugar · magnesium stearate
GL PU SO	**Ex-Lax Chocolate** Sandoz Consumer	tablet	yellow phenolphthalein, 90mg				cocoa · confectioner's sugar · hydrogenated palm kernel oil · nonfat dry milk · vanillin · lecithin
GL PU	**Ex-Lax Extra Gentle** Sandoz Consumer	tablet	yellow phenolphthalein, 65mg		docusate sodium, 75mg		acacia · croscarmellose sodium · dibasic calcium phosphate · colloidal silicon dioxide · microcrystalline cellulose · red#7 · sucrose · titanium dioxide · magnesium stearate · stearic acid · talc ·
GL PU	**Ex-Lax Gentle Nature Natural** Sandoz Consumer	tablet	sennosides A & B, 20mg				alginic acid · calcium phosphate dibasic · magnesium stearate · microcrystalline cellulose · silicon dioxide · starch · sodium lauryl sulfate · stearic acid
GL PU	**Ex-Lax Maximum Relief Formula** Sandoz Consumer	tablet	yellow phenolphthalein, 135mg				acacia · alginic acid · blue#1 · carnauba wax · colloidal silicon dioxide · dibasic calcium phosphate · microcrystalline cellulose · povidone · starch · sucrose · titanium dioxide · magnesium stearate · sodium benzoate · sodium lauryl sulfate · stearic acid · talc

See Chapter 12, "Laxative Products," for more information about these products.

LAXATIVE PRODUCTS - continued

	Product Manufacturer/Supplier	Dosage Form	Stimulant	Bulk	Emollient/ Lubricant	Other Laxatives	Other Ingredients
GL PU	**Ex-Lax Regular Strength** Sandoz Consumer	tablet	yellow phenolphthalein, 90mg				acacia · alginic acid · carnauba wax · colloidal silicon dioxide · dibasic calcium phosphate · iron oxides · microcrystalline cellulose · starch · sucrose · titanium dioxide · magnesium stearate · sodium benzoate · sodium lauryl sulfate · stearic acid · talc
**	**Feen-A-Mint** Schering-Plough HealthCare	tablet	bisacodyl, 5mg				
	Femilax G & W Labs	tablet	phenolphthalein, 65mg		docusate sodium, 100mg		
	Fiber Goldline Labs	tablet		calcium polycarbophil, 625mg			
	Fiberall Ciba Self-Medication	tablet		calcium polycarbophil, 1250mg			crospovidone · dextrose · flavors · yellow#10 aluminum lake · magnesium stearate
	Fiberall, Fruit & Nut Ciba Self-Medication	wafer		psyllium hydrophilic mucilloid, 3.4g		glycerin	baking powder · brown sugar · butter flavor · cinnamon · corn syrup · crisp rice · dried ground apricots · flour · granulated sugar · granulated walnuts · margarine · molasses · oats · salt · vegetable oil · soybean oil · cottonseed oil · water · wheat bran · lecithin
PU	**Fiberall, Natural** Ciba Self-Medication	powder		psyllium hydrophilic mucilloid, 3.4g			citric acid · flavor · wheat bran · polysorbate 60
	Fiberall, Oatmeal Raisin Ciba Self-Medication	wafer		psyllium hydrophilic mucilloid, 3.4g		glycerin	wheat bran · baking powder · cinnamon · cinnamon flavor · cloves · corn syrup · flour · granulated sugar · molasses · oats · raisins · vegetable oil · soybean oil · cottonseed oil · water · lecithin
SO	**Fiberall, Orange** Ciba Self-Medication	powder		psyllium hydrophilic mucilloid, 3.4g			wheat bran · citric acid · flavor · saccharin · polysorbate 60 · yellow#6 lake · beta carotene

See Chapter 12, "Laxative Products," for more information about these products.

LAXATIVE PRODUCTS - continued

	Product Manufacturer/Supplier	Dosage Form	Stimulant	Bulk	Emollient/ Lubricant	Other Laxatives	Other Ingredients
GL LA PU SO SU	**FiberCon** Lederle Consumer	tablet		calcium polycarbophil, 625mg			calcium carbonate · caramel · crospovidone · hydroxypropyl methylcellulose · microcrystalline cellulose · povidone · silica gel · magnesium stearate
AL LA PR SO SL PE	**Fleet Babylax** C. B. Fleet	liquid				glycerin	
SO	**Fleet Bisacodyl Enema** C. B. Fleet	enema	bisacodyl, 10mg				
GL PU SO	**Fleet Glycerin Adult Size** C. B. Fleet	suppository				glycerin	
GL PU SO PE	**Fleet Glycerin Child Size** C. B. Fleet	suppository				glycerin	
AL LA PR SO	**Fleet Glycerin Rectal Applicators** C. B. Fleet	liquid				glycerin, 7.5ml	
PU	**Fleet Laxative** C. B. Fleet	tablet	bisacodyl, 5mg				
GL PU	**Fleet Laxative** C. B. Fleet	suppository	bisacodyl, 10mg				
**	**Fleet Magnesium Citrate Prep Kit 4** C. B. Fleet	powder · suppository · tablet	bisacodyl, 20mg/4tablets · bisacodyl, 10mg (suppository)			magnesium citrate, 18.7g (powder)	
**	**Fleet Magnesium Citrate Prep Kit 5** C. B. Fleet	enema · powder · tablet	bisacodyl, 20mg/4tablets			magnesium citrate, 18.7g (powder)	
**	**Fleet Magnesium Citrate Prep Kit 6** C. B. Fleet	enema · powder · tablet	bisacodyl, 20mg/4tablets · bisacodyl, 10mg (enema)			magnesium citrate, 18.7g (powder)	
PR	**Fleet Mineral Oil Enema** C. B. Fleet	enema			mineral oil, 100%		
AL LA PR SO SL	**Fleet Mineral Oil Oral Lubricant** C. B. Fleet	liquid			mineral oil, 100%		

See Chapter 12, "Laxative Products," for more information about these products.

LAXATIVE PRODUCTS - continued

	Product Manufacturer/Supplier	Dosage Form	Stimulant	Bulk	Emollient/ Lubricant	Other Laxatives	Other Ingredients
	Fleet Prep Kit 1 C. B. Fleet	liquid · suppository · tablet	bisacodyl, 20mg/4tablets · bisacodyl, 10mg (suppository)			sodium phosphate oral solution, 45ml (liquid) (total sodium, 4950mg/45ml) · glycerin (liquid)	flavor (liquid) · saccharin (liquid)
	Fleet Prep Kit 2 C. B. Fleet	enema · liquid · tablet	bisacodyl, 20mg/4tablets			sodium phosphate oral solution, 45ml (liquid) (total sodium, 4950mg/45ml) · glycerin (liquid)	flavor (liquid) · saccharin (liquid)
	Fleet Prep Kit 3 C. B. Fleet	enema · liquid · tablet	bisacodyl, 20mg/4tablets · bisacodyl, 10mg (enema)			sodium phosphate oral solution, 45ml (liquid) (total sodium, 4950mg/45ml) · glycerin (liquid)	flavor (liquid) · saccharin (liquid)
	Fleet Ready-to-Use Enema C. B. Fleet	enema				monobasic sodium phosphate, 19g/118ml · dibasic sodium phosphate, 7g/118ml (total sodium, 4.4g/118ml)	
PE	**Fleet Ready-to-Use Enema for Children** C. B. Fleet	enema				monobasic sodium phosphate, 9.5g/59ml · dibasic sodium phosphate, 3.5g/59ml (total sodium, 2.2g/59ml)	
LA SL PE	**Fletcher's Castoria** Mentholatum	liquid	senna concentrate, 166.5mg/5ml			glycerin	alcohol, 3.5% · flavor · sucrose · water
LA SL PE	**Fletcher's, Children's Cherry** Mentholatum	suspension	yellow phenolphthalein, 0.3%			glycerin	citric acid · FD&C red#40 · flavor · magnesium aluminum silicate · methylparaben · sucrose · water · xanthan gum · sodium benzoate
SO	**Garfields Tea** Alvin Last	cut plant	senna, 610mg/1/2tsp	psyllium seed husks · buckthorn bark			anise seed · fennel seed
	Genasoft Goldline Labs	capsule			docusate sodium, 100mg		

See Chapter 12, "Laxative Products," for more information about these products.

LAXATIVE PRODUCTS - continued

	Product Manufacturer/Supplier	Dosage Form	Stimulant	Bulk	Emollient/ Lubricant	Other Laxatives	Other Ingredients
	Genasoft Plus Goldline Labs	capsule	casanthranol, 30mg		docusate sodium, 100mg		
	GenFiber Goldline Labs	powder		psyllium hydrophilic mucilloid, 3.4g/7g			dextrose
	Gentlax S Blair Labs	tablet	senna concentrate, 187mg		docusate sodium, 50mg		
GL PU SO	**Gentle Laxative** Hudson	tablet	bisacodyl, 5mg				
	Glycerin Multisource	suppository				glycerin	sodium stearate
AL LA	**Haleys M-O, Flavored or Regular** Bayer Consumer	emulsion			mineral oil, 25%	magnesium hydroxide, 6%	
	Hydrocil Instant Solvay Ph'cals	powder		psyllium, 95%			povidone · polyethylene glycol
SO	**Innerclean Herbal** Alvin Last	cut plant · tablet	senna leaves	psyllium seed husks · buckthorn bark			anise seed · fennel seed
SO	**Kasof** Roberts Ph'cal	capsule			docusate potassium, 240mg	glycerin	gelatin · methylparaben · polyethylene glycol · propylparaben · purified water · red#40 · blue#1 · sorbitol · yellow#10
AL LA PR SO SL	**Kellogg's Tasteless Castor Oil** BIRA	liquid	castor oil, 100%				
SO	**Kondremul** Ciba Self-Medication	emulsion			mineral oil, 55%	glycerin	acacia · benzoic acid · carrageenan · ethyl vanillin · mapleine triple oil · purified water · vanillin
SU	**Konsyl** Konsyl Ph'cals	powder		psyllium mucilloid, 100%			sodium, <4mg
	Konsyl Fiber Konsyl Ph'cals	tablet		calcium polycarbophil, 625mg (equivalent to polycarbophil, 500mg)			
	Konsyl-D Konsyl Ph'cals	powder		psyllium hydrophilic mucilloid, 50%			dextrose, 50% · sodium, <4mg
	Konsyl-Orange Konsyl Ph'cals	powder		psyllium hydrophilic mucilloid, 28%			sucrose, 67% · sodium, 2.4mg
	Lax-Pills G & W Labs	tablet	phenolphthalein, 90mg				
GL PU SO	**Laxative & Stool Softner** Hudson	softgel	casanthranol, 30mg		docusate sodium, 100mg		

See Chapter 12, "Laxative Products," for more information about these products.

LAXATIVE PRODUCTS - continued

	Product Manufacturer/Supplier	Dosage Form	Stimulant	Bulk	Emollient/ Lubricant	Other Laxatives	Other Ingredients
AL LA PR SL	**Liqui-Doss** Ferndale Labs	emulsion			mineral oil		
GL PU SO	**Mag-Ox 400** Blaine Ph'cals	tablet				magnesium oxide, 400mg (elemental magnesium, 241.3mg or 19.86mEq)	
	Magnesium Citrate Multisource	solution				magnesium citrate, 1.74g/oz	
GL LA PU SO	**Medilax** Mission Pharmacal	tablet	phenolphthalein, 120mg				aspartame
DY LA PU	**Metamucil Fiber, Apple Crisp or Cinnamon Spice** Procter & Gamble	wafer		psyllium hydrophilic mucilloid, 3.4g/2 wafers			ascorbic acid · brown sugar (Apple Crisp) · cinnamon · corn oil · flavors · fructose · lecithin · modified food starch · molasses · oat hull fiber · sodium bicarbonate · sucrose · nutmeg · oats (Cinnamon Spice) · water · wheat flour
GL LA PU SU	**Metamucil Original Texture, Effervescent Sugar Free** Procter & Gamble	individual packet		psyllium hydrophilic fiber, 3.4g/packet			aspartame · calcium carbonate · citric acid · flavoring · potassium bicarbonate · silicon dioxide · sodium bicarbonate · phenylketonurics: contains phenylalanine, 28mg/dose (Lemon-Lime); 30mg/dose (Orange)
** GL LA PU SO	**Metamucil Original Texture, Orange** Procter & Gamble	powder		psyllium hydrophilic mucilloid, 3.4g/tsp			citric acid · FD&C yellow#6 · flavoring · sucrose
DY GL LA PU	**Metamucil Original Texture, Regular Flavor** Procter & Gamble	powder		psyllium hydrophilic mucilloid, 3.4g/tsp			dextrose · sodium, 3mg/tsp
GL LA PU SO	**Metamucil Smooth Texture, Citrus or Orange** Procter & Gamble	powder		psyllium hydrophilic mucilloid, 3.4g/tsp			citric acid · D&C yellow#10 · FD&C yellow#6 · flavoring · sucrose

See Chapter 12, "Laxative Products," for more information about these products.

LAXATIVE PRODUCTS - continued

	Product Manufacturer/Supplier	Dosage Form	Stimulant	Bulk	Emollient/ Lubricant	Other Laxatives	Other Ingredients
GL LA PU SO	**Metamucil Smooth Texture; Sugar Free, Citrus or Orange** Procter & Gamble	individual packet		psyllium hydrophilic mucilloid, 3.4g/packet			aspartame · citric acid · D&C yellow#10 · FD&C yellow#6 · flavoring · maltodextrin · phenylketonurics: contains phenylalanine, 25mg/dose
** GL LA PU SO	**Metamucil Smooth Texture; Sugar Free, Citrus or Orange** Procter & Gamble	powder		psyllium hydrophilic mucilloid, 3.4g/tsp			aspartame · citric acid · D&C yellow#10 · FD&C yellow#6 · flavoring · maltodextrin · phenylketonurics: contains phenylalanine, 25mg/dose
DY GL LA PU SO	**Metamucil Smooth Texture; Sugar Free, Regular Flavor** Procter & Gamble	powder		psyllium hydrophilic mucilloid, 3.4g/tsp		magnesium sulfate	citric acid, 1% · maltodextrin
**	**Milk of Magnesia** Schein Ph'cal	suspension				magnesium hydroxide, 405mg/5ml	citric acid · purified water
	Milk of Magnesia Pharmaceutical Assoc.	suspension				magnesium hydroxide, 400mg/5ml	
AL DY LA	**Milk of Magnesia** Roxane Labs	suspension				magnesium hydroxide, 390mg/5ml	citric acid · methylparaben · propylparaben · sodium hypochlorite solution
	Milk of Magnesia Cascara Roxane Labs	suspension	cascara sagrada (equivalent to fluidextract, 5ml)			magnesium hydroxide, 390mg/5ml	sorbitol · alcohol · methylparaben · propylparaben
	Milk of Magnesia Cascara Pharmaceutical Assoc.	suspension	cascara aromatic fluidextract, 5ml			magnesium hydroxide, 400mg/5ml	alcohol, 3-3.3%
	Milk of Magnesia Cascara Concentrate Pharmaceutical Assoc.	suspension	cascara aromatic fluidextract, 5ml			magnesium hydroxide, 800mg/5ml	alcohol, 6-6.7%
	Milk of Magnesia Concentrate Pharmaceutical Assoc.	suspension				magnesium hydroxide, 1200mg/5ml	

See Chapter 12, "Laxative Products," for more information about these products.

LAXATIVE PRODUCTS - continued

	Product Manufacturer/Supplier	Dosage Form	Stimulant	Bulk	Emollient/ Lubricant	Other Laxatives	Other Ingredients
AL	**Milk of Magnesia Concentrate** Roxane Labs	suspension				magnesium hydroxide, 1165mg/5ml · glycerin	sorbitol solution, 29% · sugar, 8% · lemon · citric acid · benzyl alcohol (bulk formulation only) · sodium carboxymethylcellulose · sodium hexametaphosphate · sodium citrate · sodium hypochlorite (total sodium, 0.45 mEq/5ml) · vanillin
LA SO	**Milkinol** Schwarz Pharma	emulsion			mineral oil		butylated hydroxyanisole · emulsifier · color · flavor
	Mineral Oil Multisource	liquid			mineral oil		
	Modane Savage Labs	tablet	phenolphthalein, 130mg				acacia · calcium carbonate · calcium sulfate · corn starch · dibasic calcium phosphate · FD&C red#40 aluminum lake · lactose · povidone · shellac · sucrose · titanium dioxide · water · white wax · magnesium stearate · sodium benzoate · talc
	Modane Bulk Savage Labs	powder		psyllium hydrophilic mucilloid, 50%			dextrose, 50% · sodium, 2mg/tsp · potassium, 37mg/tsp
	Modane Plus Savage Labs	tablet	phenolphthalein, 60mg		docusate sodium, 100mg		acacia · calcium carbonate · calcium sulfate · croscarmellose sodium · FD&C yellow#6 aluminum lake · microcrystalline cellulose · povidone · shellac · silica gel · sucrose · titanium dioxide · water · carnauba wax · magnesium stearate · sodium benzoate · talc
	Modane Soft Savage Labs	capsule			docusate sodium, 100mg (sodium, 0.27mEq/dose)	glycerin	gelatin · methylparaben · propylene glycol · propylparaben · sorbitol · water · polyethylene glycol 400
	Natural Bulk Schein Ph'cal	granule		psyllium hydrophilic mucilloid, 3.4g/tsp			

See Chapter 12, "Laxative Products," for more information about these products.

LAXATIVE PRODUCTS - continued

	Product Manufacturer/Supplier	Dosage Form	Stimulant	Bulk	Emollient/ Lubricant	Other Laxatives	Other Ingredients
	Natural Bulk, Orange Flavor Schein Ph'cal	granule		psyllium hydrophilic mucilloid, 3.4g/tsp			sucrose · citric acid · FD&C yellow#6 lake · orange flavor · sodium, <0.01g
	Natural Fiber, Citrus or Orange Goldline Labs	powder		psyllium hydrophilic mucilloid, 3.5g/tbsp			
	Nature's Remedy Block Drug	tablet	cascara sagrada, 150mg · aloe, 100mg				calcium stearate · FD&C blue#2 · FD&C yellow#6 · hydroxypropyl cellulose · lactose · hydroxypropyl methylcellulose · microcrystalline cellulose · titanium dioxide · polyethylene glycol
**	**Neoloid** Kenwood Labs	oil	castor oil, 36.4%				sodium benzoate, 0.2% · potassium sorbate · mint flavoring
	Perdiem Ciba Self-Medication	granule	senna (cassia pod concentrate), 0.74g/tsp	psyllium, 3.25g/tsp			sodium, 1.8mg/tsp · potassium, 35.5mg/tsp · acacia · iron oxides · natural flavors · paraffin · sucrose · talc
	Perdiem Fiber Ciba Self-Medication	granule		psyllium, 4g/tsp			sodium, 1.8mg/tsp · potassium, 36.1mg/tsp · acacia · iron oxides · natural flavors · paraffin · sucrose · titanium dioxide · talc
GL	**Peri-Colace** Roberts Ph'cal	capsule	casanthranol, 30mg		docusate sodium, 100mg		
	Peri-Colace Roberts Ph'cal	syrup	casanthranol, 10mg/5ml		docusate sodium, 20mg/5ml		
	Peri-Dos Goldline Labs	capsule	casanthranol, 30mg		docusate sodium, 100mg		
**	**Phillips'** Bayer Consumer	gelcap	phenolphthalein, 90mg		docusate sodium, 83mg		
AL LA	**Phillips' Milk of Magnesia** Bayer Consumer	suspension				magnesium hydroxide, 400mg/5ml	cherry, mint, or original flavor
GL	**Phillips' Milk of Magnesia** Bayer Consumer	chewable tablet				magnesium hydroxide, 311mg	mint flavor
AL LA	**Phillips' Milk of Magnesia Concentrate** Bayer Consumer	suspension				magnesium hydroxide, 800mg/5ml	strawberry flavor

See Chapter 12, "Laxative Products," for more information about these products.

LAXATIVE PRODUCTS - continued

	Product Manufacturer/Supplier	Dosage Form	Stimulant	Bulk	Emollient/ Lubricant	Other Laxatives	Other Ingredients
	Phospho-soda Buffered Saline, Ginger-Lemon & Unflavored C. B. Fleet	liquid				monobasic sodium phosphate, 2.4g/5ml (sodium, 550mg/5ml) · dibasic sodium phosphate, 0.9g/5ml	flavor
	Pro-Cal-Sof Vangard Labs	capsule			docusate calcium, 240mg		
	Pro-Sof Vangard Labs	capsule			docusate sodium, 100mg; 250mg		
	Pro-Sof Plus Vangard Labs	capsule	casanthranol, 30mg		docusate sodium, 100mg		
GL LA PU SO	**Prulet** Mission Pharmacal	chewable tablet	phenolphthalein, 60mg				flavor
LA PR SU SL	**Purge** Fleming	liquid	castor oil, 95%				lemon-flavored base
	Regulace Republic Drug	gelcap	casanthranol, 30mg		docusate sodium, 100mg		
	Regulax SS Republic Drug	gelcap			docusate sodium, 100mg; 200mg		
SO	**Reliable Gentle Laxative** Goldline Labs	tablet	bisacodyl, 5mg				
	Sani-Supp G & W Labs	suppository				glycerin	sodium stearate
	Senna-Gen Goldline Labs	tablet	senna concentrate, 217mg				
	Senokot Purdue Frederick	suppository	senna concentrate, 652mg				
	Senokot Purdue Frederick	syrup	senna concentrate, 8.8mg sennosides/5ml				alcohol, 7%
	Senokot Purdue Frederick	tablet	senna concentrate, 8.6mg sennosides				sodium, 0.007mEq/dose
	Senokot Purdue Frederick	granule	senna concentrate, 15mg sennosides/tsp				sodium, 0.06mEq/dose
** AL PE	**Senokot Children's** Purdue Frederick	syrup	senna concentrate, 8.8mg sennosides/5ml				methylparaben · potassium sorbate · propylparaben · sucrose · water · chocolate flavor

See Chapter 12, "Laxative Products," for more information about these products.

LAXATIVE PRODUCTS - continued

	Product Manufacturer/Supplier	Dosage Form	Stimulant	Bulk	Emollient/ Lubricant	Other Laxatives	Other Ingredients
	Senokot-S Purdue Frederick	tablet	senna concentrate, 8.6mg sennosides		docusate sodium, 50mg		sodium, 0.15mEq
	SenokotXTRA Purdue Frederick	tablet	senna concentrate, 17mg sennosides				sodium, 0.014mEq/dose
	Senolax Schein Ph'cal	tablet	senna concentrate, 187mg				dicalcium phosphate · microcrystalline cellulose · colloidal silica · magnesium stearate
	Serutan Menley & James Labs	granule		psyllium hydrophilic mucilloid, 2.5mg/tsp			saccharin sodium · sucrose · caramel color · corn starch · invert sugar · oat flour · wheat germ · acacia · sodium carboxymethylcellulose · magnesium stearate
**	**Sof·lax** C. B. Fleet	gelcap			docusate sodium, 100mg		
**	**Sof·lax Overnight** C. B. Fleet	gelcap	casanthranol, 30mg		docusate sodium, 100mg		
GL PU SO	**Stool Softner** Hudson	softgel			docusate sodium, 100mg		
SO	**Surfak 240mg** Pharmacia & Upjohn	softgel			docusate calcium, 240mg	glycerin	alcohol, up to 3% · corn oil · FD&C blue#1 · FD&C red#40 · gelatin · methylparaben · propylparaben · sorbitol
GL SO SU	**Swiss Kriss** Modern Products	powder · tablet	senna, 52.5%	oat bran · psyllium seed husks			
AL LA PR SO SL	**Therevac Plus** Jones Medical	enema			docusate sodium, 283mg	glycerin	benzocaine, 20mg · PEG-400
AL LA PR SL	**Therevac-SB** Jones Medical	enema			docusate sodium, 283mg	glycerin	PEG-400
GL LA SU	**Unilax** B. F. Ascher	capsule	yellow phenolphthalein, 130mg		docusate sodium, 230mg		
GL PU SO	**Uro-Mag** Blaine Ph'cals	capsule				magnesium oxide, 140mg (elemental magnesium, 84.5mg or 6.93mEq)	
DY GL LA PU SO	**V-Lax** Century Ph'cals	powder		psyllium hydrophilic mucilloid, 50%			dextrose, 50%

See Chapter 12, "Laxative Products," for more information about these products.

LAXATIVE PRODUCTS - continued

Product Manufacturer/Supplier	**Dosage Form**	**Stimulant**	**Bulk**	**Emollient/ Lubricant**	**Other Laxatives**	**Other Ingredients**
Woman's Gentle Laxative Goldline Labs	tablet	yellow phenolphthalein, 65mg		docusate sodium, 100mg		

** New listing

See Chapter 12, "Laxative Products," for more information about these products.

ORAL REHYDRATION SOLUTIONS

	Product Manufacturer/Supplier	Osmolarity (mOsm/L)	Carbohydrates (g/L)	Electrolytes (mEq/L)	Other Ingredients
** DY GL LA PU	**Infalyte** Mead Johnson Nutritionals	200	rice syrup solids, 30	sodium, 50 · chloride, 45 · citrate, 34 · potassium, 25	
** PE	**Naturalyte, Bubblegum or Unflavored** Unico	270	dextrose, 25	sodium, 45 · potassium, 20 · chloride, 35 · citrate, 30	
** PE	**Naturalyte, Fruit Flavored or Grape** Unico	270	dextrose, 20 · fructose, 5	sodium, 45 · potassium, 20 · chloride, 35 · citrate, 30	
** PE	**Pedialyte** Ross Products/Abbott Labs	249	dextrose, 25	sodium, 45 · potassium, 20 · chloride, 35 · citrate, 30	water
DY GL LA PU PE	**Pediatric Electrolyte** Goldline Labs		dextrose, 25	citrates, 48 · sodium, 45 · chloride, 35 · potassium, 20	
**	**Rehydralyte** Ross Products/Abbott Labs	304	dextrose, 25	sodium, 75 · potassium, 20 · chloride, 65 · citrate, 30	water
** PE	**Revital Ice Freezer Pops** Clear Mountain Labs		3/62.5ml (dextrose, crystalline fructose, sucrose)	sodium, 45 · chloride, 35 · citrate, 30 · potassium, 20	filtered water · natural flavors · citric acid · cellulose gum · may contain: sodium sorbate and/or sodium benzoate

** New listing

See Chapter 13, "Antidiarrheal Products," for more information about these products.

ANTIDIARRHEAL PRODUCTS

	Product Manufacturer/Supplier	Dosage Form	Adsorbent	Other Active Ingredients	Other Ingredients
**	**Dairy Ease [a]** Blistex	caplet			lactase, 3000 FCC units · colloidal silicon dioxide · dibasic calcium phosphate · magnesium stearate · microcrystalline cellulose · pregelatinized starch
**	**Dairy Ease [a]** Blistex	chewable tablet			lactase, 3000 FCC units · dibasic calcium phosphate · mannitol · colloidal silicon dioxide · magnesium stearate
**	**Dairy Ease [a]** Blistex	drops			water · glycerol · lactase enzyme
GL PU SO	**Diar Aid** Thompson Medical	caplet		loperamide HCl, 2mg	corn starch · lactose · magnesium stearate · microcrystalline cellulose
	Diarrhea and Cramp Relief Goldline Labs	suspension	attapulgite, 600g/15ml		
LA SL	**Diasorb** Columbia Labs	liquid	attapulgite, 750mg/5ml (activated nonfibrous)		
GL PU	**Diasorb** Columbia Labs	tablet	attapulgite, 750mg (activated nonfibrous)		
	Donnagel Wyeth-Ayerst Labs	chewable tablet	attapulgite, 600mg		D&C yellow#10 aluminum lake · FD&C blue#1 aluminum lake · flavors · magnesium stearate · mannitol · saccharin sodium · sorbitol · water
	Donnagel Wyeth-Ayerst Labs	suspension	attapulgite, 600mg/5ml		alcohol, 1.4% · benzyl alcohol · citric acid · FD&C blue#1 · flavors · magnesium aluminum silicate · methylparaben · phosphoric acid · propylene glycol · propylparaben · saccharin sodium · sorbitol · titanium dioxide · water · xanthan gum · carboxymethylcellulose sodium
	Equalactin Numark Labs	chewable tablet	polycarbophil, 500mg		citric acid · flavor · glycine · magnesium stearate · microcrystalline cellulose · sorbitol · stearic acid · povidone
	Imodium A-D McNeil Consumer	caplet		loperamide HCl, 2mg	dibasic calcium phosphate · magnesium stearate · microcrystalline cellulose · colloidal silicon dioxide · FD&C blue#1 · D&C yellow#10
	Imodium A-D McNeil Consumer	liquid		loperamide HCl, 1mg/5ml	alcohol, 5.25% · citric acid · flavors · glycerin · methylparaben · propylparaben · purified water
DY GL LA SL	**K-C** Century Ph'cals	suspension	pectin, 260mg/30ml	kaolin 5.2g/30ml · bismuth subcarbonate, 260mg/30ml	
DY GL LA SL	**Kao-Spen** Century Ph'cals	suspension	pectin, 260mg/30ml	kaolin, 5.2g/30ml	
	Kaodene A-D Pfeiffer Ph'cals	caplet		loperamide HCl, 2mg	

See Chapter 13, "Antidiarrheal Products," for more information about these products.

ANTIDIARRHEAL PRODUCTS - continued

	Product Manufacturer/Supplier	Dosage Form	Adsorbent	Other Active Ingredients	Other Ingredients
	Kaodene NN (Non-Narcotic) Pfeiffer Ph'cals	suspension	pectin, 195mg/30ml	kaolin, 3.89g/30ml · bismuth subsalicylate, 30mg/30ml	
DY LA SU SL	**Kaolin Pectin** Roxane Labs	suspension	pectin, 130.2mg/30ml	kaolin, 5.7g/30ml	glycerin, 1.75% · carboxymethylcellulose sodium, 0.4% · lime/mint flavor · saccharin sodium, 0.025% · methylparaben · propylparaben · magnesium aluminum silicate · sodium hypochlorite solution
LA SL	**Kaopectate** Pharmacia & Upjohn	liquid	attapulgite, 750mg/15ml		flavors · glucono-delta-lactone · magnesium aluminum silicate · methylparaben · sorbic acid · sucrose · titanium dioxide · xanthan gum · purified water
GL PU SO	**Kaopectate** Pharmacia & Upjohn	caplet	attapulgite, 750mg		croscarmellose sodium · hydroxypropyl cellulose · hydroxypropyl methylcellulose · methylparaben · pectin · propylene glycol · propylparaben · sucrose · titanium dioxide · zinc stearate · may also contain talc
LA SL PE	**Kaopectate, Children's** Pharmacia & Upjohn	liquid	attapulgite, 300mg/7.5ml		FD&C red#40 · flavors · glucono-delta-lactone · magnesium aluminum silicate · methylparaben · sorbic acid · sucrose · titanium dioxide · xanthan gum · purified water
** SO SU	**Lactaid [a]** McNeil Consumer	drops			glycerin · water · lactase enzyme
**	**Lactaid [a]** McNeil Consumer	caplet			mannitol · cellulose · lactase enzyme (lactase, 3000 FCC units) · magnesium stearate · dextrose · sodium citrate
**	**Lactaid Extra Strength [a]** McNeil Consumer	caplet			mannitol · cellulose · lactase enzyme (lactase, 4500 FCC units) · magnesium stearate · dextrose · sodium citrate
**	**Lactrase [a]** Schwarz Pharma	capsule			lactase, 250mg · malto-dextrin · magnesium stearate · gelatin · titanium dioxide · yellow iron oxide
GL PU	**Maalox Anti-Diarrheal** Ciba Self-Medication	caplet		loperamide HCl, 2mg	corn starch · lactose · magnesium stearate · microcrystalline cellulose · FD&C blue#1 · D&C yellow#10
	Parepectolin Rhône-Poulenc Rorer Ph'cals	suspension	attapulgite, 600mg/15ml		flavors · glucono-delta-lactone · magnesium aluminum silicate · methylparaben · sorbic acid · sucrose · titanium dioxide · xanthan gum · purified water
DY PU	**Pepto Diarrhea Control** Procter & Gamble	caplet		loperamide HCl, 2mg	corn starch · lactose · magnesium stearate · microcrystalline cellulose
GL PU	**Pepto-Bismol** Procter & Gamble	chewable tablet		bismuth subsalicylate, 262.5mg	calcium carbonate · flavor · magnesium stearate · mannitol · povidone · D&C red#27 aluminum lake · saccharin sodium · talc
**	**Pepto-Bismol** Procter & Gamble	caplet		bismuth subsalicylate, 262.5mg	calcium carbonate · microcrystalline cellulose · mannitol · sodium starch glycolate · povidone · magnesium stearate · D&C red#27 aluminum lake · silicon dioxide · polysorbate 80

See Chapter 13, "Antidiarrheal Products," for more information about these products.

ANTIDIARRHEAL PRODUCTS - continued

	Product Manufacturer/Supplier	Dosage Form	Adsorbent	Other Active Ingredients	Other Ingredients
LA SU SL	**Pepto-Bismol Maximum Strength** Procter & Gamble	liquid		bismuth subsalicylate, 1050mg/30ml	benzoic acid · flavor · magnesium aluminum silicate · methylcellulose · D&C red#22 · D&C red#28 · saccharin sodium · salicylic acid · sodium salicylate · sorbic acid · water
LA SU SL	**Pepto-Bismol Original Strength** Procter & Gamble	liquid		bismuth subsalicylate, 525mg/30ml	benzoic acid · flavor · magnesium aluminum silicate · methylcellulose · D&C red#22 · D&C red#28 · saccharin sodium · salicylic acid · sodium salicylate · sorbic acid · water
GL PU	**Pepto-Bismol, Cherry** Procter & Gamble	chewable tablet		bismuth subsalicylate, 262.39mg	adipic acid · calcium carbonate · flavors · magnesium stearate · mannitol · povidone · D&C red#27 aluminum lake · FD&C red#40 aluminum lake · saccharin sodium · talc
LA SO SL	**Percy Medicine** Merrick	liquid		bismuth subnitrate, 959mg/10ml · calcium hydroxide, 21.9mg/10ml · potassium carbonate, 5.6mg/10ml	distilled water · ethyl alcohol, 5% · glycerin · gum arabic · rhubarb fluid extract · sugar · flavors · natural color
	Pink Bismuth Goldline Labs	chewable tablet		bismuth subsalicylate, 262mg	
GL PU	**Rheaban** Pfizer Consumer	caplet	activated attapulgite, 750mg		carnauba wax · croscarmellose sodium · D&C yellow#10 aluminum lake · D&C blue#1 aluminum lake · hydroxypropyl cellulose · hydroxypropyl methylcellulose · methylparaben · pectin · pharmaceutical glaze · propylene glycol · propylparaben · sucrose · titanium dioxide · zinc stearate · talc

** New listing
[a] This preparation can be added to milk products and/or taken with milk to prevent osmotic diarrhea.

See Chapter 13, "Antidiarrheal Products," for more information about these products.

HEMORRHOIDAL PRODUCTS

	Product Manufacturer/Supplier	Dosage Form	Anesthetic	Vasoconstrictor [a]	Astringent	Protectant	Other Ingredients
	Americaine Hemorrhoidal Ciba Self-Medication	ointment	benzocaine, 20%				benzethonium chloride, 0.1% · polyethylene glycol 300 · polyethylene glycol 3350
	Anusert G & W Labs	suppository		phenylephrine, 0.25%		hard fat, 88.7%	
	Anusol Warner Wellcome Consumer	ointment	pramoxine HCl, 1%		zinc oxide, 12.5%	mineral oil, 46.7% · cocoa butter · kaolin · peruvian balsam	polyethylene wax · benzyl benzoate · dibasic calcium phosphate · glyceryl monooleate · glyceryl monostearate · polyethylene wax
**	**Anusol** Warner Wellcome Consumer	suppository	benzyl alcohol			topical starch, 51%	partially hydrogenated soy bean oil · sorbitan tristearate · tocopheryl · acetate
	Balneol Solvay Ph'cals	lotion				mineral oil · lanolin oil	propylene glycol · glyceryl stearate/PEG-100 stearate · PEG-40 stearate · laureth-4, PEG-4 dilaurate · sodium acetate · carbomer 934 · triethanolamine · methylparaben · dioctyl sodium sulfosuccinate · fragrance · acetic acid
	Calmol 4 Mentholatum	suppository				cocoa butter, 80% · zinc oxide, 10%	glyceryl stearate · methylparaben · propylparaben · bismuth subgallate
	Fleet Medicated Wipes C. B. Fleet	pad			witch hazel, 50%	glycerin, 10%	methylparaben · benzalkonium chloride
**	**Fleet Pain-Relief** C. B. Fleet	pad	pramoxine HCl, 1%			glycerin, 12%	
	Hem-Prep G & W Labs	ointment · suppository		phenylephrine, 0.25%	zinc oxide, 11%	petrolatum, 89% · hard fat, 89% (suppository)	
	Hemorid for Women Thompson Medical	cream	pramoxine HCl, 1%	phenylephrine HCl, 0.25%		petrolatum, 30% · mineral oil, 20%	water · stearyl alcohol · cetyl alcohol · methylparaben · propylparaben · polysorbate 80 · aloe vera gel
**	**Hemorid for Women** Thompson Medical	ointment	pramoxine HCl, 1%	phenylephrine HCl, 0.25%		petrolatum, 82.15% · mineral oil, 12.5%	aloe · white wax
	Hemorid for Women Thompson Medical	suppository		phenylephrine HCl, 0.25%	zinc oxide, 231mg	hard fat, 88.25%	aloe

See Chapter 14, "Hemorrhoidal Products," for more information about these products.

HEMORRHOIDAL PRODUCTS - continued

	Product Manufacturer/Supplier	Dosage Form	Anesthetic	Vasocon-strictor [a]	Astringent	Protectant	Other Ingredients
**	**Hydrosal Hemorrhoidal** Hydrosal	ointment	benzyl alcohol, 1.4%	ephedrine sulfate, 0.2%	zinc oxide, 5%	lanolin, 14.25% · petrolatum, 22.5% · mineral oil, 14.25%	aloe · water · sorbitan sesquioleate · D&C red#33 · ceresin wax
	Hygenic Cleansing Schein Ph'cal	pad			witch hazel, 50%	glycerin, 10%	alcohol, 7% · water · methylparaben · benzalkonium chloride
	Lanacane Creme Combe	cream	benzocaine, 6%				benzethonium chloride, 0.1% · water-washable base
	Medicone E. E. Dickinson	ointment	benzocaine, 20%			light mineral oil · white petrolatum	
	Medicone E. E. Dickinson	suppository		phenylephrine HCl, 0.25%		hard fat, 88.7%	corn starch · methylparaben · propylparaben
	Nupercainal Ciba Self-Medication	ointment	dibucaine, 1%				acetone · sodium bisulfite · water · lanolin · white petrolatum · light mineral oil
	Nupercainal Ciba Self-Medication	suppository			zinc oxide, 0.25g	cocoa butter, 2.1g	acetone sodium bisulfite · bismuth subgallate
	Pazo Bristol-Myers Products	suppository		ephedrine sulfate, 0.2%	zinc oxide, 5%		hydrogenated vegetable oil
	Pazo Bristol-Myers Products	ointment	camphor, 2%	ephedrine sulfate, 0.2%	zinc oxide, 5%	lanolin, 5% · petrolatum	
	Preparation H Whitehall-Robins Healthcare	suppository				cocoa butter, 79% · shark liver oil, 3%	ascorbyl palmitate · benzoic acid · BHA · corn oil · disodium edetate · glycerin · methylparaben · PEG-12 dilaurate · propylparaben · tocopherol · water · wax
	Preparation H Whitehall-Robins Healthcare	ointment		phenylephrine HCl, 0.25%		petrolatum, 71.9% · mineral oil, 14% · shark liver oil, 3%	beeswax · benzoic acid · BHA · corn oil · lanolin alcohol · methylparaben · paraffin · propylparaben · thyme oil · tocopherol · water · lanolin · glycerin

See Chapter 14, "Hemorrhoidal Products," for more information about these products.

HEMORRHOIDAL PRODUCTS - continued

	Product Manufacturer/Supplier	Dosage Form	Anesthetic	Vasoconstrictor [a]	Astringent	Protectant	Other Ingredients
	Preparation H Whitehall-Robins Healthcare	cream		phenylephrine HCl, 0.25%		petrolatum, 18% · glycerin, 12% · shark liver oil, 3%	BHA · carboxymethyl cellulose · sodium · cetyl alcohol · citric acid · disodium edetate · glyceryl oleate · glyceryl stearate · methylparaben · propyl gallate · propylparaben · simethicone · sodium benzoate · sodium lauryl sulfate · stearyl alcohol · tocopherol · xanthan gum · water · lanolin · propylene glycol
**	**Procto Foam** Schwarz Pharma	foam	pramoxine HCl, 1%				butane · cetyl alcohol · glyceryl monostearate · methylparaben · PEG-100 stearate · polyoxyethylene 23 lauryl ether · polyoxyl 40 stearate · propane · propylene glycol · propylparaben · purified water · trolamine
**	**Prompt Relief** Goldline Labs	suppository				cocoa butter, 79% · shark liver oil, 3%	
**	**Prompt Relief** Goldline Labs	ointment				petrolatum, 79.3% · shark liver oil, 3%	
	Sani G & W Labs	pad			witch hazel, 50%	glycerin, 10%	
	Sooth-It Health Care Products	pad			witch hazel, 50%	glycerin	alcohol, 7% · water · aloe vera · sodium citrate · citric acid · benzalkonium chloride · methylparaben · sodium hydroxide
	Sooth-It Plus Health Care Products	pad	pramoxine HCl, 1%		witch hazel, 21% · witch hazel extract	glycerin, 26.5%	aloe vera · benzalkonium chloride · citric acid · methylparaben · purified water · sodium hydroxide
	Tronolane Ross Products/Abbott Labs	cream	pramoxine HCl, 1%		zinc oxide	glycerin	beeswax · cetyl alcohol · cetyl esters wax · methylparaben · propylparaben · sodium lauryl sulfate
	Tronolane Ross Products/Abbott Labs	suppository			zinc oxide, 5%	hard fat, 95%	

See Chapter 14, "Hemorrhoidal Products," for more information about these products.

HEMORRHOIDAL PRODUCTS - continued

	Product Manufacturer/Supplier	Dosage Form	Anesthetic	Vasoconstrictor [a]	Astringent	Protectant	Other Ingredients
	Tronothane Hydrochloride Abbott Labs	cream	pramoxine HCl, 1%			glycerin	cetyl alcohol · cetyl esters wax · sodium lauryl sulfate · methylparaben · propylparaben
	Tucks Warner Wellcome Consumer	pad			witch hazel, 50%	glycerin	alcohol · propylene glycol · sodium citrate · diazolidinyl urea · citric acid · methylparaben · propylparaben
**	**Tucks Clear** Warner Wellcome Consumer	gel	benzyl alcohol		witch hazel, 50%	glycerin, 10%	carbomer 9748 · disodium edetate · propylene glycol · sodium hydroxide
	Vaseline Pure Petroleum Jelly Chesebrough-Pond's	ointment				white petrolatum, 100%	
**	**Wyanoids Relief Factor** Wyeth-Ayerst Labs	suppository				cocoa butter, 79% · shark liver oil, 3% · glycerin	ascorbyl palmitate · benzoic acid · BHA · corn oil · disodium edetate · methylparaben · PEG-12 dilaurate · propylparaben · tocopherol · water · white wax

** New listing

[a] Patients who are taking monoamine oxidase inhibitors or who have diabetes, hyperthyroidism, hypertension, cardiovascular disease, or difficulty in urination due to prostate enlargement should not use products containing a vasoconstrictor without first consulting a physician.

See Chapter 14, "Hemorrhoidal Products," for more information about these products.

ANTHELMINTIC PRODUCTS

	Product Manufacturer/Supplier	Dosage Form	Active Ingredients	Other Ingredients
LA SL	**Antiminth** Pfizer Consumer	suspension	pyrantel pamoate, 250mg/5ml	caramel-currant flavor · citric acid · glycerin · lecithin · magnesium aluminum silicate · polysorbate · povidone · simethicone emulsion · sodium benzoate · sorbitol solution
	Ascarel Pfeiffer Ph'cals	liquid	pyrantel pamoate, 50mg/ml	
LA SU PE	**Pin-X** Effcon Labs	liquid	pyrantel pamoate, 50mg/1ml	citric acid · lecithin · methylparaben · povidone · propylparaben · saccharin sodium · sodium benzoate · glycerin · magnesium aluminum silicate · polysorbate 80 · propylene glycol · purified water
	Reese's Pinworm Reese Chemical	liquid	pyrantel pamoate, 144mg/ml	
	Reese's Pinworm Reese Chemical	caplet	pyrantel pamoate, 180mg	

** New listing

See Chapter 15, "Anthelmintic Products," for more information about these products.

EMETIC PRODUCTS

	Product Manufacturer/Supplier	Dosage Form	Active Ingredients	Other Ingredients
**	**Ipecac** Multisource	syrup	powdered ipecac	alcohol, 1.5-1.75% · glycerin · purified water

** New listing

See Chapter 16, "Emetic and Antiemetic Products," for more information about these products.

GASTRIC DECONTAMINANT PRODUCTS

	Product Manufacturer/Supplier	Dosage Form	Activated Charcoal	Other Ingredients
**	**Actidose with Sorbitol** Paddock Labs	liquid	25g/120ml; 50g/240ml	sorbitol
**	**Actidose-Aqua** Paddock Labs	liquid	15g/72ml; 25g/120ml; 50g/240ml	
** DY GL SU	**CharcoAid** Requa	suspension	30g/120ml	sorbitol, 70%
** DY GL SU	**CharcoAid 2000** Requa	suspension	50g/240ml	water
**	**Charcoal Plus DS** Kramer Labs	tablet	250mg	sugar powder · stearic acid · gum arabic · calcium sulfate · sugar cane · gelatin · talc · red#40 aluminum lake · titanium dioxide · povidone · sodium benzoate
DY GL	**CharcoCaps** Requa	caplet	260mg	sugar, 300mg · cycopodium clavatum · cinchona officionalis · sulfur · carbo vegetabilus
DY GL	**CharcoCaps** Requa	tablet	250mg	sugar, 250mg
DY GL SU	**CharcoCaps** Requa	capsule	260mg	
**	**Liqui Char** Jones Medical	liquid	25g/4fl oz	water
**	**Liqui Char** Jones Medical	liquid	25g/4fl oz	sorbitol, 27g/4fl oz

** New listing

See Chapter 16, "Emetic and Antiemetic Products," for more information about these products.

ANTIEMETIC PRODUCTS

	Product Manufacturer/Supplier	Dosage Form	Active Ingredients	Other Ingredients
PU	**Bonine** Pfizer Consumer	chewable tablet	meclizine HCl, 25mg	raspberry flavor · corn starch · FD&C red#40 · lactose · magnesium stearate · purified siliceous earth · saccharin · talc
	Calm-X Republic Drug	tablet	dimenhydrinate, 50mg	
**	**Cola** Unico	syrup	phosphoric acid	high fructose corn syrup and/or sucrose · water · caramel color · natural flavors · caffeine
GL PU SO	**Dramamine** Pharmacia & Upjohn	chewable tablet	dimenhydrinate, 50mg	aspartame · citric acid · FD&C yellow#5 · flavor · magnesium stearate · methacrylic acid copolymer · sorbitol · FD&C yellow#6
PU SO	**Dramamine II Less Drowsy Formula** Pharmacia & Upjohn	tablet	meclizine HCl, 25mg	colloidal silicon dioxide · corn starch · lactose · D&C yellow#10 aluminum lake · microcrystalline cellulose · magnesium stearate
GL PU SO	**Dramamine Original** Pharmacia & Upjohn	tablet	dimenhydrinate, 50mg	colloidal silicon dioxide · croscarmellose sodium · lactose · magnesium stearate · microcrystalline cellulose
AL LA SL PE	**Dramamine, Children's** Pharmacia & Upjohn	liquid	dimenhydrinate, 12.5mg/5ml	FD&C red#40 · flavor · glycerin · methylparaben · sucrose · water
	Emetrol, Cherry or Lemon Mint Pharmacia & Upjohn	liquid	phosphoric acid, 21.5g/5ml	dextrose, 1.87g/5ml · fructose, 1.87g/5ml · FD&C red#40 (Cherry) · D&C yellow#10 (Lemon Mint) · flavors · glycerin · methylparaben · purified water
AL	**Especol** Pfeiffer Ph'cals	solution	phosphorated carbohydrate solution	
	Marezine Martin Himmel	tablet	cyclizine HCl, 50mg	cellulose · lactose · starch · hydrogenated vegetable oil · magnesium stearate · silicon dioxide
DY GL SO SU	**Nauzene** Alva-Amco Pharmacal	tablet	diphenhydramine HCl, 25mg	lactose microcrystalline cellulose · stearic acid · magnesium stearate
	Triptone Del Ph'cals	tablet	dimenhydrinate, 50mg	

** New listing

See Chapter 16, "Emetic and Antiemetic Products," for more information about these products.

OSTOMY APPLIANCES

	Product Manufacturer/Supplier	Product Form	Size (in)	Quantity	Comments
**	**Active Life Drainable Pouches with Stomahesive Skin Barrier** ConvaTec	pouch	10 · 12	10/bx	one piece · stoma opening sizes: 0.75"-2.5"
**	**Adhesive Drainable Pouches** Hollister	pouch	12 · 16	50/bx	standard adhesive · transparent odor-barrier film · opening sizes: 1"-3"
**	**Closed-End Adhesive Pouches** Bard	pouch	5 x 8 · 5.5 x 8 · 6.5 x 10	10/pk	odorproof · rustlefree · extra gauge · one piece · rounded corners
**	**Cool Comfort Nu-Support Belts** Nu-Hope Labs	belt	width: 3, 4, 6, 9 · circumference: petite/youth 16-27, adult 28-52	1/bx	lightweight, ventilated elastic · hinged horizontally for contoured fit · standard pouch opening is 2 3/8"
**	**Drainable Adhesive Pouches** Bard	pouch	regular, 6 x 11 3/16 · mini, 5 x 9 1/4	10/pk	odorproof · rustlefree · extra gauge · one piece · regular available in plain or wide opening
**	**Karaya Seal Drainable Pouches** Hollister	pouch	9 · 12 · 16	30/bx	Karaya 5 seal ring and microporous adhesive · opening sizes: 1"-2" and 1"-3"
** PE	**Little Ones Active Life Drainable Pouches** ConvaTec	pouch	6	15/bx	transparent · one piece · stoma opening sizes: 5/16"-2"
** PE	**Little Ones Sur-Fit Drainable Pouches** ConvaTec	pouch	6	10/bx	transparent · flange sizes: 1.25" and 1.75"
**	**Nu-Flex Adult Oval or Round Drainable Pouches** Nu-Hope Labs	pouch	11	1/pk	transparent · stoma sizes: 0.5"-2" (Round) and "trim to fit" (Oval)
**	**Nu-Flex Adult Oval or Round Urinary Pouches** Nu-Hope Labs	pouch	11	1/pk	one piece · transparent · 3.5" adhesive foam pad (Round) · stoma sizes: 0.5"-2" (Round) and "trim to fit" (Oval)
**	**Nu-Flex Brief or Mini Urinary Pouches** Nu-Hope Labs	pouch	7 (Mini) · 8 (Brief)	1/pk	one piece · transparent · 3" adhesive foam pad · stoma sizes: 0.5"-2"
**	**Nu-Self Adult or Brief Drainable Pouches** Nu-Hope Labs	pouch	7.5 (Brief) · 11 (Adult)	1/pk	opaque · stoma sizes: 0.5"-2" · 3.5" adhesive foam pad (Adult)
**	**Sheer Plus Drainable Pouches** Smith & Nephew	pouch	11 · 12.25 · 12.5	10/pk	clear or opaque · one piece · 4" x 4" adhesive face plate on free-floating collar with barrier · odor proof · Pre-Fit or Trim 'n' Fit openings
**	**Stoma Urine Bags** Bard	bag	adult 6 x 13.25 · medium 6.5 x 10.25 · pediatric 5.2 x 8.5	5/pk	adhesive · one piece
**	**Sur-Fit Drainable Pouches** ConvaTec	pouch	10 · 12	10/bx	flange sizes: 1.25"-2.75"

See Chapter 17, "Ostomy Care Products," for more information about these products.

OSTOMY APPLIANCES - continued

	Product Manufacturer/Supplier	Product Form	Size (in)	Quantity	Comments
**	**Torbot Belts** Torbot	belt	Elastic Web: 1 1/8 width, up to 45 · Reliabelt: 5 width; small, medium, large · Rubber: adjustable, for wet environment · Versatile: 2 or 3 width	1/pk	4 types for various sizes and uses
**	**Torbot Foam Pads** Torbot	pad	diameter: 2 11/16-4 7/8 · thickness: 1/16, 1/8	1/pk	use with cement between faceplate and skin for greater comfort · does not allow leakage · available in black or white foam
**	**Torbot Plastic Pouches, Opaque White** Torbot	pouch	10 · 12	1/pk	lined · heavy duty · odorproof · reusable; average life of 2 weeks
**	**Torbot Plastic Pouches, Transparent** Torbot	pouch	9 · 10 · 11	1/pk	lightweight, clear vinyl · reusable; average life of one week or until odor is detected
**	**Torbot Plastic Urinary Pouches, Opaque White** Torbot	pouch	10 · 12	1/pk	lined · heavy duty · odorproof · reusable; average life of 2 weeks · small, narrower spout for special urinal outlet
**	**Torbot Plastic Urinary Pouches, Transparent** Torbot	pouch	pediatric 6.5 · 9 · 10 · 11	1/pk	lightweight, clear vinyl · includes small spout fitted for urinal valve and stem · reusable; average life of one week or until odor is detected
**	**Torbot Rubber Pouches** Torbot	pouch	9 · 10 · 11 · 12	1/pk	recommended for use by ostomates with loose drainage · high quality butyl rubber · for longer term usage · available in black or white, folded or welded seam, and lightweight or medium weight
**	**Torbot Rubber Urinary Pouches** Torbot	pouch	pediatric 5.5 · 9 · 10 · 11 · 12	1/pk	high quality butyl rubber · for longer term usage · small, narrower spout for special urinal outlet · available in black or flesh pink, with metal or plastic valve and stem
**	**Urostomy Pouches** Hollister	pouch	12 · 16	20/bx	Karaya 5 seal ring · standard adhesive · transparent odor-barrier film · opening sizes: 1"-2"
**	**VPI Non-Adhesive Colostomy Systems** VPI	pouch	closed-end: 6 · open-end: 8	2/pk · 10/pk	reusable system · for single patient use only · closed-end set includes pouches, o-ring seal, and belt · open-end set includes pouches, o-ring seal, belt, and drain tail closure · flange sizes: 1 7/8", 2 3/8", 2 7/8"
**	**VPI Non-Adhesive Ileostomy Systems** VPI	pouch	300cc · 500cc	1-4/pk	reusable system · for single patient use only · set includes pouch, o-ring seal, belt, and drain tail closure
**	**VPI Non-Adhesive Urostomy Systems** VPI	pouch	300cc · 500cc · 800cc · 1100cc	1/pk	reusable system · for single patient use only · set includes pouch, o-ring seal, and belt

** New listing

See Chapter 17, "Ostomy Care Products," for more information about these products.

OSTOMY ACCESSORIES

	Product Manufacturer/Supplier	Ingredients
	Adhesive Disk Products	
	A-Ds Transdermal Patch Torbot	medical grade adhesive
**	**Blanchard Karaya Wafers** Blanchard	karaya gum powder, 70% · glycerin, 30%
	Lan-Tex Torbot	hydrophilic polymer combined with synthetic rubber polymer
	Stomaseal 3M Health Care	acrylate adhesive · polyethylene film
	Universal Adhesive Gaskets Smith & Nephew	rubber-based adhesive
	Cement Products	
	Liquid Cement Perry Products	rubber base · ethyl ether, 24% · alcohol, 5% · nitromersol, 0.005%
	Mastisol Ferndale Labs	gum mastic
	Skin-Bond Cement Smith & Nephew	natural rubber · hexane
	Skin-Bond Cement (Nonflammable) Smith & Nephew	natural rubber · trichloroethane
	Solvent Products	
	Atlantic Adhesive Remover Torbot	naphtha petroleum
	Detachol Ferndale Labs	paraffin hydrocarbons
	Remove Adhesive Remover Smith & Nephew	C10-11 isoparaffin · aloe extract · benzyl alcohol
	Uni-Solve Adhesive Remover Smith & Nephew	1, 1, 1-trichloroethane · naphtha
	Appliance Deodorizer Products	
	Banish II Liquid Deodorant Smith & Nephew	zinc ricinoleate
	Liquid Deodorant Perry Products	water · alcohol · fragrance
	Odo-Way Appliance Deodorant Tablets Smith & Nephew	dicalcium phosphate · magnesium stearate · chloride
	Oxychinol Ferndale Labs	potassium oxyquinoline sulfate
	QAD Tablets Torbot	quaternary ammonium compound

See Chapter 17, "Ostomy Care Products," for more information about these products.

OSTOMY ACCESSORIES - continued

Product Manufacturer/Supplier	Ingredients
Super Banish Appliance Deodorant Smith & Nephew	silver nitrate · ethylene thiourea
Internal Deodorizer Products	
CharcoCaps Caplets, Capsules, or Tablets Requa	activated charcoal, 260mg (caplet, capsule) · activated charcoal, 250mg (tablet) · sugar, 300mg (caplet, capsule)
Devrom Chewable Tablets Parthenon	bismuth subgallate
Skin Protective Products	
Barri-Care Moisture Barrier Ointment Care-Tech Labs	chloroxylenol, 0.8% · vitamins A, D3, E · mineral oil · petrolatum · milk protein · propylparaben · paraffin · methylparaben · propylene glycol · potassium hydroxide
Care-Creme Cream Care-Tech Labs	chloroxylenol, 0.8% · cetyl alcohol · cod liver oil · lanolin oil · lanolin alcohol · propylene glycol · vitamins A, D3, and E
Formula A Stretchable Karaya Washers & Sheets Smith & Nephew	karaya gum powder · propylene glycol
Pro Cute Ferndale Labs	stearic acid · cetyl alcohol · forlan-LM · ceraphyl 230 · glycerin · triethanolamine · deltyl prime · PVP · sorbic acid · silicone · perfume · menthol · dowicil 200
Skin-Prep Protective Dressing Smith & Nephew	poly MVE/MA n-butyl monoester
Tincture of Benzoin Multisource	tincture of benzoin
Triple Care Cream Smith & Nephew	petrolatum · zinc oxide · aloe · allantoin
Triple Care Extra Protective Barrier Smith & Nephew	chloroxylenol · zinc oxide · petrolatum · karaya · methylcellulose · mineral oil · glycerin
Uni-Salve Ointment Smith & Nephew	petrolatum · benzethonium chloride · chloroxylenol · vitamins A&D
Velvet Fresh Powder Care-Tech Labs	corn starch · tricalcium phosphate · fragrance

** New listing

See Chapter 17, "Ostomy Care Products," for more information about these products.

INSULIN PREPARATIONS

Product Manufacturer/Supplier	Species Source [a]	Onset (h)	Peak (h)	Duration (h)	Preservative	Purity (ppm of proinsulin)	Stability at Room Temp. (mo)	Zinc (mg/ 100 U)	Protein (mg/ 100 U)
Rapid Acting									
Humulin R (Regular Human Insulin) Eli Lilly	h	0.5	2-4	6-8	metacresol	<1	1	0.01-0.04	
Novolin R (Regular Human Insulin) Novo Nordisk Ph'cals	h	0.5	2.5-5	8	metacresol	<1	1, in use	trace	
Novolin R PenFill (Regular Human Insulin, 1.5ml cartridge) Novo Nordisk Ph'cals	h	0.5	2.5-5	8	metacresol	<1	1, in use	trace	
Novolin R Prefilled (Reg. Human Insulin, 1.5ml syringe) Novo Nordisk Ph'cals	h	0.5	2.5-5	8	metacresol	<1	1, in use	trace	
Regular (Purified Pork) Novo Nordisk Ph'cals	p	0.5	2.5-5	8	phenol	<1	1, in use	trace	
Regular Iletin I Eli Lilly	b · p	0.5	2-4	6-8	metacresol	<10	1	0.01-0.04	
Regular Iletin II (Purified Pork) Eli Lilly	p	0.5	2-4	6-8	metacresol	<1	1	0.01-0.04	
Velosulin BR (Buffered Reg. Human Insulin, semi-synthetic) Novo Nordisk Ph'cals	h	0.5	1-3	8	metacresol, 0.3%	<1	1, in use	trace	
Intermediate Acting									
Humulin L (Lente Human Insulin Zinc Suspension) Eli Lilly	h	1-3	6-12	18-24	methylparaben	<1	1	0.12-0.25	none
Humulin N (NPH Human Insulin Isophane Suspension) Eli Lilly	h	1-2	6-12	18-24	phenol · metacresol	<1	1	0.01-0.04	protamine, 0.3-0.5
Iletin I Lente (Zinc Suspension) Eli Lilly	b · p	1-3	6-12	18-24	methylparaben	<10	1	0.12-0.25	none
Iletin I NPH (Isophane Suspension) Eli Lilly	b · p	1-2	6-12	18-26	phenol · metacresol	<10	1	0.01-0.04	protamine, 0.3-0.6
Iletin II Lente (Zinc Suspension, Purified Pork) Eli Lilly	p	1-3	6-12	18-24	methylparaben	<1	1	0.12-0.25	none

See Chapter 18, "Diabetes Care Products and Monitoring Devices," for more information about these products.

INSULIN PREPARATIONS - continued

Product Manufacturer/Supplier	Species Source [a]	Onset (h)	Peak (h)	Duration (h)	Preservative	Purity (ppm of proinsulin)	Stability at Room Temp. (mo)	Zinc (mg/ 100 U)	Protein (mg/ 100 U)
Iletin II NPH (Isophane Suspension, Purified Pork) Eli Lilly	p	1-2	6-12	18-26	phenol · metacresol	<1	1	0.01-0.04	protamine, 0.3-0.6
Lente (Zinc Suspension, Purified Pork) Novo Nordisk Ph'cals	p	2.5	7-15	22	methylparaben	<1	1, in use	0.15	
Novolin L (Lente Human Insulin Zinc Suspension) Novo Nordisk Ph'cals	h	2.5	7-15	22	methylparaben	<1	1, in use	0.15	
Novolin N (NPH Human Insulin Isophane Suspension) Novo Nordisk Ph'cals	h	1.5	4-12	24	phenol · metacresol	<1	1, in use	trace	protamine, 0.35
Novolin N PenFill (NPH Human Insulin Isophane Susp., 1.5ml) Novo Nordisk Ph'cals	h	1.5	4-12	24	phenol · metacresol	<1	0.25 (7 days), in use	trace	protamine, 0.35
Novolin N Prefilled (NPH Human Insulin Iso. Susp., 1.5ml) Novo Nordisk Ph'cals	h	1.5	4-12	24	phenol · metacresol	<1	0.25 (7 days), in use	trace	protamine, 0.35
NPH (Isophane, Purified Pork) Novo Nordisk Ph'cals	p	1.5	4-12	24	phenol · metacresol	<1	1, in use	trace	protamine, 0.35
Mixed (Intermediate/Rapid Acting)									
Humulin 50/50 (50% NPH Isophane Suspension, 50% Regular) Eli Lilly	h	within 1hr	2-12	up to 24	phenol · metacresol	<1	1	0.01-0.04	protamine, 0.27
Humulin 70/30 (70% NPH Isophane Suspension, 30% Regular) Eli Lilly	h	within 1hr	2-12	up to 24	phenol · metacresol	<1	1	0.01-0.04	protamine, 0.3-0.5
Novolin 70/30 (70% NPH Human Iso. Susp., 30% Regular Human) Novo Nordisk Ph'cals	h	0.5	2-12	24	phenol · metacresol	<1	1, in use	trace	protamine, 0.25
Novolin 70/30 PenFill (70% NPH Human, 30% Reg. Human; 1.5ml) Novo Nordisk Ph'cals	h	0.5	2-12	24	phenol · metacresol	<1	0.25 (7 days), in use	trace	protamine, 0.25

See Chapter 18, "Diabetes Care Products and Monitoring Devices," for more information about these products.

INSULIN PREPARATIONS - continued

Product Manufacturer/Supplier	Species Source [a]	Onset (h)	Peak (h)	Duration (h)	Preservative	Purity (ppm of proinsulin)	Stability at Room Temp. (mo)	Zinc (mg/ 100 U)	Protein (mg/ 100 U)
Novolin 70/30 Prefilled (70% NPH Human, 30% Reg Hum.; 1.5ml) Novo Nordisk Ph'cals	h	0.5	2-12	24	phenol · metacresol	<1	0.25 7 days), in use	trace	protamine, 0.25
Long Acting									
Humulin U (Ultralente Human Insulin Extended Zinc Susp.) Eli Lilly	h	4-6	8-20	24-28	methylparaben	<1	1	0.12-0.25	

** New listing
[a] b=beef, p=pork, h=human insulin derived through recombinant DNA biotechnology. Insulins with a combination of beef and pork contain 70% beef and 30% pork.

See Chapter 18, "Diabetes Care Products and Monitoring Devices," for more information about these products.

INSULIN SYRINGES AND RELATED PRODUCTS

	Product Manufacturer/Supplier	Comments
	Syringes	
**	**Autopen** Owen Mumford	pen-like injection device · 6" long, 7 oz. in weight · uses a prefilled, replaceable, 1.5ml cartridge of insulin · two models: delivers 2 to 32 units in 2-unit increments, or delivers 1 to 16 units in 1-unit increments · dial-a-dose selector offers both visual and audio indication of setting · one-handed insulin delivery button
	B-D Micro-Fine IV Syringe Becton Dickinson Consumer	28 gauge, disposable · 3/10, 1/2, or 1cc · for U-100 insulin · packages of 10 in boxes of 100 · capped at both needle and plunger ends for sterility and protection · single scale, single unit markings for precise dosage measurement · large bold numbers · lubricated needle · zero dead space · flat plunger tip
	B-D Ultra-Fine Syringe Becton Dickinson Consumer	29 gauge, disposable · 3/10, 1/2, or 1cc · for U-100 insulin · packages of 10 in boxes of 100 · capped at both needle and plunger ends for sterility and protection · single scale, single unit markings for precise dosage measurement · large bold numbers · lubricated needle · zero dead space · flat plunger tip
	Monoject Ultra Comfort 29 Syringe Can-Am Care	29 gauge, disposable · 3/10, 1/2, or 1cc · for U-100 insulin · individually packaged in tamper-evident, sterile peel packs of five; 30 or 100 count boxes · bold numbers · zero dead space · flat plunger tip · permanently attached, advanced laser-welded needle · improved lubricant
	Monoject Ultra Comfort Syringe Can-Am Care	28 gauge, disposable · 1/2 or 1cc · for U-100 insulin · individually packaged in tamper-evident, sterile peel packs of five; 30 or 100 count boxes · bold numbers · zero dead space · flat plunger tip · permanently attached, advanced laser-welded needle · improved lubricant
	NovoFine 30 Needle Novo Nordisk Ph'cals	30 gauge, disposable · beveled needle tip · siliconized throughout the length · ensures minimal friction with skin · 1/3 inch (8mm) long · for single use only, 100/box · disposable needles specifically designed for use with NovoNordisk insulin delivery systems · protective outer cap, smooth plastic needle cap, and a protective tab · should not be used if protective tab is missing or damaged
**	**NovoPen1.5** Novo Nordisk Ph'cals	lightweight, durable dial-a-dose insulin delivery device · made from stainless steel and high-impact plastic · 6" long, 1.4 oz. in weight · uses 1.5ml cartridges of Novolin human insulin · delivers 1 to 40 units in 1-unit increments · uses the NovoFine 30 disposable needle
**	**Terumo Syringe** Terumo	29 gauge, disposable · 1/4, 1/2, or 1cc · for U-100 insulin · individually sterile wrapped in boxes of 100 · 1/4cc is the only insulin syringe available with 1/2 unit scale markings · 1/2cc has single unit scale markings, and the 1cc has scale markings every two units · large, bold numbers · lubricated needle · zero dead space · tapered hub/flush fit plunger tip · latex free
	Related Products	
**	**Autoject** Owen Mumford	plastic spring-loaded syringe injector to be positioned over skin · press device against injection site, then push button to simultaneously insert needle and inject insulin
**	**Autoject 2** Owen Mumford	plastic spring-loaded syringe injector to be positioned over skin · press device against injection site then push button to simultaneously insert needle and inject insulin · fits most brands and sizes of disposable syringes · can be adjusted for depth of needle penetration · internal syringe cocking device · observation window shows when injection is complete · safety lock prevents accidental discharge
**	**Autoject Mini** Owen Mumford	plastic spring-loaded syringe injector to be positioned over skin · same features as Autoject 2, but in a compact, lightweight size · can be pre-loaded for later use · can deliver doses of 1ml or less
**	**B-D Home Sharps Container** Becton Dickinson Consumer	container for safe disposal of syringes and lancets · leak-proof, puncture-resistant plastic with snap-on lid · red-colored with biohazard symbol · small opening for depositing of syringes and lancets helps prevent children from reaching inside · compact size for easy storage
	B-D Magni-Guide Becton Dickinson Consumer	magnifies entire syringe scale calibrations 2 times to make them easier to read · helps guide syringe needle into insulin vial · syringe is slipped into curved channel of Magni-Guide · insulin vial is snapped into collar at opposite end
	B-D Safe-Clip Becton Dickinson Consumer	clips and stores more than one year's supply of used syringe needles for safe and easy disposal
	Count-a-Dose Jordan Medical	syringe filling device · empty B-D Lo-Dose 1/2cc syringe is secured in easy-to-locate platform · click wheel activates slide to ensure accurate dosage in 1-unit increments · slide moves syringe plunger to control insulin intake · "click" heard and felt as each insulin unit is filled · holds 1 insulin vial, or 2 vials for mixing insulins
	Holdease Meditec	needle guide and syringe/vial holder · unit holds syringe and insulin together in easy-to-handle unit while user fills syringe

See Chapter 18, "Diabetes Care Products and Monitoring Devices," for more information about these products.

INSULIN SYRINGES AND RELATED PRODUCTS - continued

	Product Manufacturer/Supplier	Comments
	Inject-Ease Palco Labs	plastic spring-loaded syringe injector to be positioned over skin · press device against site, push button to simultaneously insert needle and inject insulin · fits most brands and sizes of disposable syringes · can be adjusted for depth of needle penetration
	Instaject Jordan Medical	combination insulin injector and blood lancet device · button-activated · self-contained as injector · fits most brands and sizes of disposable syringes · can be adjusted for depth of needle penetration
	Insuflon Chronimed	small, flexible teflon catheter to be inserted subcutaneously · allows the patient to inject insulin for several days without repeated skin punctures
**	**Insul-eze** Palco Labs	syringe loading device with magnifier · assists patients with impaired vision or manual dexterity problems · magnifies syringe calibration · sits on any flat surface, horizontally or vertically · holds all types of insulin bottles
	Insulgage Meditec	permanent, precalibrated device; purchased according to dose (from 2 to 85 units) · dose marked in Inkprint, raised numbers, Braille and raised numbers, or Braille · two gauges can be used for mixed dosages
**	**Load-Matic** Palco Labs	syringe loading device · allows visually-impaired patients to measure dosage by touch alone · using B-D 1cc syringe, dosage may be set in single-unit or ten-unit increments; dosage may then be used repeatedly without further adjustment
	Monoject Injectomatic Can-Am Care	metal spring-loaded syringe injector · press device against selected injection site to insert needle, then press syringe plunger to inject insulin · increases injection-site alternatives · 1/2cc size for 1/2cc and 3/10cc syringes, 1cc size for 1cc syringes · used only with Monoject disposable syringes and a 90-degree injection angle
	TruHand Whittier Medical	syringe/vial holder with magnifier · easy-to-use device · click sound is heard when insulin vial is locked in place · user fills the syringe while reading enlarged scale markings · insulin vials may be interchanged to allow for mixed dosages
	Wright Prefilled Syringe Case LLW Enterprises	impact-resistant polypropylene case for carrying one prefilled insulin syringe · resembles a fountain pen with clip · holds most types of disposable syringes · case interior holds syringe's plunger in personalized preset position · 90-day product replacement warranty

** New listing

See Chapter 18, "Diabetes Care Products and Monitoring Devices," for more information about these products.

This page intentionally left blank.

GLUCOSE AND KETONE TEST PRODUCTS

	Product Manufacturer/Supplier	Product Form	Biological Fluid Tested	Active Ingredients
	Acetest Bayer Diagnostics	tablet	urine · blood	nitroprusside-glycine · buffer
	Albustix Bayer Diagnostics	strip	urine	tetrabromphenol blue · buffer
	Bili-Labstix Bayer Diagnostics	stick	urine	see Multistix 10 SG
	Chemstrip 2GP Boehringer Mannheim	strip	urine	glucose: tetramethylbenzidine · glucose oxidase · peroxidase · protein: tetrachlorophenol · tetrabromosulfophthalein
**	**Chemstrip 2LN** Boehringer Mannheim	strip	urine	see Chemstrip 10 with SG
**	**Chemstrip 4 the OB** Boehringer Mannheim	strip	urine	see Chemstrip 10 with SG
**	**Chemstrip 6** Boehringer Mannheim	strip	urine	see Chemstrip 10 with SG
**	**Chemstrip 7** Boehringer Mannheim	strip	urine	see Chemstrip 10 with SG
	Chemstrip 8 Boehringer Mannheim	strip	urine	see Chemstrip 10 with SG
	Chemstrip 9 Boehringer Mannheim	strip	urine	see Chemstrip 10 with SG
	Chemstrip 10 with SG Boehringer Mannheim	strip	urine	specific gravity: EGTA · ethyleneglycol-bis (aminoethylether) tetraacetic acid · bromthymol blue · pH: bromthymol blue · methyl red · phenolphthalein · leukocytes: indoxylcarbonic acid ester · diazonium salt · nitrite: 3-hydroxy-1,2,3,4-tetrahydro-7,8-benzoquinoline · sulfanilamide · protein: tetrachlorophenol-tetrabromosulfophthalein · glucose: tetramethylbenzidine · glucose oxidase · peroxidase · ketones: sodium nitroferricyanide · glycine · urobilinogen: 4-methoxybenzene-diazonium-tetrafluoroborate · bilirubin: 2,6-dichlorobenzene-diazonium-tetrafluoroborate · blood: tetramethylbenzidine · 2,5-dimethyl-2,5-dihydroperoxthexane
	Chemstrip bG Boehringer Mannheim	strip	blood	glucose oxidase · peroxidase · o-tolidine · tetramethylbenzidine
	Chemstrip K Boehringer Mannheim	strip	urine	sodium nitroferricyanide · glycine
	Chemstrip uG Boehringer Mannheim	strip	urine	glucose oxidase (aspergillus niger) · peroxidase (horseradish) · tetramethylbenzidine
	Chemstrip uGK Boehringer Mannheim	strip	urine	glucose oxidase (aspergillus niger) · peroxidase (horseradish) · tetramethylbenzidine · sodium nitroferricyanide · glycine
	Clinistix Bayer Diagnostics	strip	urine	glucose oxidase · peroxide o-tolidine
	Clinitest Bayer Diagnostics	tablet	urine	copper reduction

See Chapter 18, "Diabetes Care Products and Monitoring Devices," for more information about these products.

Indication of Product Deterioration	Test Time (sec)	Drug Interference	Comments [a]
tan-to-brown discoloration or darkening	30	some false (+)	tests for ketones · requires dropper and clean, white paper
discoloration or darkening of reagent area	60	some false (+) · some masking of color development	tests for protein · match strip to color blocks
see Multistix 10 SG	see Multistix 10 SG	see Multistix 10 SG	tests for glucose, protein, pH, blood, ketones, and bilirubin
discoloration of test area	60 (dip & read)	phenazopyridine	tests for glucose and protein
discoloration of test area	60 (dip & read)	see Chemstrip 10 with SG	tests for leukocytes and nitrite
discoloration of test area	60 (dip & read)	see Chemstrip 10 with SG	tests for leukocytes, protein, glucose, and blood
discoloration of test area	60 (dip & read)	see Chemstrip 10 with SG	tests for leukocytes, pH, protein, glucose, ketones, and blood
discoloration of test area	60 (dip & read)	see Chemstrip 10 with SG	tests for leukocytes, pH, protein, glucose, ketones, bilirubin, and blood
discoloration of test area	1-60 (dip & read)	see Chemstrip 10 with SG	tests for leukocytes, pH, protein, glucose, ketones, urobilinogen, bilirubin, and blood
see Chemstrip 10 with SG	see Chemstrip 10 with SG	see Chemstrip 10 with SG	tests for leukocytes, nitrite, pH, protein, glucose, ketones, urobilinogen, bilirubin, and blood
discoloration of test area	60 (dip & read)	phenazopyridine · mesna	tests for specific gravity, pH, leukocytes, nitrite, protein, glucose, ketones, urobilinogen, bilirubin, and blood
darkening of test area when compared to "unused" color block on side of vial	120	dopamine or methyldopa in concentration of 10mg/dL will cause false (-)	tests for glucose in capillary blood · requires drop of blood on both zones of the test strip · requires cotton ball to wipe off blood after 60 seconds · can be read visually after 60 additional seconds or used with an Accu-Chek II, IIm, or III meter
discoloration of test area	60 (dip & read)	mesna	tests for ketones
discoloration of test area	60 (dip & read)		tests for glucose
discoloration of test area	60 (dip & read)	mesna	tests for glucose and ketones
tan or dark test area	10	no false (+) · some false (-) (levodopa, ascorbic acid, aspirin)	tests for glucose · convenient for type II diabetics · not quantitative
deep blue tablet	15	false (+) in presence of reducing agents · no false (-)	tests for glucose · use either 2-drop or 5-drop method · for use by type I diabetics · most reliable at high glucose levels · use for "sliding scale" · packaged with water dropper and test tube

GLUCOSE AND KETONE TEST PRODUCTS - continued

	Product Manufacturer/Supplier	Product Form	Biological Fluid Tested	Active Ingredients
	Combistix Bayer Diagnostics	strip	urine	see Hema-Combistix
	Dextrostix Bayer Diagnostics	strip	blood	see Clinistix
	Diastix Bayer Diagnostics	strip	urine	glucose oxidase · peroxidase · potassium iodide · chromogen
**	**Glucofilm** Bayer Diagnostics	strip	blood	glucose oxidase · peroxidase · tetramethylbenzidine
	Glucostix Bayer Diagnostics	strip	blood	glucose oxidase · peroxidase · ortho-tolidine dihydrochloride
	Hema-Combistix Bayer Diagnostics	strip	urine	pH: methyl red · bromthymol blue · protein: tetrabromphenol blue · buffer · glucose: glucose oxidase · peroxidase · potassium iodide · buffer · blood: disopropylbenzene dihydroperoxide · 5,5'-tetramethylbenzidine · buffer
	Keto-Diastix Bayer Diagnostics	strip	urine	glucose oxidase · nitroprusside
	Ketostix Bayer Diagnostics	strip	urine	nitroprusside
	Labstix Bayer Diagnostics	strip	urine	glucose oxidase · nitroprusside
	Micral Boehringer Mannheim	strip	urine	anti-human albumin IgG (mouse) · labeled with colloidal gold · fixed albumin
	Multistix Bayer Diagnostics	strip	urine	see Multistix 10 SG
	Multistix 2 Bayer Diagnostics	stick	urine	see Multistix 10 SG
	Multistix 7 Bayer Diagnostics	stick	urine	see Multistix 10 SG
	Multistix 8 SG Bayer Diagnostics	stick	urine	see Multistix 10 SG
	Multistix 9 SG Bayer Diagnostics	stick	urine	see Multistix 10 SG
	Multistix 10 SG Bayer Diagnostics	strip	urine	glucose: glucose oxidase · peroxidase · potassium iodide · buffer · bilirubin: 2,4-dichloroaniline diazonium salt · buffer · ketone: sodium nitroprusside · buffer · specific gravity: bromthymol blue · poly (methyl vinyl ether/maleic anhydride) · sodium hydroxide · blood: disopropylbenzene dihydroperoxide · 5.5'-tetramethylbenzidine · buffer · pH: methyl red · bromthymol blue · protein: tetrabromphenol blue · buffer · urobilinogen: p-diethylaminobenzaldehyde · nitrite: p-arsanilic acid · 1,2,3,4-tetrahydrobenzo(h)-quinolin-3-ol · buffer · leukocytes: derivatized pyrrole amino acid ester · diazonium salt · buffer

See Chapter 18, "Diabetes Care Products and Monitoring Devices," for more information about these products.

Indication of Product Deterioration	Test Time (sec)	Drug Interference	Comments [a]
see Hema-Combistix	see Hema-Combistix	see Hema-Combistix	tests for glucose, protein, and pH
test area does not resemble "0" on color chart	60	no false (+) · some false (-)	tests for glucose · useful in screening · accurate if read by Dextrometer · can use to correlate blood and urine levels
variation from light blue or "neg" on color chart	30	no false (+) · some complete false (-) (levodopa, ascorbic acid, aspirin)	tests for glucose · under-reading possible at high glucose levels · for use by both type I and type II diabetics
discoloration or darkening of reagent areas	60	some slightly lower results	tests for glucose
discoloration or darkening of reagent area	120	some slightly lower results	tests for glucose · blot after 30 seconds, read after 90 additional seconds
discoloration or darkening of test area	proper read time is critical for optimal results · glucose: 30 · blood: 60 · protein and pH: up to 120	no false (+) for glucose · some false (+) · some false (-) · color may be masked	tests for glucose, pH, protein, and blood
green glucose area; darkened ketone area	15-30	no false (+) for glucose · some false (-)	tests for glucose and ketones
tan or brown	15	false (+) possible but rare (levodopa)	tests for acetoacetic acid · useful in determining whether or not a diabetic is developing ketoacidosis
discoloration of test area	30-60 (dip & read)	no false (+) for glucose · some false (-)	tests for blood, pH, glucose, ketones, and protein
variation from white to red	5 (dip) · 60 (read)	oxytetracycline	tests for human albumin
see Multistix 10 SG	see Multistix 10 SG	see Multistix 10 SG	tests for glucose, protein, pH, bilirubin, and urobilinogen
see Multistix 10 SG	see Multistix 10 SG	see Multistix 10 SG	tests for nitrite and leukocytes
see Multistix 10 SG	see Multistix 10 SG	see Multistix 10 SG	tests for glucose, protein, pH, blood, ketones, nitrite, and leukocytes
see Multistix 10 SG	see Multistix 10 SG	see Multistix 10 SG	tests for glucose, protein, pH, blood, ketones, nitrite, leukocytes, and specific gravity
see Multistix 10 SG	see Multistix 10 SG	see Multistix 10 SG	tests for glucose, protein, pH, blood, ketones, bilirubin, nitrite, and specific gravity
discoloration or darkening of test area	proper read time is critical for optimal results · glucose & bilirubin: 30 · ketone: 40 · specific gravity: 45 · urobilinogen, blood, & nitrite: 60 · leukocytes: 120 · pH & protein: up to 120	no false (+) for glucose · some false (+) · some false (-) · color may be masked	test for glucose, bilirubin, ketones, specific gravity, blood, pH, protein, urobilinogen, nitrite, and leukocytes

GLUCOSE AND KETONE TEST PRODUCTS - continued

	Product Manufacturer/Supplier	Product Form	Biological Fluid Tested	Active Ingredients
	Multistix SG Bayer Diagnostics	stick	urine	see Multistix 10 SG
	N-Multistix Bayer Diagnostics	strip	urine	see Multistix 10 SG
	N-Multistix SG Bayer Diagnostics	stick	urine	see Multistix 10 SG
**	**Supreme** Chronimed	strip	blood	
	Uristix Bayer Diagnostics	strip	urine	see Multistix 10 SG
**	**Uristix 4** Bayer Diagnostics	strip	urine	see Multistix 10 SG

** New listing
[a] Protect all products from light, heat, and moisture.

See Chapter 18, "Diabetes Care Products and Monitoring Devices," for more information about these products.

Indication of Product Deterioration	Test Time (sec)	Drug Interference	Comments [a]
see Multistix 10 SG	see Multistix 10 SG	see Multistix 10 SG	tests for glucose, protein, pH, blood, ketones, bilirubin, urobilinogen, leukocytes, and specific gravity
see Multistix 10 SG	see Multistix 10 SG	see Multistix 10 SG	tests for glucose, protein, pH, blood, ketones, bilirubin, and nitrite
see Multistix 10 SG	see Multistix 10 SG	see Multistix 10 SG	tests for glucose, protein, pH, blood, ketones, bilirubin, urobilinogen, nitrite, and specific gravity
	60		tests for glucose · apply blood to test areas; turn strip over after 60 seconds; read by comparing color of strip's reverse side to color chart · may also be used with a Supreme meter
discoloration of test area	30-60 (dip & read)	no false (+) for glucose · some false (-)	tests for glucose and protein; useful to determine if protein is in urine (diabetic nephropathy)
discoloration of test area	30-60 (dip & read)	no false (+) for glucose · some false (-)	tests for glucose, protein, nitrite, and leukocytes

BLOOD GLUCOSE METERS

	Product Manufacturer/Supplier	Test Strip	Method	Test Time (sec)	Range (mg/dL)
	Accu-Chek Advantage Boehringer Mannheim	Accu-Chek Advantage	no timing, no wiping, no cleaning	40	20-600
	Accu-Chek Easy Boehringer Mannheim	Accu-Chek Easy	no timing, no wiping, visual confirmation	15-60	20-500
**	**Accu-Chek III** Boehringer Mannheim	Chemstrip bG	wiping required, visual confirmation	120	20-500
**	**Accu-Chek Instant** Boehringer Mannheim	Accu-Chek Instant	no timing, no wiping, visual confirmation	12	20-500
	CheckMate Plus Cascade Medical	CheckMate Plus	no timing, no wiping	30-70	25-500
**	**Diascan Partner** Home Diagnostics	Diascan	wipe	90	10-600
	Diascan-S Home Diagnostics	Diascan	wipe, visual confirmation	90	10-600
	ExacTech Card Model MediSense	ExacTech	no timing, no wiping, no cleaning; 3-step process	30	40-450
	Glucometer Elite Bayer Diagnostics	Glucometer Elite	no timing, no wiping	60	40-500
	Glucometer Encore Bayer Diagnostics	Glucometer Encore	no timing, no wiping	15-60	10-600
**	**Glucometer M+** Bayer Diagnostics	Glucofilm	wipe	60	20-500
	MediSense 2 Card Model MediSense	MediSense 2	no timing, no wiping, no cleaning	20	20-600
	MediSense 2 Pen Model MediSense	MediSense 2	no timing, no wiping	20	20-600
	One Touch Basic LifeScan	Genuine One Touch	no timing, no wiping; 3-step process	45	0-600
**	**One Touch Profile** LifeScan	Genuine One Touch	no timing, no wiping; 3-step process	45	0-600
**	**Precision Q·I·D** MediSense	Precision Q·I·D Microflo	no timing, no wiping; 2-step process; hand-held	20	20-600

See Chapter 18, "Diabetes Care Products and Monitoring Devices," for more information about these products.

Memory Capacity	Calibration	Warranty	Battery	Dimensions (in) (L x W x H)	Weight (oz)	Comments
100 tests; with time and date	lot-specific code chip	3 years	(2) 3-volt lithium	3.6 x 2.4 x 0.6	3	shows time and date · new strip requires 30% less blood than previous strip
350 tests; with time and date, ave./min./max. event markers	lot-specific code chip	3 years	6-volt alkaline	4.5 x 2.5 x 0.75	3.4	shows time and date · 7-day test average · event markers · 7-day max./min. value · control marker
20 tests; with time and date	lot-specific code strip	2 years	6-volt alkaline	5.5 x 2.7 x 0.8	5.4	shows time and date · test strips may also be read visually
9 tests	push-button	3 years	(4) 1.5-volt alkaline	4 x 2.2 x 0.6	1.76	
255 tests; with time and date	automatic	lifetime	(2) 3-volt lithium	6.3 x 1.1 x 0.7	1.8	built-in lancing device · activity markers code test results · word prompts in 6 languages · data port for CheckLink software
10 tests				3.1 x 8.4 x 0.61	7.8	voice instructions guide user through test procedure · error codes announced · minimal cleaning required
10 tests	single button	2 years	J-type 6-volt alkaline (1,500 tests)	3.1 x 5.2 x 0.6	4.8	extreme temperature warnings
1 test	2 steps with calibrator bar	4 years	non-replaceable (4,000 tests)	2.15 x 3.65 x 0.375	1.5	credit card size
10 tests	code strip	5 years	(2) 3-volt lithium (DL or CR 2032)	3.38 x 2.5 x 0.5	1.75	after blood touches the test strip, the blood is drawn into a chamber within the strip for automatic sampling
10 tests	push-button	3 years	non-replaceable (15,000 tests)	4.3 x 2.5 x 0.7	3.6	test strips have easy-grip feature
300 tests; with 14-day average and number of tests/day	push-button	3 years	(2) AA alkaline	5.6 x 3.1 x 0.9	8	volume control · user may set alarms
125 downloadable tests, 10 recallable tests	1 step with calibrator bar	4 years	non-replaceable (4,000 tests)	2.15 x 3.65 x 0.375	1.5	credit card size
125 downloadable tests, 10 recallable tests	1 step with calibrator bar	4 years	non-replaceable (4,000 tests)	5.4 x 0.1	1.1	pen shape/size
1 test	built-in single button	3 years	J-type 6-volt alkaline	4.75 x 2.63 x 1.06	4.8	prompts in English or Spanish · alerts user when the meter requires cleaning
250 tests; with time and date, 14- and 30-day averages by time of day or activity	built-in single button	5 years	(2) AAA alkaline	4.3 x 2.6 x 1.2	4.5	shows time and date · 15 event labels · screen prompts, in any one of 19 languages, alert user in response to test results · alerts user the meter requires cleaning · records insulin type/dosage and carbohydrates · In Touch diabetes management software available, IBM Windows format
125 downloadable tests, 10 recallable tests	1 step with calibrator bar	4 years	non-replaceable (4,000 tests)	3.82 x 1.89 x 0.57	1.4	extra large display · test strip ensures correct blood sampling · Precision Link diabetes management software available, Windows format

BLOOD GLUCOSE METERS - continued

Product Manufacturer/Supplier	Test Strip	Method	Test Time (sec)	Range (mg/dL)
Supreme Chronimed	Supreme	no timing, no wiping	55	40-400
Ultra+ Home Diagnostics	Ultra+	no timing, no wiping, visual confirmation	45	0-600

** New listing

See Chapter 18, "Diabetes Care Products and Monitoring Devices," for more information about these products.

Memory Capacity	Calibration	Warranty	Battery	Dimensions (in) (L x W x H)	Weight (oz)	Comments
	single button	3 years	J-type 6-volt alkaline	5 x 2.25 x 0.75	4.5	color chart may serve as a visual-read backup
2 tests	single button	2 years	J-type 6-volt alkaline	2.8 x 3.9 x 1.2	4.7	

BLOOD SUGAR ELEVATING PRODUCTS

	Product Manufacturer/Supplier	Dosage Form	Comments
	B-D Glucose Becton Dickinson Consumer	chewable tablet	glucose, 5g; 19cal · orange flavor
	DEX4 Glucose Can-Am Care	chewable tablet	dextrose, 4g; 15cal · grape, lemon, orange, or raspberry flavor · vitamin C · convenient plastic tube of 10 tablets or bottle of 50 tablets
	DextroEnergy Glucose Aero Assemblies	chewable tablet	dextrose, 3g; 12.5cal · vitamin C · black currant, lemon, orange, original, or raspberry flavor · 14 tablets/pack
DY	**Glutose** Paddock Labs	gel	glucose, 15g (dextrose solution, 40%); 60cal · lemon flavor · tube of 15g or 45g
DY	**Glutose** Paddock Labs	chewable tablet	glucose, 5g; 20cal · lemon flavor
GL	**Insta-Glucose** ICN Ph'cals	gel	carbohydrate, 24g; 96cal · cherry flavor · convenient plastic tube of one unit dose
	Monojel Glucose Can-Am Care	gel	glucose, 10g (dextrose, 40%); 46cal · orange flavor · individual foil packet

See Chapter 18, "Diabetes Care Products and Monitoring Devices," for more information about these products.

MISCELLANEOUS DIABETES PRODUCTS

	Product Manufacturer/Supplier	Comments
	Carrying Cases	
	Control Injection Monitor Kit IMK-1A Mustang	carrying case holds a one-week supply of syringes and swabs, plus two insulin vials and a needle break-off disk · is also a syringe storage box for patient to verify if shots have been taken · dimensions: 12" x 8" x 1.75"
	Control Injection Monitor Kit IMK-1B Mustang	carrying case designed for use by physically/visually impaired patients · holds a one-week supply of prefilled syringes, plus swabs and a needle break-off disk · is also a syringe storage box for patient to verify if shots have been taken · dimensions: 12" x 8" x 1.75"
**	**Daily Diabetic's Case** Medport	compact version of Diabetic's Travel Organizer · organizes a 3-day supply · includes one refreezable ice pack · can be attached to a belt or carried by the strap · dimensions: 6.75" x 5.5" x 2.5"
**	**Dia-Pak Jr.** Atwater Carey	compact version of Dia-Pak Original · optional adjustable waist belt · dimensions: 6" x 5" x 1.5"
**	**Dia-Pak Mini** Atwater Carey	smallest version of Dia-Pak Original · semi-rigid case protects 2 pre-drawn insulin syringes, a small glucose meter, and a few additional supplies; compatible with all insulin pen systems · optional refreezable cold gel packs · clips to belt · dimensions: 2" x 6" x 1"
**	**Dia-Pak Original** Atwater Carey	water-resistant, nylon-fabric carrying case for daily supplies · organizes a 2-week supply · optional refreezable cold gel packs with insulating insert · optional adjustable waist belt or adjustable shoulder strap · dimensions: 6" x 8" x 2.5"
**	**Diabetic's Travel Organizer** Medport	insulated, water-resistant, nylon-fabric carrying case for daily supplies · organizes a 2-week supply · includes 2 refreezable ice packs · one side of case keeps supplies cool, the other side keeps supplies at room temperature · includes removable pouch used for safe storage of medical waste until disposal · carried by handle · dimensions: 9" x 6" x 2.5"
**	**Diabetic's Traveler and Diabetic's Traveler II** Entry 21	insulated, water-resistant, nylon-vinyl carrying cases for daily supplies · keep insulin cold for up to 10 hours · include refreezable ice pack · Traveler includes adjustable shoulder strap; dimensions: 9" x 8" x 2.5" · Traveler II dimensions: 6" x 7" 2.5"
**	**Diabetic's Wallet** Medport	smallest version of Diabetic's Travel Organizer · rigid case protects 4 pre-drawn insulin syringes, a small glucose meter, and a few additional supplies · includes one refreezable ice pack · dimensions: 9" x 3" x 0.75"
**	**DK Organizer** Cases Plus	carrying case for daily supplies · watertight, hard shell exterior · made from ABS plastic · lightweight, durable, dust proof, shock-resistant · foam interior with molded compartments protects supplies · carried by handle or optional shoulder strap · dimensions: 9" wide x 7.5" tall x 3.2" deep · also available are DK Plus Organizer 9" x 7.5" x 6" and DK Max Organizer 14" x 10.5" x 6"
**	**Insul-Tote** Palco Labs	foam-insulated nylon-fabric carrying case for daily supplies · includes a refreezable gel pack · available in a back-opening model or a top-opening model with shoulder strap · both models' dimensions: 7" x 7" x 3"
**	**Insul-Tote Junior** Palco Labs	smaller version of Insul-Tote · includes adjustable hip strap · dimensions: 6" x 4.5" x 3"
	Insulin Protector Medicool	insulated nylon-fabric carrying case for daily supplies · keeps insulin cool for up to 16 hours · cooler component may be prerefrigerated to keep insulin cool, or unrefrigerated to prevent insulin from freezing in extremely cold conditions · comes with 2 refreezable cooler packs · dimensions: 7.75" x 4" x 2.5"
	ProtectAll Medicool	insulated nylon-fabric carrying case for daily supplies · removable cooler compartment accommodates 2 insulin vials or a pen system and 2 pen vials, keeping them cool for up to 12 hours · additional storage compartments and pockets · carried around the waist or over the shoulder with strap that adjusts up to 52 inches
**	**Thermakit** Jordan Medical	thermal styrofoam case for insulin · holds 2 insulin vials and 2 insulin syringes · dimensions: 2" x 6" x 2"
	Computer Software	
**	**Diabetes Works** ITA Software	requires IBM-compatible PC with Windows · five computer programs packaged together: Insulin Therapy Analysis v2.1 pharmacologically predicts user's glucose results, Diabetes Easy Internet Access uses America Online, Glucose Plotter v1.4 uploads data from One Touch II and One Touch Profile meters, Diabetes Diet Analyzer examines three meals plus snacks, and Dear Diary v2.5 accepts personal journaling of graphs/tables and events/comments

See Chapter 18, "Diabetes Care Products and Monitoring Devices," for more information about these products.

MISCELLANEOUS DIABETES PRODUCTS - continued

	Product Manufacturer/Supplier	Comments
**	**Glucotrac** Kaufman Assoc.	DOS computer program · user follows on-screen instructions · provides running monthly averages of fasting, a.m., p.m., and nighttime glucose test results · creates graphs which represent a pictoral overview of blood glucose control
**	**Level** HealthWare	Windows-based computer program · uploads data from One Touch II and One Touch Profile meters · provides detailed graphing of numerous trends all on a single page (shows many interrelationships) · provides total health profile including exercise history, caloric intake, mental stress level, illness, etc. · three data fields are left available for tracking data of personal choice · fully guaranteed
**	**MedMaster** Generation Software	Windows-based computer program · uploads data from Boehringer Mannheim and LifeScan meters · tracks and reports data including test results, meals, activities, averages and trend analysis, medication, diary and appointment entries, and graphing · includes comprehensive 138-pp. user manual
**	**Mellitus Manager** MetaMedix	requires IBM-compatible 386 (or higher) PC with Windows and at least 4 megabytes of memory · uploads data from Accu-Chek, MediSense, and One Touch meters · creates graphs and tables
	Lancets and Lancing Devices	
**	**Auto-Lancet** Palco Labs	lancing device · pen shape · regular deep penetration endcaps that screw on
**	**Autolet Lite** Owen Mumford	lancing device · mechanized lancet ejection eliminates risk of accidental injury · uses shallow, regular, and deep penetration platforms
	Autolet Lite Clinisafe Owen Mumford	professional lancing device for clinically safer blood sampling · ejection of both Unilet lancet and platform after each use at the push of a button · shallow, regular, and deep penetration platforms
**	**B-D Lancet Device** Becton Dickinson Consumer	lancing device · pen shape · uses B-D Ultra-Fine lancets and others
	B-D Ultra Fine Lancet Becton Dickinson Consumer	lancet · 28 gauge needle · fits most lancing devices · boxes of 100 and 200
**	**Carelet Safety** Gainor Medical	lancet · needle automatically retracts after use/exposure · single use only
	Cleanlet Gainor Medical	lancet · 25 gauge needle · snap-on protective cap virtually eliminates accidental needle sticks · needle tip snaps securely into protective cap for safe disposal after a single use
PE	**Cleanlet Kids** Gainor Medical	lancet · 25 gauge (0.5mm) needle · snap-on protective cap virtually eliminates accidental needle sticks · needle tip snaps securely into protective cap for safe disposal after a single use · comes in 6 bright colors per box
	Dialet Home Diagnostics	lancing device · pen shape · comes with one regular, one deep puncture endcap · for safety, blue dot appears when device is armed
	E-Z Ject Can-Am Care	lancet · needle has a comfortable "junior" lite angle · fits most lancing devices · boxes of 100 and 200 · ivory-colored or assorted colors
**	**E-Z Let** Palco Labs	lancet · tri-beveled needle point · fits most lancing devices · boxes of 100 and 200
**	**Gentle-let 1** Ulster Scientific	lancing device · needle retracts automatically for disposal after single use · normal or extra spring pressure
**	**Gentle-let, GP style** Ulster Scientific	lancet · fits most lancing devices
**	**Gentle-let-PC** Ulster Scientific	lancing device · pen shape
	Glucolet Bayer Diagnostics	lancing device with clip · pen shape · regular and deep penetration endcaps
	Haemolance Chronimed	lancing device · 21 gauge needle · built-in needle protection · needle retracts automatically for disposal after single use

See Chapter 18, "Diabetes Care Products and Monitoring Devices," for more information about these products.

MISCELLANEOUS DIABETES PRODUCTS - continued

	Product Manufacturer/Supplier	Comments
**	**Hemalet** Home Diagnostics	lancing device with clip · pen shape
**	**Lady Lite** Medicore	lancet · delicate, fine needle tip, designed for the feminine fingertip · cap is rose-shaped · fits most lancing devices · boxes of 200
**	**Medi-Lance II** Medicore	lancet · fits most lancing devices · boxes of 200
	Medi-Let Medicore	lancing device · patented lancet ejector arm · uses platforms with two penetration depths
	MediSense Lancing Device MediSense	lancing device · pen shape · uses Ultra TLC lancets · provides controlled depth of penetration
	Monoject Monojector Can-Am Care	lancing device with clip · pen shape
	Monolet Can-Am Care	lancet · the original "universal fit" design · tri-beveled needle point · 100-count box
	Penlet II LifeScan	lancing device · pen shape · "hands-off" lancet removal system to minimize possibility of accidental lancet needle sticks · comes with LifeScan lancets and two different endcaps to control the depth of penetration
**	**Soft Touch II** Boehringer Mannheim	lancing device · pen shape · regular and deep penetration endcaps that screw on · uses Soft Touch lancets and others
**	**Softclix** Boehringer Mannheim	lancing device · pen shape · adjustable dial allows for six lancet penetration depths · device's design reduces the lancet's lateral motion when entering the skin · uses Softclix lancets
**	**Unilet and Unilet G.P.** Owen Mumford	lancet · 21 gauge, 0.81mm diameter needle · Unilet G.P. fits more lancing devices than Unilet · Unilet in 200-count boxes · Unilet G.P. in boxes of 100 and 200
**	**Unilet Superlite and Unilet G.P. Superlite** Owen Mumford	lancet · 23 gauge, 0.66mm diameter needle · needle has just two cutting faces · Unilet G.P. Superlite fits more lancing devices than Unilet Superlite · boxes of 30, 100, and 200
**	**Unilet Universal ComforTouch** Owen Mumford	lancet · 26 gauge, 0.45mm diameter needle · needle has just two cutting faces · fits all major lancing devices · cap fits back over needle tip for safe disposal after a single use · boxes of 100 and 200
	Unistik 2 Owen Mumford	lancing device · lancet is concealed before and after use · self-contained lancet needle automatically retracts for disposal after single use · provides controlled depth of lancet penetration (regular or deep) · boxes of 50 and 100
	Medical Identification	
**	**CareCard Medical Card** CareCard	national emergency information system · provides a comprehensive medical history to paramedics and emergency medical technicians on-scene, as well as to the hospital where the patient will be received · provides complete information for hospital admittance · provides parental release allowing immediate treatment of minors · support products include wallet card, sports shoe card, and police certificate · one-time $20 membership fee
**	**Goldware Jewelry** Goldware	bracelets, pendants, watch charm with medical insignia on the front · 14K gold or sterling silver · custom engraved on the back with emergency medical information
**	**Identifind Iron-on Labels** Identifind	permanent · pre-printed with custom emergency medical information · large-print name tags available
**	**Med-I-Dent Jewelry** Med-I-Dent	bracelets, charms, lockets, pendants · 14K gold, sterling silver, vermeil/gold over silver, gold plated brass · all contain a waterproof medical history booklet that patient keeps current (using special pen provided) · custom engraving also available
**	**Medic Alert Jewelry** Medic Alert	bracelets, neck chains/tags with medical insignia on the front · stainless steel, sterling silver, gold-filled, or 14K gold · custom engraved on the back with emergency medical information and company's 24-hour hotline telephone number · around-the-world service available · membership fee starts at $35
**	**MediCheck Identification** MediCheck	bracelets, neck tags, wallet cards · stainless steel; wallet cards made of aluminum · custom engraved with emergency medical information · $15 donation requested

See Chapter 18, "Diabetes Care Products and Monitoring Devices," for more information about these products.

MISCELLANEOUS DIABETES PRODUCTS - continued

	Product Manufacturer/Supplier	Comments
	Meter Accessories	
**	**Digi-Voice Deluxe and Mini-DV** Science Products	voice module which talks user through glucose meter self-test procedure · plugs into the datajack of the One Touch II meter · repeat feature · comes with earphones and audio cassette tape instructions · the Mini-DV is a smaller version
**	**Smart Dot** Pharmacy Counter	blood collector-dropper places a droplet from the finger onto the target area of the glucose meter's test strip · attaches to the One Touch Basic or One Touch II meter
**	**Transfer-Ease** Transfer-Ease	pipette transfers blood sample from the finger to the target area of the glucose meter's test strip · unbreakable, disposable · packaged with easy-to-follow directions

** New listing

See Chapter 18, "Diabetes Care Products and Monitoring Devices," for more information about these products.

This page intentionally left blank.

VITAMIN PRODUCTS

	Product Manufacturer/Supplier	Vitamin A (IU)	Vitamin D (IU)	Vitamin E (IU)	Ascorbic Acid (C) (mg)	Thiamine (B1) (mg)	Riboflavin (B2) (mg)	Niacin (mg)
** DY GL LA PU SO SU	**A-D3-E with Selenium Tablets** Freeda Vitamins	10000	400	100				
GL PU	**ABC Plus Tablets** Hudson	5000 (as acetate and beta carotene)	400	30	60	1.5	1.7	niacinamide, 20
**	**Acerola Chewable Tablet** Goldline Labs				300			
GL PU	**Adavite-M Tablets** Hudson	5000 (as acetate and beta carotene)	400	30	90	3	3.4	20
** SU	**Advanced Stress Formula Plus Zinc Tablets** Sundown			30	500	10	10	100
** SU	**Advanced Stress Formula, w/ or w/o Iron, Tablets** Sundown			30	500	10	10	100
GL PU SU	**Akorn Antioxidants Caplets** Akorn	5000		200	400			
	Allbee C-800 + Iron Tablets Whitehall-Robins Healthcare			45	800	15	17	100
	Allbee C-800 Tablets Whitehall-Robins Healthcare			45	800	15	17	100

See Chapter 19, "Nutritional Products," for more information about these products.

Pyridoxine HCl (B6) (mg)	Cyanocobalamin (B12) (mcg)	Folic Acid (mcg)	Pantothenic Acid (mg)	Iron (elemental) (mg)	Calcium (elemental) (mg)	Phosphorus (mg)	Magnesium (mg)	Other Ingredients
								selenium, 50mcg
2	6	400	10 (as d-calcium pantothenate)	18 (as fumarate)	162 (as dicalcium phosphate)	109	100 (as oxide)	boron, 150mg · potassium, 40mg · chloride, 36.3mg · vitamin K, 25mcg · zinc, 15mg · manganese, 2.5mg · copper, 2mg · silicon, 2mg · iodine, 150mcg · biotin, 30mcg · chromium, 25mcg · molybdenum, 25mcg · selenium, 20mcg · tin, 10mcg · vanadium, 10mcg · nickel, 5mcg
								citrus bioflavonoid complex, 5mg
3	9	400	10 (as d-calcium pantothenate)	27 (as fumarate)	40 (as calcium phosphate)	31	100 (as oxide)	zinc, 15mg · chloride, 7.5mg · potassium, 7.5mg · manganese, 5mg · copper, 2mg · iodine, 150mcg · biotin, 30mcg · molybdenum, 15mcg · chromium, 15mcg · selenium, 10mcg
5	12	400	20					zinc, 24mg · copper, 3mg · biotin, 45mcg
5	12	400	20	27 or 0				biotin, 45mcg
								zinc, 40mg · l-glutathione, 5mg · sodium pyruvate, 3mg · copper, 2mg · selenium, 40mcg · cellulose · stearic acid · magnesium stearate · silicon dioxide
25	12	400	25	27				modified starch · hydrolyzed protein · hydroxypropyl methylcellulose · stearic acid · povidone · silicon dioxide · artificial color · lactose · magnesium stearate · polyethylene glycol 400 or 4000 · vanillin · gelatin · polysorbate 20 or 80 · sorbic acid · sodium benzoate · may also contain: hydroxypropyl cellulose · propylene glycol
25	12		25					modified starch · hydrolyzed protein · hydroxypropyl methylcellulose · stearic acid · artificial color · silicon dioxide · lactose · magnesium stearate · povidone · polyethylene glycol 400 or 4000 · vanillin · gelatin · polysorbate 20 or 80 · sorbic acid · sodium benzoate · may also contain: hydroxypropyl cellulose · propylene glycol

VITAMIN PRODUCTS - continued

	Product Manufacturer/Supplier	Vitamin A (IU)	Vitamin D (IU)	Vitamin E (IU)	Ascorbic Acid (C) (mg)	Thiamine (B1) (mg)	Riboflavin (B2) (mg)	Niacin (mg)
	Allbee with C Caplets Whitehall-Robins Healthcare				300	15	10.2	50
** GL PU SO	**Androvite for Men Tablets** Optimox	4166.7 (as beta carotene and palmitate)	66.7	66.7	166.7	8.3	8.3	8.3 (niacinamide)
	Antioxidant Advanced Formula Tablets Vitaline	12500 (as beta carotene)		200	500		10	
	Antioxidant Formula Gelcaps Goldline Labs	5000 (as beta carotene)		1	250			
GL PU SO SU	**Antioxidant Formula Softgels** Hudson	25000 (as beta carotene)		400	500			
GL PU SO SU	**Antioxidant Vitamin & Mineral Formula Softgels** Hudson	20000 (as beta carotene)		250	400			
**	**Apatate Liquid or Tablets** Kenwood Labs					15		
**	**Apatate with Fluoride Liquid** Kenwood Labs					15		
	Avail Tablets Menley & James Labs	5000	400	30	90	2.25	2.55	niacinamide, 20
** SU	**B 100 "11" B Factors Tablets or Timed-Release Tablets** Sundown					100	100	100
** SU	**B 100% RDA Complex Tablets** Sundown					1.5	1.7	20
** SU	**B 150 "11" B Factors Timed-Release Tablets** Sundown					75	75	75
** SU	**B 50 "11" B Factors Tablets** Sundown					50	50	50

See Chapter 19, "Nutritional Products," for more information about these products.

Pyridoxine HCl (B6) (mg)	Cyanocobalamin (B12) (mcg)	Folic Acid (mcg)	Pantothenic Acid (mg)	Iron (elemental) (mg)	Calcium (elemental) (mg)	Phosphorus (mg)	Magnesium (mg)	Other Ingredients
5			10					microcrystalline cellulose · corn starch · hydroxypropyl methylcellulose · magnesium stearate · silicon dioxide · propylene glycol · lactose · methacrylic acid · triethyl citrate · titanium dioxide · polysorbate 20 · artificial flavor · saccharin sodium · sodium sorbate
0.167	20.8	66.7	16.7	3			83.3 (as oxide)	zinc, 8.3mg · manganese, 1.7mg · copper, 0.3mg · chromium, 33.3mcg · selenium, 33.3mcg · iodine, 25mcg
								selenium, 50mcg
								zinc, 7.5mg · manganese, 1.5mg · copper, 1mg · selenium
								selenium, 50mcg
								carrot powder, 1mg · broccoli powder, 1mg · spinach powder, 1mg · selenium, 50mcg
0.5	25							
0.5	25							sodium fluoride, 0.5mg
3	9	400		18	400		100	zinc, 22.5mg · iodine, 150mcg · chromium, 15mcg · selenium, 15mcg
100	100	400	100					biotin, 100mcg · PABA · inositol · choline · alfalfa (tablets) · watercress · parsley · lecithin (timed-release tablets) · rice bran
2	6	400	10					choline · inositol complex · PABA
75	75	200	75					biotin, 75mcg · PABA · inositol · choline · alfalfa · watercress · parsley · rice bran
50	50	400	50					biotin, 50mcg · choline · bitartrate, 50mg · inositol complex, 50mg · PABA, 50mg · alfalfa · watercress · rice bran · parsley

VITAMIN PRODUCTS - continued

	Product Manufacturer/Supplier	Vitamin A (IU)	Vitamin D (IU)	Vitamin E (IU)	Ascorbic Acid (C) (mg)	Thiamine (B1) (mg)	Riboflavin (B2) (mg)	Niacin (mg)
** SU	**B 50 Complex Capsules or Tablets** Sundown					50	50	50
** SU	**B Complex Maxi Softgels** Sundown					7.5	8.5	100
** SU	**B Complex Maxi Tablets** Sundown					15	17	200
** SU	**B Complex Tablets** Sundown					1.5	1.7	20
** SU	**B Complex with C Tablets** Sundown				500	15	10	100
** SU	**B-C Complex Capsules** Sundown				300	15	10	50
	B-Complex 100 Regular and Controlled Time Release Tablets Vitaline					100	100	niacinamide, 100
	B-Complex 50 Regular and Controlled Time Release Tablets Vitaline					50	50	niacinamide, 50
	B-Complex with Minerals Liquid Pharmaceutical Assoc.					5mg/30ml	2.5mg/30ml	niacinamide, 50mg/30ml
	Beminal-500 Tablets Whitehall-Robins Healthcare				500	25	12.5	niacinamide, 100mg
** SU	**Beta Carotene Softgels** Sundown	10000; 25000 (as beta carotene)						
GL PU SO SU	**Brewers Yeast Tablets** Hudson					0.06	0.02	0.2
** SU	**Buffered C Tablets** Sundown				500			
PU SO PE	**Bugs Bunny Complete Vitamins Plus Minerals Chewable Tablets** Bayer Consumer	5000 (as acetate and beta carotene)	400	30	60	1.5	1.7	20

See Chapter 19, "Nutritional Products," for more information about these products.

Pyridoxine HCl (B6) (mg)	Cyanocobalamin (B12) (mcg)	Folic Acid (mcg)	Pantothenic Acid (mg)	Iron (elemental) (mg)	Calcium (elemental) (mg)	Phosphorus (mg)	Magnesium (mg)	Other Ingredients
50	50	400	500					biotin, 50mcg · PABA · inositol · choline · rice bran · watercress · parsley · lecithin (capsules) · alfalfa (tablets)
10	30	200	50					choline · inositol · PABA
20	60	400	10					choline · inositol complex · PABA
2	6	400						
5	10		20					
5			10 (as calcium pantothenate)					tartrazine
100	100	400	100					choline bitartrate, 100mg · inositol, 100mg · PABA, 30mg · biotin, 100mcg
50	50	100	50					choline bitartrate, 50mg · inositol, 50mg · PABA, 30mg · biotin, 50mcg
1mg/30ml	1mcg/30ml		10mg/30ml	15mg/30ml (as gluconate)			2mg/30ml	alcohol, 18% · choline, 100mg/30ml · inositol, 100mg/30ml · manganese, 2mg/30ml · zinc, 2mg/30ml · iodine, 100mcg/30ml
10	5		20 (as calcium pantothenate)					calcium carboxymethyl cellulose · ethylcellulose · FD&C blue#2 lake · FD&C red#40 lake · FD&C yellow#6 · flavor · iron oxide · lactose · magnesium stearate · mannitol · microcrystalline cellulose · pharmaceutical glaze · polyethylene glycol · starch · talc · titanium dioxide
					25			rose hips
2	6	400	10	18	100	100	20	zinc, 15mg · copper, 2mg · biotin, 40mcg · iodine, 150mcg

VITAMIN PRODUCTS - continued

	Product Manufacturer/Supplier	Vitamin A (IU)	Vitamin D (IU)	Vitamin E (IU)	Ascorbic Acid (C) (mg)	Thiamine (B1) (mg)	Riboflavin (B2) (mg)	Niacin (mg)
PU SO PE	**Bugs Bunny Plus Iron Chewable Tablets** Bayer Consumer	2500 (as acetate and beta carotene)	400	15	60	1.05	1.2	13.5
PU SO PE	**Bugs Bunny with Extra C Children's Chewable Tablets** Bayer Consumer	2500 (as acetate and beta carotene)	400	15	250	1.05	1.2	13.5
GL PU SO SU	**C & E Softgels** Hudson			400	500			
	C Buffered Powder Vitaline				2270/tsp			
**	**C Chewable Tablets** Sundown				250			
**	**C Color Free or Regular Timed-Release Capsules** Sundown				500			
** SU	**C Plus Tablets** Sundown				500; 1000			
**	**C Rolla Chewable Tablets** Sundown				500			
** SU	**C Tablets** Sundown				500; 1000			
** SU	**C Timed-Release Tablets** Sundown				1000; 1500			
** DY GL LA PU SO SU	**C Vitamin Tablets** Freeda Vitamins				100; 250; 500; 1000			
** DY GL LA PU SO SU	**C Vitamin Timed-Release Tablets** Freeda Vitamins				500; 1000			
**	**C with Rose Hips Chewable Tablets** Sundown				500			
** GL PU	**Calcet Plus Tablets** Mission Pharmacal	5000 (as acetate)	400	30	500 (as calcium ascorbate and ascorbic acid)	2.25	2.55	niacinamide, 30
**	**Cecon Solution** Abbott Labs				100/ml			

See Chapter 19, "Nutritional Products," for more information about these products.

Pyridoxine HCl (B6) (mg)	Cyanocobalamin (B12) (mcg)	Folic Acid (mcg)	Pantothenic Acid (mg)	Iron (elemental) (mg)	Calcium (elemental) (mg)	Phosphorus (mg)	Magnesium (mg)	Other Ingredients
1.05	4.5	300		15				sorbitol · flavor
1.05	4.5	300						sorbitol · aspartame · xylitol · flavor
								rose hips powder, 20mg
					500/tsp		200/tsp	potassium bicarbonate, 50mg/tsp
								flavor · sucrose
								rose hips · citrus bioflavonoids · hesperidin · rutin · acerola
								acerola · rose hips · citrus flavonoids · rutin · hesperidin · sucrose · flavor
								rose hips · citrus bioflavonoids · rutin · hesperidin · acerola
								rose hips · flavor · sucrose
3	9	0.8	15 (as d-calcium pantothenate)	18 (as fumarate)	152.8 (as ascorbate and carbonate)			zinc, 15mg (zinc sulfate, dried) · sugar · povidone · color · magnesium stearate · croscarmellose · food glaze · carnauba wax · beeswax · sodium benzoate
								propylene glycol

VITAMIN PRODUCTS - continued

	Product Manufacturer/Supplier	Vitamin A (IU)	Vitamin D (IU)	Vitamin E (IU)	Ascorbic Acid (C) (mg)	Thiamine (B1) (mg)	Riboflavin (B2) (mg)	Niacin (mg)
GL PU	**Ceebevim Caplets** Hudson				300	15	10.2	niacinamide, 50
GL PU SO PE	**Centrum Jr. Shamu and His Crew + Extra C Chew. Tablets** Lederle Consumer	5000	400	30	300	1.5	1.7	20
GL PU PE	**Centrum Jr. Shamu and His Crew + Extra Calcium Chew. Tablets** Lederle Consumer	5000	400	30	60	1.5	1.7	20
GL PU SO PE	**Centrum Jr. Shamu and His Crew + Iron Chew. Tablets** Lederle Consumer	5000	400	30	60	1.5	1.7	20

See Chapter 19, "Nutritional Products," for more information about these products.

Pyridoxine HCl (B6) (mg)	Cyanocobalamin (B12) (mcg)	Folic Acid (mcg)	Pantothenic Acid (mg)	Iron (elemental) (mg)	Calcium (elemental) (mg)	Phosphorus (mg)	Magnesium (mg)	Other Ingredients
5			10 (as d-calcium pantothenate)					
2	6	400	10	18	108	50	40	zinc, 15mg · copper, 2mg · manganese, 1mg · iodine, 150mcg · biotin, 45mcg · molybdenum, 20mcg · chromium, 20mcg · vitamin K, 10mcg · sugar · sorbitol · microcrystalline cellulose · citric acid · food starch · monoglyceride · diglyceride · gelatin · modified food starch · stearic acid · artificial flavors · FD&C red#40 · FD&C yellow#6 · FD&C blue#2 · aspartame · silicon dioxide · magnesium stearate · partially hydrogenated coconut oil · dextrose · lactose · acacia
2	6	400	10	18	160	50	40	zinc, 15mg · copper, 2mg · manganese, 1mg · iodine, 150mcg · biotin, 45mcg · molybdenum, 20mcg · chromium, 20mcg · vitamin K, 10mcg · sugar · sorbitol · food starch · microcrystalline cellulose · citric acid · monoglyceride · diglyceride · gelatin · modified food starch · stearic acid · artificial flavors · FD&C red#40 · FD&C yellow#6 · FD&C blue#2 · silicon dioxide · aspartame · magnesium stearate · partially hydrogenated coconut oil · dextrose · lactose · acacia
2	6	400	10	18	108	50	40	zinc, 15mg · copper, 2mg · manganese, 1mg · iodine, 150mcg · biotin, 45mcg · vitamin K, 10mcg · molybdenum, 20mcg · chromium, 20mcg · sugar · sorbitol · citric acid · food starch · microcrystalline cellulose · monoglyceride · diglyceride · gelatin · stearic acid · artificial flavors · modified food starch · FD&C red#40 · FD&C yellow#6 · FD&C blue#2 · aspartame · silicon dioxide · magnesium stearate · partially hydrogenated coconut oil · dextrose · lactose · acacia

VITAMIN PRODUCTS - continued

	Product Manufacturer/Supplier	Vitamin A (IU)	Vitamin D (IU)	Vitamin E (IU)	Ascorbic Acid (C) (mg)	Thiamine (B1) (mg)	Riboflavin (B2) (mg)	Niacin (mg)
DY GL LA GE	**Centrum Liquid** Lederle Consumer	2500/15ml	400/15ml	30/15ml	60/15ml	1.5/15ml	1.7/15ml	20/15ml
GL LA PU SO GE	**Centrum Silver Tablets** Lederle Consumer	5000	400	45	60	1.5	1.7	20
GL PU SO SU	**Centrum Tablets** Lederle Consumer	5000	400	30	60	1.5	1.7	20
	Certagen Liquid Goldline Labs	2500/15ml	400/15ml	30/15ml	60/15ml	1.5/15ml	1.7/15ml	20/15ml
SO	**Certagen Tablets** Goldline Labs	5000 (with beta carotene)	400	30	60	1.5	1.7	niacinamide, 20
GL PU SU	**Chelated Calcium Magnesium Tablets** Hudson							
GL PU SU	**Chelated Calcium Magnesium Zinc Tablets** Hudson							

See Chapter 19, "Nutritional Products," for more information about these products.

Pyridoxine HCl (B6) (mg)	Cyanocobalamin (B12) (mcg)	Folic Acid (mcg)	Pantothenic Acid (mg)	Iron (elemental) (mg)	Calcium (elemental) (mg)	Phosphorus (mg)	Magnesium (mg)	Other Ingredients
2/15ml	6/15ml		10/15ml	9/15ml				zinc, 3mg/15ml · manganese, 2.5mg/15ml · biotin, 300mcg/15ml · iodine, 150mcg/15ml · chromium, 25mcg/15ml · molybdenum, 25mcg/15ml · alcohol, 6.7% · flavors · BHA · citric acid · eidetic acid · glycerin · polysorbate 80 · sodium benzoate · sucrose
3	25	400	10	4	200	48	100	potassium, 80 mg · chloride, 72mg · zinc, 15mg · manganese, 3.5mg · copper, 2mg · silicon, 2mg · molybdenum, 160mcg · iodine, 150mcg · boron, 150mcg · chromium, 130mcg · biotin, 30mcg · selenium, 20mcg · vanadium, 10mcg · vitamin K, 10mcg · nickel, 5mcg · microcrystalline cellulose · gelatin · modified food starch · maltodextrin · crospovidone · hydroxypropyl methylcellulose · titanium dioxide · magnesium stearate · stearic acid · silicon dioxide · dextrose · triethyl citrate · polysorbate 80 · FD&C blue#2 · FD&C yellow#6 · FD&C red#40
2	6	400	10	18	162	109	100	potassium 80mg · chloride, 72mg · zinc, 15mg · manganese, 3.5mg · copper, 2mg · silicon, 2mg · molybdenum, 160mcg · iodine, 150mcg · boron, 150mcg · chromium, 65mcg · biotin, 30mcg · vitamin K, 25mcg · selenium, 20mcg · tin, 10mcg · vanadium, 10mcg · nickel, 5mcg · microcrystalline cellulose · gelatin · crospovidone · hydroxypropyl methylcellulose · titanium dioxide · magnesium stearate · stearic acid · silicon dioxide · triethyl citrate · polysorbate 80 · FD&C yellow#6 · lactose
2/15ml	6/15ml		10/15ml	9/15ml				biotin, 300mcg/15ml · chromium · iodine · manganese · molybdenum · zinc
2	6	400	10	18	162	125	100	biotin, 30mcg · copper · zinc · iodine · manganese · potassium · chloride · chromium · molybdenum · selenium · nickel · tin · silicon · vanadium · boron · vitamin K1
					500 (as carbonate and oyster shell)		250 (as oxide and gluconate)	
					333.3		133.3	zinc, 8.3mg

VITAMIN PRODUCTS - continued

	Product Manufacturer/Supplier	Vitamin A (IU)	Vitamin D (IU)	Vitamin E (IU)	Ascorbic Acid (C) (mg)	Thiamine (B1) (mg)	Riboflavin (B2) (mg)	Niacin (mg)
GL PU SO PE	**Children's Chewable Vitamins with Extra C Tablets** Hudson	2500 (as acetate and beta carotene)	400	15	250 (as ascorbic acid and sodium ascorbate)	1.05	1.2	niacinamide, 13.5
SO PE	**Children's Multiple Vitamin Chewable Tablets** Vangard Labs	1250 (as acetate and beta carotene)	400	15	60	1.05	1.2	13.5
** PE	**Circus Chews Complete Chewable Tablets** Sundown	5000 (beta carotene, 2500)	400	30	60	1.5	1.7	20
** PE	**Circus Chews with Beta Carotene Chewable Tablets** Sundown	2500 (beta carotene, 1250)	400	15	60	1.05	1.2	13.5
** PE	**Circus Chews with Calcium Chewable Tablets** Sundown	2500 (beta carotene, 1250)	400	15	60	1.05	1.2	13.5
** PE	**Circus Chews with Extra Vitamin C Tablets** Sundown	2500 (beta carotene, 1250)	400	15	250	1.05	1.2	13.5
** PE	**Circus Chews with Iron** Sundown	2500 (beta carotene, 1250)	400	15	60	1.05	1.2	13.5
	Cod Liver Oil Concentrate Capsules Schering-Plough HealthCare	10000	400					
** SU	**D-alpha Tocopherol Softgels** Sundown			400; 1000				
SO	**Daily Multiple Vitamin Tablets** Vangard Labs	5000	400	30	60	1.5	1.7	20
** SU	**Daily Multiple Vitamins & Minerals Tablets** Sundown	5000 (with beta carotene)	400	15	60	1.5	1.7	20
** SU	**Daily Multiple Vitamins, w/ or w/o Iron, Tablets** Sundown	5000 (with beta carotene)	400		60	1.5	1.7	20
GL PU SO SU	**Daily Plus Iron & Calcium Tablets** Hudson	5000 (as acetate and beta carotene)	400	30	60	1.5	1.7	niacinamide, 20

See Chapter 19, "Nutritional Products," for more information about these products.

Pyridoxine HCl (B6) (mg)	Cyanocobalamin (B12) (mcg)	Folic Acid (mcg)	Pantothenic Acid (mg)	Iron (elemental) (mg)	Calcium (elemental) (mg)	Phosphorus (mg)	Magnesium (mg)	Other Ingredients
1.05	4.5	300						
1.05	4.5	300						
2	6	0.4	10	18	100	100	20	zinc, 15mg · copper, 2mg · iodine, 150mcg · biotin, 40mcg · flavor · sucrose · dextrose · aspartame
1.05	4.5	0.3						dextrose
1.05	4.5	0.3			200			flavor · sucrose · dextrose · aspartame
1.05	4.5	0.3						flavor · sucrose · dextrose
1.05	4.5	0.3		15				flavor · dextrose · sucrose
2	6	400	10					
2	6	400	10	18	100	100	100	potassium, 38mg · chloride, 34mg · zinc, 15mg · manganese, 2.5mg · copper, 2mg · iodine, 150mcg · biotin, 10mcg · chromium, 10mcg · molybdenum, 10mcg · selenium, 10mcg · vitamin K, 5mcg
1	1	400	1	18 or 0				tartrazine (with Iron)
2	6	400	10 (as d-calcium pantothenate)	27 (as fumarate)	450 (as carbonate)			zinc, 15mg · zinc oxide

VITAMIN PRODUCTS - continued

	Product Manufacturer/Supplier	Vitamin A (IU)	Vitamin D (IU)	Vitamin E (IU)	Ascorbic Acid (C) (mg)	Thiamine (B1) (mg)	Riboflavin (B2) (mg)	Niacin (mg)
GL PU SO SU	**Daily Vitamins Plus Minerals Tablets** Hudson	5000 (as acetate and beta carotene)	400	30	60	1.5	1.7	20
	Dayalets Filmtabs Tablets Abbott Labs	5000	400	30	60	1.5	1.7	20
	Dayalets Plus Iron Filmtabs Tablets Abbott Labs	5000	400	30	60	1.5	1.7	20
	Decagen Tablets Goldline Labs	9000	400	30mg	90	10	10	20
	Dexatrim Caffeine Free Plus Vitamins Thompson Medical	caplet: 5000 (as acetate and beta carotene)	caplet: 400	caplet: 30	caplet: 60 · timed-release caplet: 180	caplet: 1.5	caplet: 1.7	caplet: niacinamide, 20
** DY GL PU SU	**DiabeVite Tablets** R & D Labs	625 (as beta carotene)	100	100	250	1.5	1.7	20
**	**DiaVite Plus Caplets** Jordan Medical	2000 (beta carotene, 10000)	600	800	500	1.5	1.7	niacinamide, 20
GL PU SO	**Dolomite Tablets** Hudson							
GL PU SO PE	**Ecee Plus Tablets** Edwards Ph'cals			200	100			
	Econo B & C Caplets Vangard Labs				300	15	10.2	50
	Enviro-Stress Slow Release Tablets Vitaline			30	600	50	50	niacinamide, 100

See Chapter 19, "Nutritional Products," for more information about these products.

Pyridoxine HCl (B6) (mg)	Cyanocobalamin (B12) (mcg)	Folic Acid (mcg)	Pantothenic Acid (mg)	Iron (elemental) (mg)	Calcium (elemental) (mg)	Phosphorus (mg)	Magnesium (mg)	Other Ingredients
2	6	400	10 (as d-calcium pantothenate)	18 (as fumarate)	130 (as dicalcium phosphate)	100	100 (as oxide)	potassium, 37.5mg · chloride, 34mg · zinc, 15mg · manganese, 2.5mg · copper, 2mg · iodine, 150mcg · biotin, 30mcg · chromium, 10mcg · molybdenum, 10mcg · selenium, 10mcg
2	6	400						cellulose · hydroxypropyl methylcellulose · povidone · hydroxypropyl cellulose · magnesium stearate · FD&C red#40 · silicon dioxide · FD&C yellow#6 · vanillin
2	6	400		18				cellulose · hydroxypropyl methylcellulose · povidone · hydroxypropyl cellulose · FD&C yellow#6 · magnesium stearate · silicon dioxide · FD&C blue#2 · vanillin · titanium dioxide
5	10	400	20	30				chromium · copper · iodine · potassium · manganese · molybdenum · selenium · zinc, 15mg · vitamin K, 25mcg · biotin, 45mcg
caplet: 2	caplet: 6	caplet: 400	caplet: 10 (as calcium pantothenate)	caplet: 18 (as fumarate)	caplet: 162 (as dicalcium phosphate)		caplet: 100 (as oxide)	caplet: zinc, 15mg · copper, 2mg · potassium iodide, 150mcg · timed-release caplet: phenylpropanolamine HCl, 75mg
2	6	800	10				100	zinc, 15mg · manganese, 2.5mg · copper, 2mg · biotin, 300mcg · chromium, 200mcg · selenium, 25mcg
2	6	400	10	15	80	20	400	citrus bioflavinoids, 50mg · inositol, 50mg · zinc, 15mg · vanadyl sulfate, 6.5mg · manganese, 2.5mg · copper, 2mg · iodine, 150mcg · chromium, 50mcg · biotin, 30mcg · vitamin K, 25mcg · molybdenum, 25mcg · selenium, 25mcg
					130		78	
							70	zinc sulfate, 80mg
5			10					tartrazine
50	25	400	50				60	zinc, 30mg · PABA, 5mg · selenium, 25mcg

VITAMIN PRODUCTS - continued

	Product Manufacturer/Supplier	Vitamin A (IU)	Vitamin D (IU)	Vitamin E (IU)	Ascorbic Acid (C) (mg)	Thiamine (B1) (mg)	Riboflavin (B2) (mg)	Niacin (mg)
GL PU SO SU	**Eye-Vites Tablets** Hudson	5000 (as beta carotene)		30	60			
** SU	**Eyetamins Tablets** Sundown	5000 (as beta carotene)		30	60			
SO	**Family Tabs Advanced Formula** Schein Ph'cal	2500 (as acetate and beta carotene)	400	30	60	1.5	1.7	20
	Femiron Multivitamins and Iron Tablets Menley & James Labs	5000	400	15	60	1.5	1.7	20
** SU	**Fish Liver Oil Softgels** Sundown	8000 (as fish liver oil)						
PU SO PE	**Flintstones Children's Chewable Tablets** Bayer Consumer	2500 (as acetate and beta carotene)	400	15	60	1.05	1.2	13.5
PU SO PE	**Flintstones Complete Chewable Tablets** Bayer Consumer	5000 (as acetate and beta carotene)	400	30	60	1.5	1.7	20
PE	**Flintstones Plus Extra C Children's Chewable Tablets** Bayer Consumer	2500 (as acetate and beta carotene)	400	15	250	1.05	1.2	13.5
PU SO PE	**Flintstones Plus Iron Chewable Tablets** Bayer Consumer	2500 (as acetate and beta carotene)	400	15	60	1.05	1.2	13.5
** SU	**Formula for Life Tablets** Sundown	7500 (beta carotene, 3750)	400	30	100	3	3.4	20
** GL PU	**Fosfree Tablets** Mission Pharmacal	1500 (as acetate)	150		50	5	2	niacinamide, 10
DY GL LA PU SO SU	**Freedavite Tablets** Freeda Vitamins	5000 (with beta carotene)	400	3	60	5	3	niacinamide, 25

See Chapter 19, "Nutritional Products," for more information about these products.

Pyridoxine HCl (B6) (mg)	Cyanocobalamin (B12) (mcg)	Folic Acid (mcg)	Pantothenic Acid (mg)	Iron (elemental) (mg)	Calcium (elemental) (mg)	Phosphorus (mg)	Magnesium (mg)	Other Ingredients
								zinc, 40mg · copper, 2mg · selenium, 40mcg
								zinc, 40mg · copper, 2mg · selenium, 40mcg
2	6	400	10	27 (as fumarate)	450			zinc, 15mg
2	6	400	10	20				FD&C red#40 · FD&C blue#2 · calcium carbonate · microcrystalline cellulose · starch · alginic acid
1.05	4.5	300						sucrose
2	6	400	10	18	100	100	20	zinc, 15mg · copper, 2mg · iodine, 150mcg · biotin, 40mcg · sorbitol
1.05	4.5	300						sucrose · fructose
1.05	4.5	300		15				sucrose
3	10	400	10	18	150	117	100	potassium, 30mg · chloride, 27.2mg · chromium, 25mcg · molybdenum, 25mcg · selenium, 25mcg · zinc, 22.5mg · manganese, 5mg · copper, 2mg · choline bitartrate, 1000mcg · inositol, 1000mcg · iodine, 150mcg · biotin, 30mcg · vitamin K, 25mcg · silicon, 10mcg · tin, 10mcg · vanadium, 10mcg · nickel, 5mcg · rutin · citrus bioflavonoids · hesperidin · lecithin · wheat germ · kelp · amino acids
3	2		1 (as d-calcium pantothenate)	14.5 (as gluconate)	175.5 (as lactate, gluconate, and carbonate)			sugar · polyethylene glycol · color · croscarmellose · povidone · food glaze · magnesium stearate · carnauba wax · beeswax · sodium benzoate
2	2		5 (as calcium pantothenate)	9.9		50		choline, 10mg · inositol, 10mg · potassium gluconate, 5mg · manganese gluconate, 2mg · magnesium gluconate, 2mg · copper gluconate, 0.2mg · zinc gluconate, 0.2mg · potassium iodide, 0.1mg · selenium, 35mcg

VITAMIN PRODUCTS - continued

	Product Manufacturer/Supplier	Vitamin A (IU)	Vitamin D (IU)	Vitamin E (IU)	Ascorbic Acid (C) (mg)	Thiamine (B1) (mg)	Riboflavin (B2) (mg)	Niacin (mg)
** DY GL LA PU SO SU	**Fruit C Chewable Tablets** Freeda Vitamins				100; 200; 500			
PE	**Fruity Chews Chewable Tablets** Goldline Labs	2500	400	15mg	60 (with sodium ascorbate)	1.05	1.2	13.5
PE	**Fruity Chews with Iron Chewable Tablets** Goldline Labs	2500	400	15mg	60 (with sodium ascorbate)	1.05	1.2	13.5
PE	**Garfield Complete Vitamins with Minerals Chewable Tablets** Menley & James Labs	5000	400	30	60	1.5	1.7	20
PE	**Garfield Regular Vitamins Chewable Tablets** Menley & James Labs	2500	400	15	60	1.05	1.2	13.5
PE	**Garfield Vitamins Plus Extra C Chewable Tablets** Menley & James Labs	2500	400	15	250	1.05	1.2	13.5
PE	**Garfield Vitamins Plus Iron Chewable Tablets** Menley & James Labs	2500	400	15	60	1.05	1.2	13.5
	Gen-Bee with C Caplets Goldline Labs				300	15	10.2	50
	Generet-500 Tablets Goldline Labs				500	6	6	30
	Generix-T Tablets Goldline Labs	10000	400	5.5	150	15	10	100
	Geravite Elixir Roberts Ph'cal					1/15ml	1.2/15ml	100/15ml
DY GL LA PU SO SU GE	**Geri-Freeda Tablets** Freeda Vitamins	10000 (with beta carotene)	400	15	150	15	15	niacinamide, 50
SO SU GE	**Gerimed Tablets** Fielding	5000	400	30	120	3	3	25

See Chapter 19, "Nutritional Products," for more information about these products.

Pyridoxine HCl (B6) (mg)	Cyanocobalamin (B12) (mcg)	Folic Acid (mcg)	Pantothenic Acid (mg)	Iron (elemental) (mg)	Calcium (elemental) (mg)	Phosphorus (mg)	Magnesium (mg)	Other Ingredients
1.05	4.5	300						
1.05	4.5	300		12				zinc, 8mg · copper, 0.8mg
2	6	400	10	18	100	100	20	zinc, 15mg · copper, 2mg · iodine, 150mcg · biotin, 40mcg · FD&C red#40 · FD&C blue#2 · FD&C yellow#6 · calcium phosphate · sorbitol · aspartame · flavors · gelatin · talc
1.05	4.5	300						FD&C red#40 · FD&C yellow#6 · FD&C blue#2 · FD&C blue#1 · sucrose · talc · flavors · gelatin · lactose · starch
1.05	4.5	300						FD&C red#40 · FD&C yellow#6 · FD&C blue#2 · FD&C blue#1 · sucrose · talc · flavors · gelatin · lactose · starch
1.05	4.5	300		15				FD&C red#40 · FD&C yellow#6 · FD&C blue#2 · FD&C blue#1 · sucrose · talc · flavors · gelatin · lactose
5			10					
5	25		10	105 (as sulfate)				
2	7.5		10	15				zinc, 1.5mg · copper · iodine · manganese
	10/15ml							alcohol, 15% · l-lysine, 150mg/15ml
15	15	100	15 (as calcium pantothenate)	15 (as fumarate)		100	10	choline, 50 mg · inositol, 50mg · PABA, 30mg · potassium gluconate, 30mg · l-lysine, 25mg · hesperidin complex, 10mg · betaine, 10mg · copper gluconate, 10mg · zinc gluconate, 10mg · iodine, 0.15mg · selenium, 35mcg
2	6				200	600		zinc, 15mg

VITAMIN PRODUCTS - continued

	Product Manufacturer/Supplier	Vitamin A (IU)	Vitamin D (IU)	Vitamin E (IU)	Ascorbic Acid (C) (mg)	Thiamine (B1) (mg)	Riboflavin (B2) (mg)	Niacin (mg)
	Geriot Tablets Goldline Labs				75	5	5	30
	Geritol Complete Tablets SmithKline Beecham	6000	400	30	60	1.5	1.7	20
	Geritol Extend Caplets SmithKline Beecham	3333	200	15	60	1.2	1.4	15
	Geritol Liquid SmithKline Beecham					2.5/15ml	2.5/15ml	50/15ml
DY GL LA SO SL GE	**Gevrabon Liquid** Lederle Consumer					5/ml	2.5/ml	50/ml
GL PU SO	**Gevral T Tablets** Lederle Consumer	5000	400	45	90	2.25	2.6	30
**	**Glutofac Caplets** Kenwood Labs	5000	400	75	300	15	10	50
GL PU SO	**Gynovite Plus Tablets** Optimox	833 (as palmitate)	66.7	66.7	30	1.6	1.6	3.3 (niacinamide)

See Chapter 19, "Nutritional Products," for more information about these products.

Pyridoxine HCl (B6) (mg)	Cyanocobalamin (B12) (mcg)	Folic Acid (mcg)	Pantothenic Acid (mg)	Iron (elemental) (mg)	Calcium (elemental) (mg)	Phosphorus (mg)	Magnesium (mg)	Other Ingredients
0.5	3		2	50 (as sulfate)				
2	6	400	10	18	162	125	100	potassium, 40mg · chloride, 35mg · zinc, 15mg · manganese, 2.5mg · copper, 2mg · iodine, 150mcg · silicon, 80mcg · biotin, 45mcg · vitamin K, 25mcg · chromium, 15mcg · molybdenum, 15mcg · selenium, 15mcg · tin, 10mcg · vanadium, 10mcg · nickel, 5mcg · microcrystalline cellulose · gelatin · hydrolyzed protein · stearic acid · crospovidone · hydroxypropyl methylcellulose · stearic acid glyceride · palmitic acid glyceride · polyethylene glycol · FD&C blue#2 · FD&C red#40 · FD&C yellow#6
2	2	200		10	130	100	35	zinc, 15mg · iodine, 150mcg · vitamin K, 80mcg · selenium, 70mcg · microcrystalline cellulose · stearic acid · croscarmellose sodium · silicon dioxide
0.5/15ml			2/15ml	18mg/15ml				methionine, 25mg/15ml · choline bitartrate, 50mg/15ml · invert sugar · purified water · alcohol, 12% · caramel color · citric acid · benzoic acid · natural flavors · artificial flavors · sodium hydroxide
1/ml	1/ml		10/ml	15/ml			2/ml	choline, 100mg · manganese, 2mg · zinc, 2mg · iodine, 100mcg · alcohol · citric acid · glycerin · sherry wine · sucrose
3	9	400		27	162	125	100	zinc, 22.5mg · copper, 1.5mg · iodine, 225mcg · BHA · BHT · blue#2 · gelatin · hydrolyzed protein · hydroxypropyl methylcellulose · lactose · magnesium stearate · methylparaben · microcrystalline cellulose · modified food starch · monoglyceride · diglyceride · polacrilin · polysorbate 60 · potassium sorbate · propylparaben · PVPP · red#40 · silica gel · sodium benzoate · sodium lauryl sulfate · sorbic acid · stearic acid · sucrose · titanium dioxide
50	12	400	20		50	40	100	zinc, 5mg · copper, 1mg · chromium, 200mcg · selenium, 25mcg
0.03	0.2	66.6	1.6	3	83.3 (as citrate)		100 (as oxide)	zinc, 2.5mg · manganese, 1.77mg · copper, 0.3mg · chromium, 33.3mcg · selenium, 33.3mcg · iodine, 25mcg

VITAMIN PRODUCTS - continued

	Product Manufacturer/Supplier	Vitamin A (IU)	Vitamin D (IU)	Vitamin E (IU)	Ascorbic Acid (C) (mg)	Thiamine (B1) (mg)	Riboflavin (B2) (mg)	Niacin (mg)
**	**Halls Vitamin C Lozenges** Warner-Lambert				60			
**	**Hepacolin Capsules** Kenwood Labs						2.5	niacinamide, 10
GL LA SO SU	**Herpetrol Tablets** Alva-Amco Pharmacal	313		3.75	15		4	
GL PU SO	**Hexavitamin Tablets** Upsher-Smith Labs	5000	400		75	2	3	20
**	**I.L.X. B12 Caplets** Kenwood Labs				120	2	2	niacinamide, 20
**	**I.L.X. B12 Elixir** Kenwood Labs					5	2	
** SU	**I.L.X. B12 Sugar Free Elixir** Kenwood Labs					5	2	
**	**I.L.X. Elixir** Kenwood Labs					5	2	
	Iberet Filmtab Tablets Abbott Labs				150	6	6	niacinamide, 30
	Iberet Liquid Abbott Labs				112.5/15ml	4.5/15ml	4.5/15ml	niacinamide, 22.5/15ml
	Iberet-500 Filmtab Tablets Abbott Labs				500	6	6	niacinamide, 30
	Iberet-500 Liquid Abbott Labs				375/15ml	4.5/15ml	4.5/15ml	niacinamide, 22.5/15ml
**	**ICAPS Plus Tablets** Ciba Vision	600 (as beta carotene)		60	200			
**	**ICAPS Timed-Release Tablets** Ciba Vision	7000 (as beta carotene)		100	200		20	

See Chapter 19, "Nutritional Products," for more information about these products.

Pyridoxine HCl (B6) (mg)	Cyanocobalamin (B12) (mcg)	Folic Acid (mcg)	Pantothenic Acid (mg)	Iron (elemental) (mg)	Calcium (elemental) (mg)	Phosphorus (mg)	Magnesium (mg)	Other Ingredients
								sugar · corn syrup · citric acid · sodium ascorbate · natural flavoring · color · red#40
2			1.5					choline bitartrate, 240mg · di-methionine, 110mg · inositol, 83mg · desiccated liver, 56mg · liver concentrate, 30mg · cobalamin concentrate, 1.5mcg
				19 (as sulfate)				lysine HCl, 315mg · zinc oxide, 2mg
	12			37.5 (micronized)				desiccated liver, 130mg
	10			102				liver fraction, 98mg · nicotinamide, 10mg
	10			102				liver fraction, 98mg · nicotinamide, 10mg
				70				liver concentrate, 98mg · nicotinamide, 10mg
5	25		10 (as calcium pantothenate)	105 (as sulfate)				castor oil · cellulosic polymers · corn starch · FD&C red#40 · FD&C yellow#6 · magnesium stearate · methyl acrylate-methyl methacrylate copolymers · polyethylene glycol · povidone · stearic acid · talc · titanium dioxide · vanillin
3.75/15ml	18.75/15ml			78.75/15ml (as sulfate)				dexpanthenol, 7.5mg/15ml · sorbitol · methylparaben · propylparaben · alcohol, 1% · natural and artificial flavor · water
5	25		10 (as calcium pantothenate)					castor oil · cellulose polymers · corn starch · FD&C red#40 · FD&C yellow#6 · magnesium stearate · methyl acrylate-methyl methacrylate copolymers · polyethylene glycol · propylene glycol · povidone · stearic acid · talc · titanium dioxide · vanillin
3.75/15ml	18.75/15ml			78.75/15ml (as sulfate)				dexpanthenol, 7.5mg/15ml · sorbitol · methylparaben · propylparaben · artificial flavor · glycerin · propylene glycol · sodium bicarbonate · sucrose · water
								zinc acetate, 40mg · copper, 2mg
								zinc, 40mg · copper, 2mg

VITAMIN PRODUCTS - continued

	Product Manufacturer/Supplier	Vitamin A (IU)	Vitamin D (IU)	Vitamin E (IU)	Ascorbic Acid (C) (mg)	Thiamine (B1) (mg)	Riboflavin (B2) (mg)	Niacin (mg)
** GL PU	**Iromin-G Tablets** Mission Pharmacal	4000 (as acetate)	400		100	5	2	niacinamide, 10
DY GL LA PU SO SU PE	**Jets Chewable Tablets** Freeda Vitamins				25	10		
** AL SU	**Kenwood Therapeutic Liquid** Kenwood Labs	10000	400	4.5	150	6	3	niacinamide, 6
AL DY GL LA SO SU SL	**Kovitonic Liquid** Freeda Vitamins					5/15ml		
DY GL LA PU SO SU	**KPN (Key Prenatal) Tablets** Freeda Vitamins	2667 (with beta carotene)	133.3	10	33.3	2	2	niacinamide, 10
FR	**Lipogen Caplets** Goldline Labs	1666.67 (as beta carotene)		10	20	0.33	0.33	3.33
**	**Liqui-Lea Liquid** Shaklee	5000/5ml	400/5ml	15/5ml		2.1/5ml	1.8/5ml	20/5ml
AL DY GL LA SO SU SL PE	**LKV (Liquid Kiddie Vitamins) Drops** Freeda Vitamins	2500	400	5	50	1	1	niacinamide, 10
** SU GE	**Mature Complete Tablets** Sundown	6000 (as beta carotene)	400	30	60	1.5	1.7	20
DY GL LA PU SO SU	**Maxi-Minerals Tablets** Freeda Vitamins							

See Chapter 19, "Nutritional Products," for more information about these products.

Pyridoxine HCl (B6) (mg)	Cyanocobalamin (B12) (mcg)	Folic Acid (mcg)	Pantothenic Acid (mg)	Iron (elemental) (mg)	Calcium (elemental) (mg)	Phosphorus (mg)	Magnesium (mg)	Other Ingredients
20.6	2	800	1 (as d-calcium pantothenate)	30 (as gluconate)	50 (as gluconate, lactate, and carbonate)			sugar · microcrystalline cellulose · color · magnesium stearate · croscarmellose · povidone · food glaze · carnauba wax · sodium benzoate · beeswax
5	25							l-lysine, 300mg · sorbitol base
1			6 (as calcium pantothenate)		38	29	6	potassium, 5mg · manganese, 1mg
10/15ml	30/15ml	100/15ml		350/15ml (as pyrophosphate) equivalent to 42 (elemental)				l-lysine, 10mg · d-sorbitol solution
0.83	2	266.6	3.3 (as calcium pantothenate)	11 (as fumarate)	333.3		33.3 (as oxide)	hesperidin-citrus bioflavinoids, 21.7mg · zinc (from gluconate), 3.3mg · potassium gluconate, 2mg · copper gluconate, 0.03mg · manganese gluconate, 0.033mg · iodine, 0.01mg
0.33	1.67		1.67					choline, 111.3mg · inositol, 111.3mg · copper · selenium · zinc
2/5ml	9/5ml		5/ml	18/5ml				biotin, 300mcg/5ml
1	4							panthenol, 3mg · biotin, 75mcg
2	6	400	10	18	162	125	100	potassium, 37.5mg · chloride, 34mg · zinc, 15mg · manganese, 2.5mg · copper, 2mg · iodine, 150mcg · silicon, 80mcg · biotin, 45mcg · vitamin K, 25mcg · chromium, 15mcg · molybdenum, 15mcg · selenium, 15mcg · tin, 10mcg · vanadium, 10mcg · nickel, 15mcg
				19.8 (as fumarate)	300 (as carbonate)		175 (as oxide)	zinc gluconate, 50mg · manganese gluconate, 20mg · potassium gluconate, 10mg · copper gluconate, 8mg · iodide, 0.1mg · selenium, 10 mcg

VITAMIN PRODUCTS - continued

	Product Manufacturer/Supplier	Vitamin A (IU)	Vitamin D (IU)	Vitamin E (IU)	Ascorbic Acid (C) (mg)	Thiamine (B1) (mg)	Riboflavin (B2) (mg)	Niacin (mg)
	Maxi-Vite Tablets Goldline Labs	10000	400	15	200	10	10	100
	Megaplex Tablets Legere Ph'cals	833	66	33	100	16	16	16
** SU	**Men's Multi Iron Free Tablets** Sundown			30	500	10	10	100
** GL PU	**Mission Prenatal F.A. Tablets** Mission Pharmacal	4000 (as acetate)	400		100	5	2	niacinamide, 10
** GL PU	**Mission Prenatal H.P. Tablets** Mission Pharmacal	4000 (as acetate)	400		100	5	2	niacinamide, 10
** GL PU	**Mission Prenatal Tablets** Mission Pharmacal	4000 (as acetate)	400		100	5	2	niacinamide, 10
GL LA PU	**Mission Surgical Supplement Tablets** Mission Pharmacal	5000 (as acetate)	400	45	500	2.5	2.6	niacinamide, 30
DY GL LA PU SO SU	**Monocaps Tablets** Freeda Vitamins	10000 (with beta carotene)	400	15	125	15	15	niacinamide, 41
GL PU SU	**Multi-Mineral Tablets** Hudson							
	Multimin Tablets Republic Drug	5000	400	30	60	1.5	17	20
	Multimineral Plus Tablets Vitaline							
GL SO	**Myadec High-Potency Multivitamin/Multimineral Tablets** Warner Wellcome Consumer	5000	400	30mg	60	1.7	2	20

See Chapter 19, "Nutritional Products," for more information about these products.

Pyridoxine HCl (B6) (mg)	Cyanocobalamin (B12) (mcg)	Folic Acid (mcg)	Pantothenic Acid (mg)	Iron (elemental) (mg)	Calcium (elemental) (mg)	Phosphorus (mg)	Magnesium (mg)	Other Ingredients
5	5	400	20	1.5	53.5	24.3	37	biotin · copper · iodine · manganese · zinc
16	83		16	2.5	66	16	33	choline, 116mg · potassium, 16.5mg · biotin, 16mg ·
5	12	400	20					biotin, 45mcg · zinc, 24mg · copper, 3mg
10	2	0.8	1 (as d-calcium pantothenate)	30 (as gluconate)	50 (as gluconate, lactate, and carbonate)			zinc sulfate, 15mg · sugar · microcrystalline cellulose · color · magnesium stearate · croscarmellose · food glaze · povidone · carnauba wax · sodium benzoate · beeswax
25	2	0.8	1 (as d-calcium pantothenate)	30 (as gluconate)	50 (as gluconate, lactate, and carbonate)			sugar · microcrystalline cellulose · color · magnesium stearate · croscarmellose · food glaze · povidone · carnauba wax · sodium benzoate · beeswax
3	2	0.4	1 (as d-calcium pantothenate)	30 (as gluconate)	50 (as gluconate, lactate, and carbonate)			microcrystalline cellulose · sugar · color · povidone · croscarmellose · magnesium stearate · food glaze · carnauba wax · beeswax · sodium benzoate
3.6	9		16.3 (as d-calcium pantothenate)	27 (as gluconate)				zinc, 22.5mg · sugar · color · povidone · magnesium stearate · carnauba wax · sodium benzoate · beeswax · calcium carbonate
15	15	100	15 (as calcium pantothenate)	13.5	100 (as carbonate)		100 (as oxide)	magnesium oxide, 100mg · l-lysine, 15mg · zinc gluconate, 12mg · PABA, 10mg · l-linoleic acid, 10mg · potassium gluconate, 10mg · copper gluconate, 1mg · iodine, 0.15mg · biotin, 15mcg · selenium, 10mcg
				3 (as gluconate)	166.7	75.7	66.7 (as oxide)	potassium, 12.5mg · manganese, 8.3mg · zinc, 2.5mg · copper, 0.33mg · iodine, 25mcg
2	6	400	10	18	162	125	100	potassium, 40mg · biotin, 30mcg · minerals
				3.6 (carbonyl)	200 (citrate/carbonate complex)		100	potassium, 32mg · zinc, 10.5mg · manganese, 5mg · silicon, 2.4mg · boron, 500mcg · copper, 500mcg · chromium, 50mcg · iodine, 50 mcg · molybdenum, 50mcg · selenium, 25mcg · vanadium, 25mcg
3	6	400	10	18	162	125	100	zinc, 15mg · biotin, 30mcg · vitamin K, 25mcg · chromium · copper · iodine · potassium · manganese · molybdenum · selenium · chloride · nickel · tin · silicon · vanadium · boron

VITAMIN PRODUCTS - continued

	Product Manufacturer/Supplier	Vitamin A (IU)	Vitamin D (IU)	Vitamin E (IU)	Ascorbic Acid (C) (mg)	Thiamine (B1) (mg)	Riboflavin (B2) (mg)	Niacin (mg)
DY GL LA PU SU	**Natalins Tablets** Mead Johnson Nutritionals	4000 (as preformed vitamin A, 2667 and beta carotene, 1333)	400	15	70	1.5	1.6	17
DY GL PU	**Nephro-Vite Tablets** R & D Labs				60	1.5	1.7	20
SU	**Nestabs Tablets** Fielding	5000	400	30	120	3	3	20
LA	**Niferex Daily Tablets** Central Ph'cals	5000 (as acetate)	400	30	60	1.5	1.7	niacinamide, 20mg
	Ocuvite Extra Tablets Storz Ophthalmics	6000 (as beta carotene)		50	200		3	niacinamide, 40
	Ocuvite Tablets Storz Ophthalmics	5000 (as beta carotene)		30	60			
	One Daily Plus Iron Tablets Multisource	5000	400	30	60	1.5	1.7	20
	One-A-Day 55 Plus Tablets Bayer Consumer	600 (as acetate and beta carotene)	400	60	120	4.5	3.4	20
PU SO	**One-A-Day Essential Tablets** Bayer Consumer	5000 (as acetate and beta carotene)	400	30	60	1.5	1.7	20
	One-A-Day Extras Antioxidant Softgels Bayer Consumer	5000 (as beta carotene)		200	250			
PU SO	**One-A-Day Maximum Formula Tablets** Bayer Consumer	5000 (as acetate and beta carotene)	400	30	60	1.5	1.7	20

See Chapter 19, "Nutritional Products," for more information about these products.

Pyridoxine HCl (B6) (mg)	Cyanocobalamin (B12) (mcg)	Folic Acid (mcg)	Pantothenic Acid (mg)	Iron (elemental) (mg)	Calcium (elemental) (mg)	Phosphorus (mg)	Magnesium (mg)	Other Ingredients
2.6	2.5	500		30	200		100	acacia · zinc, 15mg · copper, 1.5mg · povidone · microcrystalline cellulose · polacrilin potassium · hydroxypropyl methylcellulose · polyethylene glycol · magnesium stearate · hydroxypropyl cellulose · silicon dioxide
10	6	800	10 (as calcium pantothenate)		10		<0.30	d-biotin · lactose · cellulose · silicon dioxide · stearic acid
3	8	800		36	80			zinc, 15mg · iodine, 150mcg
2	6	400	10	18 (as polysaccharide complex)	259 (as calcium carbonate and dicalcium phosphate)	5.4	100 (as oxide)	zinc, 15mg (as zinc sulfate) · manganese, 5mg (as manganese sulfate) · copper, 2mg (as copper sulfate) · biotin, 0.3mg
								zinc, 40mg · copper, 2mg · manganese, 5mg · selenium, 40mcg · l-glutathione, 5mg · dibasic calcium phosphate · FD&C yellow#6 · hydroxypropyl methylcellulose · magnesium stearate · microcrystalline cellulose · mineral oil · polysorbate 80 · polyvinylpyrrolidone · silica gel · sodium lauryl sulfate · stearic acid · titanium dioxide · triethyl citrate
								zinc, 40mg · copper, 2mg · selenium, 40mcg · dibasic calcium phosphate · FD&C yellow#6 · hydroxypropyl methylcellulose · magnesium stearate · microcrystalline cellulose · polysorbate 80 · polyvinyl-pyrrolidone · silica gel · sodium lauryl sulfate · stearic acid · titanium dioxide · triethyl citrate
2	6	400	10	18				
6	25	400	20		220		100	vitamin B6 · biotin · vitamin K · iodine · copper · zinc · chromium · selenium · molybdenum · manganese · potassium · chloride · FD&C yellow#6
2	6	400	10					
								zinc · copper · selenium · manganese
2	6	400	10	18	130	100	100	zinc, 15mg · biotin, 30mcg · chloride · chromium · copper · iodine · potassium · manganese · molybdenum · selenium

VITAMIN PRODUCTS - continued

	Product Manufacturer/Supplier	Vitamin A (IU)	Vitamin D (IU)	Vitamin E (IU)	Ascorbic Acid (C) (mg)	Thiamine (B1) (mg)	Riboflavin (B2) (mg)	Niacin (mg)
	One-A-Day Men's Tablets Bayer Consumer	5000 (as acetate and beta carotene)	400	45	200	2.25	2.55	20
	One-A-Day Women's Tablets Bayer Consumer	5000 (as acetate and beta carotene)	400	30	60	1.5	1.7	20
	One-Tablet-Daily Tablets Goldline Labs	5000	400	30	60	1.5	1.7	20
	One-Tablet-Daily with Minerals Tablets Goldline Labs	6500 (with beta carotene)	400	30	60	1.5	1.7	20
	Opti-Gen Tablets Goldline Labs	5000 (as beta carotene)		30	60			
	Optilets-500 Filmtab Tablets Abbott Labs	5000	400	30	500	15	10	niacinamide, 100mg
	Optilets-M-500 Filmtab Tablets Abbott Labs	5000	400	30	500	15	10	niacinamide, 100mg
** GL PU SO	**Optimox Prenatal Tablets** Optimox	833.3 (as palmitate)	66.7	2	30	0.5	0.6	6.7 (niacinamide)
GL PU SO	**Optivite P.M.T. Tablets** Optimox	2083 (as beta carotene and palmitate)	16.7	16.7	250	4.2	4.2	4.2 (niacinamide)
** GL LA PU SO SU	**Os-Cal Fortified Tablets** SmithKline Beecham		125	0.8	50	1.7 (as mononitrate)	1.7	15

See Chapter 19, "Nutritional Products," for more information about these products.

Pyridoxine HCl (B6) (mg)	Cyanocobalamin (B12) (mcg)	Folic Acid (mcg)	Pantothenic Acid (mg)	Iron (elemental) (mg)	Calcium (elemental) (mg)	Phosphorus (mg)	Magnesium (mg)	Other Ingredients
3	9	400	10					calcium carbonate · gelatin · starch · cellulose · calcium silicate · hydroxypropyl methylcellulose · magnesium stearate · FD&C yellow#6 · lecithin · sodium hexametaphosphate
2	6	400	10	27	450			acacia · gelatin · microcrystalline cellulose · hydroxypropyl methylcellulose · zinc, 15mg · modified cellulose gum · magnesium stearate · FD&C yellow#5 · FD&C yellow#6 · hydroxypropyl cellulose · starch · lecithin · sodium hexametaphosphate
2	6	400	10					
2	6	400	10	18	130	100	100	biotin, 30mcg · iodine · copper · zinc · chromium · selenium · molybdenum · manganese · potassium · chloride
								zinc, 40mg · copper, 2mg · selenium
5	12		20 (as calcium pantothenate)					cellulosic polymers · corn starch · D&C yellow#10 · FD&C yellow#6 · iron oxide · polyethylene glycol · povidone · stearic acid · talc · titanium dioxide · vanillin
5	12		20 (as calcium pantothenate)	20			80	zinc, 1.5mg · copper, 2mg · iodine, 0.15mg · manganese, 1mg · polyethylene glycol · propylene glycol · povidone · cellulosic · polymers · colloidal silicon dioxide · corn starch · D&C red#7 · FD&C blue#1 · titanium dioxide · iron oxide · magnesium stearate · microcrystalline cellulose · sorbic acid
0.007	0.87	133.3	3.3	5	100 (as citrate)		100 (as oxide)	zinc, 3.2mg · manganese, 0.8mg · copper, 0.3mg · iodine, 33.3mcg · selenium, 12.5mcg · chromium, 16.7mcg
0.5	10.4	33	4.2	2.5	20.8		41.7	potassium, 7.9mg · manganese, 1.7mg · chromium, 16.6mcg · selenium, 16.6mcg · iodine, 12.5mcg
2				5 (as fumarate)	250 (as oyster shell powder)		3 (as oxide)	zinc, 0.5 (as sulfate) · manganese, 0.5 (as sulfate) · corn syrup solids · hydroxypropyl methylcellulose · calcium stearate · corn starch · mineral oil · titanium dioxide · polysorbate 80 · methylparaben · yellow#10 lake · blue#1 lake · propylparaben · carnauba wax · edetate disodium

VITAMIN PRODUCTS - continued

	Product Manufacturer/Supplier	Vitamin A (IU)	Vitamin D (IU)	Vitamin E (IU)	Ascorbic Acid (C) (mg)	Thiamine (B1) (mg)	Riboflavin (B2) (mg)	Niacin (mg)
** DY GL LA PU SO SU	**Oxi-Freeda Tablets** Freeda Vitamins	5000 (as beta carotene)		150	100	20	20	niacinamide, 40
**	**Palmitate-A 5,000 Tablets** Akorn	5000						
**	**Palmitate-A Tablets** Akorn	15000						
DY GL LA PU SO SU	**Parvlex Tablets** Freeda Vitamins				50	20	20	niacinamide, 20
**	**Perfect Antioxidant Caplet** Sundown	7500 (as beta carotene)		200	250			
GL LA PU SO SU	**Peridin-C Tablets** Beutlich, L.P. Ph'cals				200			
GL LA PU PE	**Poly-Vi-Sol Chewable Vitamins** Mead Johnson Nutritionals	2500	400	15	60	1.05	1.2	13.5
AL GL LA SO SU SL PE	**Poly-Vi-Sol Vitamin Drops** Mead Johnson Nutritionals	1500/ml	400/ml	5/ml	35/ml	0.5/ml	0.6/ml	8/ml
GL LA PU PE	**Poly-Vi-Sol with Iron Chewable Vitamins & Minerals Tablets** Mead Johnson Nutritionals	2500	400	15	60	1.05	1.2	13.5
AL GL LA SO SL PE	**Poly-Vi-Sol with Iron Vitamin Drops** Mead Johnson Nutritionals	1500/ml	400/ml	5/ml	35/ml	0.5/ml	0.6/ml	8/ml
AL PE	**Poly-Vitamin Multivitamin Supplement Infants' Drops** Schein Ph'cal	1500/ml	400/ml	5/ml	35/ml	0.5/ml	0.6/ml	8/ml

See Chapter 19, "Nutritional Products," for more information about these products.

Pyridoxine HCl (B6) (mg)	Cyanocobalamin (B12) (mcg)	Folic Acid (mcg)	Pantothenic Acid (mg)	Iron (elemental) (mg)	Calcium (elemental) (mg)	Phosphorus (mg)	Magnesium (mg)	Other Ingredients
20	10		20 (as calcium pantothenate)					l-cysteine, 75mg · glutathione, 40mg · zinc, 15mg · oceanic selenium, 50mcg
								cellulose · stearic acid · magnesium stearate · silicon dioxide
								cellulose · stearic acid · magnesium stearate · silicon dioxide
10	50	400	1 (as calcium pantothenate)	100 (as fumarate)				copper, 1.5mg · manganese gluconate, 1mg
								zinc, 7.5mg · manganese, 1.5mg · copper, 1mg · selenium, 15mcg · rose hips
								hesperidin complex, 150mg · hesperidin methyl chalcone, 50mg
1.05	4.5	300						dextrates · sugar · magnesium stearate · silicon dioxide · artificial flavor · artificial color · salt
0.4/ml	2/ml							glycerin · water · polysorbate 80 · ferrous sulfate · artificial flavor · color
1.05	4.5	300		12				zinc, 8mg · copper, 0.8mg · dextrates · sugar · magnesium stearate · stearic acid · silicon dioxide · artificial flavor · color · salt
0.4/ml				10/ml				glycerin · water · artificial flavor · color · polysorbate 80
0.4/ml	2/ml							glycerin · water · polysorbate 80 · flavor

VITAMIN PRODUCTS - continued

	Product Manufacturer/Supplier	Vitamin A (IU)	Vitamin D (IU)	Vitamin E (IU)	Ascorbic Acid (C) (mg)	Thiamine (B1) (mg)	Riboflavin (B2) (mg)	Niacin (mg)
AL PE	**Poly-Vitamin Multivitamin Supplement w/ Iron Infants' Drops** Schein Ph'cal	1500/ml	400/ml	5/ml	35/ml	0.5/ml	0.6/ml	8/ml
** SU	**Pre-Natal Multi Vitamin-Mineral Complex Tablets** Sundown	4000	400	11	100	1.5	1.7	18
PR	**Prenatal Formula Tablets** Schein Ph'cal	4000	400	11	100	1.5	1.7	18
	Prenatal-S Tablets Goldline Labs	4000	400	11	100	1.5	1.7	18
DY GL SO	**Pro-Pep Chewable Tablets** Alva-Amco Pharmacal	375	30	2.16	5	0.17	0.12	1.375
GL PU SO	**Progen Caplets** Legere Ph'cals	12500		15	500			
GL LA PU SO SU	**Protegra Antioxidant Softgels** Lederle Consumer	5000 (as beta carotene)		200	250			
DY GL LA PU SO SU	**Quintabs-M Tablets** Freeda Vitamins	10000 (with beta carotene)	400	50	300	30	30	niacinamide, 150
GL	**Rejuvex for the Mature Woman Caplets** Sunsource			30		2	2	10
	S.S.S. Tonic S.S.S. Company					1.67/15ml	0.8m/15ml	niacinamide, 6.7/15ml
	S.S.S. Vitamin Tablets S.S.S. Company			50	300	7.5	7.5	50
	Secran B Vitamin Supplement Liquid Scherer Labs					5ml		5ml

See Chapter 19, "Nutritional Products," for more information about these products.

Pyridoxine HCl (B6) (mg)	Cyanocobalamin (B12) (mcg)	Folic Acid (mcg)	Pantothenic Acid (mg)	Iron (elemental) (mg)	Calcium (elemental) (mg)	Phosphorus (mg)	Magnesium (mg)	Other Ingredients
0.4/ml				10/ml				glycerin · water · polysorbate 80 · preservatives · flavors · colors
2.6	4	800		60	200			zinc, 25mg
2.6	4	800		60	200			zinc, 25mg · croscarmellose · cellulose · cellulose gum · stearic acid · magnesium stearate · polyvinyl pyrrolidone · iron oxide · titanium dioxide · hydrous magnesium silicate · distilled acetylated monoglycerides · pharmaceutical glaze · vanillin
2.6	4	800		60	200			zinc, 25mg
0.17	0.5	30	0.78	1.2				zinc, 1mg · copper, 0.14mg · biotin, 23mcg · iodine, 9mcg · dextrose · maltodextrin · sorbitol
5							20	garlic, 75mg · zinc, 50mg · selenium, 50mcg
								zinc, 7.5mg · manganese, 1.5mg · copper, 1mg · selenium, 15mcg · gelatin · cottonseed oil · glycerin · sorbitol · calcium phosphate · lecithin · beeswax · soybean oil · FD&C red#40 · titanium dioxide · FD&C blue#1 ·
30	30	400	30 (as calcium pantothenate)	45 (as fumarate)	30 (as gluconate)		30	PABA, 30mg · potassium gluconate, 30mg · zinc gluconate, 30mg · manganese gluconate, 15mg · copper gluconate, 2mg · potassium iodide, 0.15mg · selenium, 35mcg
10			10 (as d-calcium pantothenate)				500 (as oxide)	dong quai, 200mg · boron, 3mg · manganese, 2mg · selenium, 25mcg · raw glandular powders from bovine source · microcrystalline cellulose · croscarmellose sodium · colloidal silica · stearic acid · magnesium stearate
								alcohol, 12%
12.5	12.5	200	10	50	100		50	zinc, 12mg · copper, 1.5mg · biotin, 22.5mcg
	5ml							alcohol, 15% · sodium citrate · sugar · glycerin · sherry wine concentrate · FD&C red#40 · citric acid

VITAMIN PRODUCTS - continued

	Product Manufacturer/Supplier	Vitamin A (IU)	Vitamin D (IU)	Vitamin E (IU)	Ascorbic Acid (C) (mg)	Thiamine (B1) (mg)	Riboflavin (B2) (mg)	Niacin (mg)
PE	**Sesame Street Complete Vitamins & Minerals Chewable Tablets** McNeil Consumer	2750 (as acetate and beta carotene, 495)	200	10	40	0.75	0.85	10
PE	**Sesame Street Vitamins Plus Extra C Chewable Tablets** McNeil Consumer	2750 (as acetate and beta carotene, 495)	200	10	80	0.75	0.85	10
PE	**Sesame Street Vitamins Plus Iron Chewable Tablets** McNeil Consumer	2750 (as acetate and beta carotene, 495)	200	10	40	0.75	0.85	10
	Sigtab-M Tablets Roberts Ph'cal	6000	400	45		5mg	5	niacinamide, 25mg
	Sigtabs Tablets Roberts Ph'cal	5000 (as acetate)	400	15		10.3	10	100
	Stress Formula Plus Iron Tablets Multisource			30	500	10	10	100
	Stress Formula Tablets Multisource			30	500	15	10	niacinamide, 100
	Stress Formula with Zinc Tablets Multisource			30	500	15	10	niacinamide, 100
	Stress-600 Tablets Upsher-Smith Labs			30	600	15	15	100
GL PU SO	**Stress-600 with Zinc Tablets** Upsher-Smith Labs			30	600	20	10	100

See Chapter 19, "Nutritional Products," for more information about these products.

Pyridoxine HCl (B6) (mg)	Cyanocobalamin (B12) (mcg)	Folic Acid (mcg)	Pantothenic Acid (mg)	Iron (elemental) (mg)	Calcium (elemental) (mg)	Phosphorus (mg)	Magnesium (mg)	Other Ingredients
0.7	3	200	5	10	80		20	iodine, 75mcg · biotin, 15mcg · zinc, 8mg · copper, 1mg · sucrose · natural flavors · talc · stearic acid glyceride · palmitic acid glyceride · starch · silicon dioxide · gelatin · natural coloring · lactose · potassium iodide · d-biotin
0.7	3	200	5					sucrose · talc · natural flavors · stearic acid glyceride · palmitic acid glyceride · gelatin · silicon dioxide · starch · magnesium stearate · natural coloring · dicalcium phosphate · lactose
0.7	3	200	5	10				sucrose · talc · natural flavors · stearic acid glyceride · palmitic acid glyceride · gelatin · silicon dioxide · magnesium stearate · starch · natural coloring · dicalcium phosphate · lactose
pyridoxine, 3mg	18	400	0.015	18	200	150	100	potassium chloride, 40mg · chloride, 36.3mg · zinc, 15mg · manganese sulfate, 5mg · copper, 2mg · boron, 150mcg · iodine, 150mcg · biotin, 45mcg · vitamin K1, 25mcg · chromium, 25mcg · molybdenum, 25mcg · selenium, 25mcg · vanadium, 19mcg · tin, 10mcg · nickel, 5mcg · silicon, 2mcg · microcrystalline cellulose · stearic acid · croscarmellose sodium · magnesium stearate · hydroxypropyl methylcellulose · propylene glycol
6	18	400	20 (as calcium pantothenate)					sucrose · calcium sulfate · gelatin · povidone · lacca · magnesium stearate · silica · sodium benzoate · polyethylene glycol · carnauba wax · sesame seed oil · titanium dioxide
5	12	400	20	27				biotin, 45mcg
5	12	400	20					biotin, 45mcg
5	12	400	20					zinc, 23.9mg · copper, 3mg · biotin, 45mcg
5	12	400	20					biotin, 45mcg
5	12	400	25					zinc, 23.9mg · copper, 3mg · biotin, 45mcg

VITAMIN PRODUCTS - continued

	Product Manufacturer/Supplier	Vitamin A (IU)	Vitamin D (IU)	Vitamin E (IU)	Ascorbic Acid (C) (mg)	Thiamine (B1) (mg)	Riboflavin (B2) (mg)	Niacin (mg)
GL LA PU SO SU	**Stresstabs High Potency Stress Formula + Iron Tablets** Lederle Consumer			30	500	10	10	100
GL LA PU SO SU	**Stresstabs High Potency Stress Formula Plus Zinc Tablets** Lederle Consumer			30	500	10	10	100
GL LA PU SO SU	**Stresstabs High Potency Stress Formula Tablets** Lederle Consumer			30	500	10	10	100
	Stuart Prenatal Tablets Wyeth-Ayerst Labs	4000 (as acetate and beta carotene)	400	11	100	1.5	1.7	18
GL PU SO PE	**Sunkist Multivitamins Complete Tablets** Ciba Self-Medication	5000	400	30	60	1.5	1.7	20mg
GL PU SO PE	**Sunkist Multivitamins Plus Extra C Tablets** Ciba Self-Medication	2500	400	15	250	1.1	1.2	14mg

See Chapter 19, "Nutritional Products," for more information about these products.

Pyridoxine HCl (B6) (mg)	Cyanocobalamin (B12) (mcg)	Folic Acid (mcg)	Pantothenic Acid (mg)	Iron (elemental) (mg)	Calcium (elemental) (mg)	Phosphorus (mg)	Magnesium (mg)	Other Ingredients
5	12	400	20	18				biotin, 45mcg · microcrystalline cellulose · calcium carbonate · modified food starch · stearic acid · magnesium stearate · silicon dioxide · mineral oil · FD&C yellow#6 · FD&C red#40
5	12	400	20					zinc, 23.9mg · copper, 3mg · biotin, 45mcg · microcrystalline cellulose · calcium carbonate · modified food starch · mineral oil · silicon dioxide · stearic acid · magnesium stearate · FD&C yellow#6
5	12	400	20					biotin, 45mcg · microcrystalline cellulose · calcium carbonate · modified food starch · mineral oil · magnesium stearate · silicon dioxide · FD&C yellow#6 · stearic acid
2.6	4	800		60	200			zinc, 25mg · croscarmellose sodium · hydroxypropyl methylcellulose · microcrystalline cellulose · pregelatinized starch · red iron oxide · titanium dioxide
2	6	400	10	18	100	78	20	iodine, 150mcg · biotin, 40mcg · vitamin K1, 10mcg · zinc, 10mg · manganese, 1mg · copper, 2mg · sorbitol · dicalcium phosphate · monoglyceride · diglyceride · natural flavors · stearic acid · carrageenan · starch · hydrolyzed protein · citric acid · yellow#6 · gelatin · magnesium stearate · red#40 · yellow#5 · aspartame · silica · calcium silicate · cellulose · hydrogenated vegetable oils · beta carotene
1	5	300						vitamin K1, 5mcg · sorbitol · flavors · monoglyceride · diglyceride · starch · stearic acid · hydrolyzed protein · aspartame · hydrogenated vegetable oils · yellow#6 · silica · red#40 · cellulose · yellow#5 · gelatin · beta carotene

VITAMIN PRODUCTS - continued

	Product Manufacturer/Supplier	Vitamin A (IU)	Vitamin D (IU)	Vitamin E (IU)	Ascorbic Acid (C) (mg)	Thiamine (B1) (mg)	Riboflavin (B2) (mg)	Niacin (mg)
GL PU SO PE	**Sunkist Multivitamins Plus Iron Tablets** Ciba Self-Medication	2500	400	15	60	1.1	1.2	niacinamide, 13.5mg
GL PU SO PE	**Sunkist Multivitamins Regular Tablets** Ciba Self-Medication	2500	400	15	60	1.1	1.2	niacinamide, 13.5mg
**	**Sunkist Vitamin C Caplets** Ciba Self-Medication				500			
**	**Sunkist Vitamin C Chewable Tablets** Ciba Self-Medication				60; 250; 500			
** SU	**Sunvite Multi Vitamin-Mineral Formula Tablets** Sundown	5000 (with beta carotene)	400	30	60	1.5	1.7	20
** SU	**Sunvite Platinum Multi Vitamin-Mineral Formula Tablets** Sundown	6000 (with beta carotene)	400	45	60	1.5	1.7	20
** DY GL LA PU SO SU	**Super A&D3 Tablets** Freeda Vitamins	25000	1000					

See Chapter 19, "Nutritional Products," for more information about these products.

Pyridox-ine HCl (B6) (mg)	Cyanoco-balamin (B12) (mcg)	Folic Acid (mcg)	Panto-thenic Acid (mg)	Iron (elemental) (mg)	Calcium (elemental) (mg)	Phos-phorus (mg)	Magne-sium (mg)	Other Ingredients
1	5	300		15				vitamin K1, 5mcg · sorbitol · flavors · monoglyceride · diglyceride · starch · stearic acid · carrageenan · hydrolyzed protein · aspartame · magnesium stearate · hydrolyzed vegetable oils · red#40 · silica · yellow#5 · yellow#6 · cellulose · gelatin · beta carotene
1	5	300						vitamin K1, 5mcg · sorbitol · flavors · monoglyceride · diglyceride · starch · stearic acid · hydrolyzed protein · carrageenan · hydrogenated vegetable oils · magnesium stearate · citric acid · aspartame · silica · yellow#6 · red#40 · cellulose · yellow#5 · gelatin · beta carotene
								citrus bioflavonoids · microcrystalline cellulose · cellulose · dicalcium phosphate · stearic acid · talc · magnesium stearate · silica hydrogel
								fructose (250mg · 500mg) · sorbitol · sucrose · natural flavors · citrus bioflavonoids · hydrogenated vegetable oil (250mg) · dextrin · magnesium stearate · modified food starch · silica hydrogel · lactose
2	6	400	10	18	162	125	100	potassium, 40mg · chloride, 36.3 mg · chromium, 25mcg · zinc, 15mg · manganese, 2.5mg · copper, 2mg · silicon, 2mg · iodine, 150mcg · boron, 150mcg · biotin, 30mcg · molybdenum, 25mcg · selenium, 25mcg · vitamin K-1, 25mcg · tin, 10mcg · nickel, 5mcg
3	25	200	10	9	200	48	100	potassium, 80mg · chloride, 72mg zinc, 15mg · manganese, 2.5mg · copper, 2mg · iodine, 150mcg · biotin, 30mcg · chromium, 25mcg · molybdenum, 25mcg · selenium, 25mcg · silicon, 10mcg · vanadium, 10mcg · vitamin K1, 10mcg · nickel, 5mcg

VITAMIN PRODUCTS - continued

	Product Manufacturer/Supplier	Vitamin A (IU)	Vitamin D (IU)	Vitamin E (IU)	Ascorbic Acid (C) (mg)	Thiamine (B1) (mg)	Riboflavin (B2) (mg)	Niacin (mg)
** SU	**Super C Tablets** Sundown				1000			
DY GL LA PU SO SU	**Super Dec B-100 Coated Tablets** Freeda Vitamins					100	100	niacinamide, 100
** SU	**Super Multiple 33 with Minerals Tablets** Sundown	10000 (with beta carotene)	400	25	120	15	17	100
** SU	**Super Multiple 42 with Beta Carotene Softgels** Sundown	5000 (with beta carotene)	200	15	250	7.5	8.5	50
** SU	**Super Multiple 50 Tablets** Sundown	2500 (with beta carotene)	200	30	250	12.5	12.5	25

See Chapter 19, "Nutritional Products," for more information about these products.

Pyridoxine HCl (B6) (mg)	Cyanocobalamin (B12) (mcg)	Folic Acid (mcg)	Pantothenic Acid (mg)	Iron (elemental) (mg)	Calcium (elemental) (mg)	Phosphorus (mg)	Magnesium (mg)	Other Ingredients
								citrus bioflavonoids, 500mg · rutin, 100mg · hesperidin, 100mg · acerola, 5mg · rose hips · alfalfa · cereal grass · parsley
100	100	400	100 (as calcium pantothenate)					PABA, 100mg · inositol, 100mg · d-biotin, 100mcg
20	60	400	50	6	26	13.5		choline bitartrate, 100mg · betaine HCl, 25mg · citrus bioflavonoids, 25mg · desiccated liver, 25mg · glutamic acid, 25mg · inositol, 25mg · PABA, 25mg · selenium, 25mcg · rutin, 25mg · biotin, 20mcg · zinc, 18mg · l-lysine, 10mg · hesperidin, 5mg · acerola, 1mg · copper, 0.25mg · iodine, 0.13mg · alfalfa · parsley · rice bran · watercress · lecithin · magnesium gluconate · manganese gluconate
10	30	200	12.5	5.4	8	4.5		potassium, 75mg · choline bitartrate, 50mg · desiccated liver, 25mg · citrus bioflavonoids, 12.5mg · PABA, 12.5mg · zinc, 7.5mg · amino acids, 5mg · hesperidin, 5mg · manganese, 2mg · acerola, 1mg · copper, 0.4mg · inositol, 150mcg · iodine, 75mcg · biotin, 25mcg · selenium, 12.5mcg · papaya · fish liver oil · rose hips · magnesium gluconate · lecithin · yeast
12.5	25	200	25	9	75		50	inositol, 125mg · choline bitartrate, 50mg · potassium, 25mg · amino acids, 12.5mg · betaine, 12.5mg · citrus bioflavonoids, 12.5mg · desiccated liver, 12.5mg · PABA, 12.5mg · rutin, 12.5mg · l-lysine, 7.5mg · zinc, 7.5mg · hesperidin, 2.5mg · manganese, 2.5mg · copper, 1mg · octacosanol, 187.5mcg · biotin, 150mcg · iodine, 75mcg · chromium, 25mcg · selenium, 25mcg · alfalfa · rice bran · watercress · parsley · brewers yeast · RNA · acidophilus · DNA · wheat germ · apple pectin · lecithin · kelp · yogurt culture · glutamic acid

VITAMIN PRODUCTS - continued

	Product Manufacturer/Supplier	Vitamin A (IU)	Vitamin D (IU)	Vitamin E (IU)	Ascorbic Acid (C) (mg)	Thiamine (B1) (mg)	Riboflavin (B2) (mg)	Niacin (mg)
** SU	**Super Multiple Minus Iron Tablets** Sundown	2500	200	30	250	12.5	12.5	25
DY GL LA PU SO SU	**Super Quints-50 Tablets** Freeda Vitamins					50	50	niacinamide, 50
	Surbex Filmtab Tablets Abbott Labs					6	6	niacinamide, 30mg
	Surbex With C Filmtab Tablets Abbott Labs				250	6	6	niacinamide, 30mg
	Surbex-750 with Iron Filmtab Tablets Abbott Labs			30	750	15	15	niacinamide, 100
	Surbex-750 with Zinc Abbott Labs			30	750	15	15	100
	Surbex-T Filmtab Tablets Abbott Labs				500	15	10	niacinamide, 100mg
	Surbu-Gen-T Tablets Goldline Labs				500	15	10	100

See Chapter 19, "Nutritional Products," for more information about these products.

Pyridoxine HCl (B6) (mg)	Cyanocobalamin (B12) (mcg)	Folic Acid (mcg)	Pantothenic Acid (mg)	Iron (elemental) (mg)	Calcium (elemental) (mg)	Phosphorus (mg)	Magnesium (mg)	Other Ingredients
12.5	25	200	25		75		50	inositol, 125mg · choline bitartrate, 50mg · potassium, 25mg · citrus bioflavonoids, 12.5mg · PABA, 12.5mg · rutin, 12.5mg · zinc, 7.5mg · hesperidin, 2.5mg · manganese, 2.5mg · copper, 1mg · biotin, 150mcg · iodine, 75mcg · chromium, 25mcg · selenium, 25mcg · betaine · octacosanol · beta carotene · acerola · rose hips · amino acids · DNA · RNA · stearic acid · apple pectin · bone meal · alfalfa · acidophilus · watercress · wheat germ · brewer's yeast
50	50	400	50 (as calcium pantothenate)					inositol, 50mg · PABA, 30mg · d-biotin, 50mcg · l-lysine · glycerin · l-glutamine · l-glutamic acid
2.5	5		10 (as calcium pantothenate)					cellulosic polymers · corn starch · D&C yellow#10 · dibasic calcium phosphate · FD&C yellow#6 · magnesium stearate · polyethylene glycol · povidone · propylene glycol · stearic acid · titanium dioxide · vanillin
2.5	5		10 (as calcium pantothenate)					cellulosic polymers · corn starch · D&C yellow#10 · FD&C yellow#6 · lactose · magnesium stearate · polyethylene glycol · microcrystalline cellulose · povidone · propylene glycol · titanium dioxide · vanillin
25	12	400	20 (as calcium pantothenate)	27 (as sulfate)				cellulosic polymers · colloidal silicon dioxide · FD&C red#3 · corn starch · iron oxide · magnesium stearate · microcrystalline cellulose · polyethylene glycol · povidone · vanillin
20	12	400	20					zinc, 22.5mg · cellulose · povidone · talc · magnesium stearate · titanium dioxide · polyethylene glycol · colloidal silicon dioxide · vanillin · iron oxide
5	10		20 (as calcium pantothenate)					cellulosic polymers · corn starch · D&C yellow#10 · FD&C yellow#6 · magnesium stearate · microcrystalline cellulose · polyethylene glycol · povidone · stearic acid · titanium dioxide · vanillin
5	10		20					

VITAMIN PRODUCTS - continued

	Product Manufacturer/Supplier	Vitamin A (IU)	Vitamin D (IU)	Vitamin E (IU)	Ascorbic Acid (C) (mg)	Thiamine (B1) (mg)	Riboflavin (B2) (mg)	Niacin (mg)
GL LA PU SU	**Theragran High Potency Multivitamin Caplets** Mead Johnson Nutritionals	5000 (as acetate and beta carotene)	400	30mg	90	3	3.4	20
AL DY GL LA SL	**Theragran High Potency Multivitamin Liquid** Mead Johnson Nutritionals	5000/5ml	400/5ml		200/5ml	10/5ml	10/5ml	100/5ml
GL LA PU SU	**Theragran Stress Formula High Potency Multivitamin Caplets** Mead Johnson Nutritionals			30	600	15	15	100
GL LA PU SU	**Theragran-M High Potency Vitamins with Minerals Caplets** Mead Johnson Nutritionals	5000	400	30	90	3	3.4	20
GL PU SO	**Therapeutic B Complex with Vitamin C Capsules** Upsher-Smith Labs				300	15	10.2	50
** SU	**Therapeutic M Multi Vitamins Plus Minerals Tablets** Sundown	5000 (with beta carotene)	400	30	90	3	3.4	20

See Chapter 19, "Nutritional Products," for more information about these products.

Pyridoxine HCl (B6) (mg)	Cyanocobalamin (B12) (mcg)	Folic Acid (mcg)	Pantothenic Acid (mg)	Iron (elemental) (mg)	Calcium (elemental) (mg)	Phosphorus (mg)	Magnesium (mg)	Other Ingredients
3	9	400	10					biotin, 30mcg · lactose · microcrystalline cellulose · hydroxypropyl methylcellulose · povidone · silicon dioxide · magnesium stearate · polyethylene glycol · triacetin · stearic acid · titanium dioxide · annatto · FD&C red#40
4.1/5ml	5/5ml		21.4/5ml					sucrose · water · glycerin · propylene glycol · polysorbate 80 · carboxymethyl cellulose sodium · flavors · sodium benzoate · methylparaben · ferric ammonium citrate
25	12	400	20	27				biotin, 45mcg · lactose · crospovidone · povidone · hydroxypropyl methylcellulose · magnesium stearate · silicon dioxide · stearic acid · polyethylene glycol · triacetin · titanium dioxide · FD&C red#40 · FD&C yellow#6
3	9	400	10	18	40	31	100	zinc, 15mg · chlorine, 7.5mg · potassium, 7.5mg · manganese, 3.5mg · copper, 2mg · silicon, 2mg · boron, 150mcg · iodine, 150mcg · molybdenum, 32mcg · biotin, 30mcg · chromium, 26mcg · selenium, 21mcg · tin, 10mcg · vanadium, 10mcg · nickel, 5mcg · lactose · crospovidone · hydroxypropyl methylcellulose · povidone · magnesium stearate · stearic acid · polyethylene glycol · triacetin · FD&C red#40 · titanium dioxide · FD&C blue#2 · silica gel · microcrystalline cellulose
5			10					
3	9	400	10	27	40	31	100	zinc, 15mg · chloride, 7.5mg · potassium, 7.5mg · manganese, 5mg · copper, 2mg · iodine, 150mcg · biotin, 30mcg · chromium, 15mcg · molybdenum, 15mcg · selenium, 10mcg

VITAMIN PRODUCTS - continued

	Product Manufacturer/Supplier	Vitamin A (IU)	Vitamin D (IU)	Vitamin E (IU)	Ascorbic Acid (C) (mg)	Thiamine (B1) (mg)	Riboflavin (B2) (mg)	Niacin (mg)
GL PU SO	**Therapeutic Multiple with Minerals Tablets** Upsher-Smith Labs	5500	400	30	120	3	3.4	30
GL PU SO	**Therapeutic Multivitamin Tablets** Upsher-Smith Labs	5500	400	30	120	3	3.4	30
	Therapeutic Tablets Goldline Labs	5000 (with beta carotene)	400	30mg	90	3	3.4	30
	Therapeutic-M Tablets Goldline Labs	5000 (with beta carotene)	400	30mg	90	3	3.4	30
	Theravee Hematinic Tablets Vangard Labs	8333	133	5	100	3.3	3.3	33.3
	Theravee Tablets Vangard Labs	5500	400	30	120	3	3.4	30
	Theravee-M Tablets Vangard Labs	5000	400	30	90	3	3.4	20
	Theravit M Tablets Schein Ph'cal	5000 (beta carotene, 1250)	400	30	90	3	3.4	30
	Theravite Liquid Goldline Labs	5000/5ml	400/5ml		200/5ml	10/5ml	10/5ml	100/5ml
	Theravits Tablets Schein Ph'cal	5000 (beta carotene, 1250)	400	30	90	3	3.4	30
AL GL LA SU SL PE	**Tri-Vi-Sol Vitamins A,D+C Drops** Mead Johnson Nutritionals	1500/ml	400/ml		35/ml			

See Chapter 19, "Nutritional Products," for more information about these products.

Pyridox-ine HCl (B6) (mg)	Cyanoco-balamin (B12) (mcg)	Folic Acid (mcg)	Panto-thenic Acid (mg)	Iron (elemental) (mg)	Calcium (elemental) (mg)	Phos-phorus (mg)	Magne-sium (mg)	Other Ingredients
3	9	400	10	27	40		100	zinc, 15mg · potassium, 7.5mg · chloride, 7.5mg · manganese, 5mg · copper, 2mg · iodine, 150mcg · biotin, 15mcg · chromium, 15mcg · molybdenum, 15mcg · selenium, 10mcg
3	9	400	10					biotin, 15mcg
3	9	400	10					biotin, 30mcg
3	9	400	10	27	40	31	100	zinc, 15mg · biotin, 30mcg · chlorine · chromium · copper · iodine · potassium · manganese · molybdenum · selenium
3.3	50	330	11.7	66.7			41.7	copper, 0.67mg
3	9	400	10					biotin, 15mcg
3	9	400	10	27	40	31	100	zinc, 15mg · potassium chloride, 7.5mg · manganese, 5mg · copper, 2mg · iodine, 150mcg · biotin, 30mcg · chromium · molybdenum
3	9	400	10	27	40	31	100	zinc, 15mg · manganese, 5mg · copper, 2mg · iodine, 150mcg · biotin, 35mcg · chromium 15mcg · molybdenum, 15mcg · selenium, 10mcg
4.1/5ml	5/5ml		21.4/5ml					
3	9	400	10					biotin, 35mcg · dicalcium phosphate · microcrystalline cellulose · stearic acid · cellulose gum · hydroxypropyl methylcellulose · pharmaceutical glaze · magnesium stearate · color · ethyl cellulose · acetylated monoglycerides · titanium dioxide · magnesium silicate · silica · tablet brown · ethyl vanillin
								glycerin · water · polysorbate 80 · artificial flavor · color

VITAMIN PRODUCTS - continued

	Product Manufacturer/Supplier	Vitamin A (IU)	Vitamin D (IU)	Vitamin E (IU)	Ascorbic Acid (C) (mg)	Thiamine (B1) (mg)	Riboflavin (B2) (mg)	Niacin (mg)
AL GL LA SU SL PE	**Tri-Vi-Sol With Iron Vitamin A,D+C Drops** Mead Johnson Nutritionals	1500/ml	400/ml		35/ml			
DY GL LA PU SO SU	**Ultra-Freeda Tablets** Freeda Vitamins	3333.3 (as palmitate and beta carotene, 833.3)	133.3	66.7	333.3	16.7	16.7	8.3 · niacinamide, 25
PE	**Unicap Jr. Chewable Tablets** Pharmacia & Upjohn	5000	400	15	60	1.5	1.7	20
	Unicap M Tablets Pharmacia & Upjohn	5000	400	30	60	1.5	1.7	20
	Unicap Plus Iron Tablets Pharmacia & Upjohn	5000	400	30	60	1.5	1.7	20
GE	**Unicap Senior Tablets** Pharmacia & Upjohn	5000	200	15	60	1.2	1.4	16
	Unicap Softgels Pharmacia & Upjohn	5000	400	30	60	1.5	1.7	20
	Unicap T Tablets Pharmacia & Upjohn	5000	400	30	500	10	10	100
	Unicap Tablets Pharmacia & Upjohn	5000	400	15	60	1.5	1.7	20
GL PU SO	**Unilife B6 Free Tablets** Chronimed	5000	400	30	60	1.5	1.7	20
** DY GL LA PU SO SU	**Unilife-A Gelcaps** Chronimed	15000 (as palmitate)						
	Vantrom Tablets Vangard Labs	5000	400	30	60	1.5	1.7	20

See Chapter 19, "Nutritional Products," for more information about these products.

Pyridoxine HCl (B6) (mg)	Cyanocobalamin (B12) (mcg)	Folic Acid (mcg)	Pantothenic Acid (mg)	Iron (elemental) (mg)	Calcium (elemental) (mg)	Phosphorus (mg)	Magnesium (mg)	Other Ingredients
				10/ml				glycerin · water · propylene · glycol · polysorbate 80 · artificial flavor · color
16.7	33.3	266.7	33.3	5 (as fumarate)	66.7		33.3	bioflavinoids complex, 33.3mg · choline bitartrate, 33.3mg · i-inosital, 33.3mg · PABA, 16.7mg · potassium, 11mg · zinc, 7.5mg · manganese, 3.3mg · biotin, 100mcg · chromium, 66.7mcg · iodine, 40.7mcg · selenium, 33.3mcg · molybdenum, 4.2mcg
2	6	400						sucrose · mannitol · flavor
2	6	400	10	18	60	45		zinc, 15mg · potassium, 5mg · copper, 2mg · manganese, 1mg · iodine, 150mcg · tartrazine
2	6	400	10	22.5	100			
2.2	3	400	10	10	100	77	30	zinc, 15mg · potassium, 5mg · copper, 2mg · manganese, 1mg · iodine, 150mcg
2	6	400						
6	18	400	25	18				zinc, 15mg · potassium, 5mg · copper, 2mg · manganese, 1mg · iodine, 150mcg · selenium, 10mcg
2	6	400						
	6	400	10	18				biotin, 300mg · zinc, 15mg · PABA, 5mg · copper, 2mg · chromium, 200mcg · iodine,150 mcg · molybdenum, 100mcg · selenium, 50mcg
2	6	400	10	18	162	109	100	potassium, 40mg · chloride, 36.3mg · zinc, 15mg · manganese, 2.5mg · copper, 2mg · silicon, 2mg · boron, 150mcg · iodine, 150mcg · biotin, 30mcg · chromium, 25mcg · vitamin K, 25mcg · molybdenum, 25mcg · selenium, 20mcg · tin, 10mcg · vanadium, 10mcg · nickel, 5mcg

VITAMIN PRODUCTS - continued

	Product Manufacturer/Supplier	Vitamin A (IU)	Vitamin D (IU)	Vitamin E (IU)	Ascorbic Acid (C) (mg)	Thiamine (B1) (mg)	Riboflavin (B2) (mg)	Niacin (mg)
GL PU	**Variplex-C Tablets** Hudson				500	15	10	niacinamide, 100
LA PE	**Vi-Daylin ADC Vitamins Drops** Ross Products/Abbott Labs	1500/ml	400/ml		35/ml			
LA PE	**Vi-Daylin ADC Vitamins Plus Iron Drops** Ross Products/Abbott Labs	1500/ml	400/ml		35/ml			
GL PE	**Vi-Daylin Multi-Vitamin Chewable Tablets** Ross Products/Abbott Labs	2500	400	15	60	1.05	1.2	13.5
LA PE	**Vi-Daylin Multi-Vitamin Drops** Ross Products/Abbott Labs	1500/ml	400/ml	5/ml	35/ml	0.5/ml	0.6/ml	8/ml
LA	**Vi-Daylin Multi-Vitamin Liquid** Ross Products/Abbott Labs	2500/5ml	400/5ml	15/ml	60/5ml	1.05/5ml	1.2/5ml	13.5/5ml
GL PE	**Vi-Daylin Multi-Vitamin Plus Iron Chewable Tablets** Ross Products/Abbott Labs	2500	400	15	60	1.05	1.2	13.5
LA PE	**Vi-Daylin Multi-Vitamin Plus Iron Drops** Ross Products/Abbott Labs	1500/ml	400/ml	5/ml	35/ml	0.5/ml	0.6/ml	8/ml
LA	**Vi-Daylin Multi-Vitamin Plus Iron Liquid** Ross Products/Abbott Labs	2500/5ml	400/5ml	15/ml	60/5ml	1.05/5ml	1.2/5ml	13.5/5ml
GL	**Vi-Zac Capsules** UCB Pharma	5000		50	500			
	Vicon C Capsules UCB Pharma				300	20	10	100
GL	**Vicon Plus Capsules** UCB Pharma	4000		50	150	10	5	25
GL PU	**Vioday Tablets** Hudson	5000 (as acetate and beta carotene)	400	30	60	1.5	1.7	niacinamide, 20
	Viogen-C Capsules Goldline Labs				300	20	10	100

See Chapter 19, "Nutritional Products," for more information about these products.

Pyridoxine HCl (B6) (mg)	Cyanocobalamin (B12) (mcg)	Folic Acid (mcg)	Pantothenic Acid (mg)	Iron (elemental) (mg)	Calcium (elemental) (mg)	Phosphorus (mg)	Magnesium (mg)	Other Ingredients
5	10		20					
								flavor · propylene glycol · polysorbate 80 · glycerin · water · methylparaben · propylparaben · caramel color
				10/ml				flavor · glycerin · water · polysorbate 80 · benzoic acid · methylparaben · caramel color
1.05	4.5	300						sucrose · flavor · dextrins · colors
0.4/ml	1.5/ml							alcohol, < 0.5% · flavor · glycerin · water · benzoic acid · methylparaben · disodium edetate · ferric ammonium citrate
1.05/5ml	4.5/5ml							alcohol, < 0.5% · glucose · sucrose · flavor · color · benzoic acid · methylparaben · cysteine HCl
1.05	4.5	300		12				sucrose · flavor · dextrins · mannitol · FD&C yellow#6
0.4/ml				10/ml				alcohol, < 0.5% · flavor · glycerin · water · color · benzoic acid · methylparaben
1.05/5ml	4.5/5ml			10/5ml				alcohol, < 0.5% · flavor · glucose · sucrose · propylparaben · benzoic acid · methylparaben · cysteine HCl
								zinc, 18mg
5			20				7	zinc, 18mg
2			10				7	zinc, 18mg · manganese, 1.8mg
2	6	400	10 (as d-calcium pantothenate)					
5			20				50	zinc, 50mg · tartrazine

VITAMIN PRODUCTS - continued

	Product Manufacturer/Supplier	Vitamin A (IU)	Vitamin D (IU)	Vitamin E (IU)	Ascorbic Acid (C) (mg)	Thiamine (B1) (mg)	Riboflavin (B2) (mg)	Niacin (mg)
** PE	**Vita-Lea for Children Tablets** Shaklee	2500 (as palmitate)	400	30	60	1.5	1.7	20
** PE	**Vita-Lea for Infants & Toddlers Powder** Shaklee	1250/5ml	100/5ml	5/5ml	20/5ml	0.35/5ml	0.4/5ml	4.5/5ml
**	**Vita-Lea, with or without Iron, Tablets** Shaklee	5000 (as palmitate)	400	60	120	1.5	1.7	20
	Vital B-50 Tablets Goldline Labs					50	50	50
DY GL LA PU SO SU PE	**Vitalets Chewable Tablets, Flavored or Unflavored** Freeda Vitamins	5000	400	5	60	2.5	0.9	niacinamide, 20

See Chapter 19, "Nutritional Products," for more information about these products.

Pyridox-ine HCl (B6) (mg)	Cyanoco-balamin (B12) (mcg)	Folic Acid (mcg)	Panto-thenic Acid (mg)	Iron (elemental) (mg)	Calcium (elemental) (mg)	Phos-phorus (mg)	Magne-sium (mg)	Other Ingredients
2	6	400	10	10	200 (as dicalcium phosphate)	160	80 (as oxide)	zinc, 10mg · manganese, 1.5mg · copper, 1mg · biotin, 300mcg · iodine, 90mcg · chromium, 50mcg · molybdenum, 50mcg · selenium, 20mcg · vitamin K, 10mcg · sorbitol · fructose · natural flavors · vegetable juice extracts · citric acid · inositol · choline bitartrate · mixed tocopherols · rice bran powder · rose hips powder · alfalfa powder · acerola extract · grapefruit bioflavonoid · hesperidin complex · lemon bioflavonoid · orange bioflavonoid · sea kelp powder
0.35/5ml	1.5/5ml	100/5ml	2.5/5ml	5/5ml	80/5ml		20/5ml	zinc, 4mg · copper, 500mcg · manganese, 500mcg · biotin, 75mcg · iodine, 35mcg · molybdenum, 12.5mcg · chromium, 10mcg · selenium, 10mcg · vitamin K, 5mcg · dextrose · trace mineral rice protein hydrolysate · inositol · choline bitartrate · acerola extract · mixed tocopherols
2	6	400	10	18 (as fumarate) or 0	450 (as dicalcium phosphate)	350	200 (as oxide)	zinc, 15mg · manganese, 3.5mg · copper, 2mg · boron, 1mg · biotin, 300mcg · molybdenum, 160mcg · iodine, 150mcg · chromium, 130mcg · vitamin K, 80mcg · selenium, 70mcg · nickel, 15mcg · tin, 10mcg · vanadium, 2mcg · microcrystalline cellulose · hydroxypropyl methylcellulose · croscarmellose sodium · spirulina · inositol · choline bitartrate · alfalfa powder · grapefruit bioflavonoid · hesperidin complex · lemon bioflavonoid · mixed tocopherols · orange bioflavonoid · rice bran powder · rose hips powder · acerola extract · hydroxylated soy lecithin · carnauba wax
50	50	100	50					PABA, 50mg · choline bitartrate, 50mg · inositol, 50mg · bromelain, 20mg · d-biotin, 50mcg
2	5		3 (as calcium pantothenate)	10 (as fumarate)	200 (as phosphate)			manganese gluconate, 1mg · biotin, 25mcg

VITAMIN PRODUCTS - continued

	Product Manufacturer/Supplier	Vitamin A (IU)	Vitamin D (IU)	Vitamin E (IU)	Ascorbic Acid (C) (mg)	Thiamine (B1) (mg)	Riboflavin (B2) (mg)	Niacin (mg)
AL GL LA SO SU SL	**Vitalize Liquid** Scot-Tussin Pharmacal					10/5ml		
** SU	**Women's One Daily Multiple Vitamin Tablets** Sundown	5000 (with beta carotene)	400	30	60	1.5	1.7	20
	Z-Bec Tablets Whitehall-Robins Healthcare			45	600	15	10.2	100
	Zymacap Capsules Roberts Ph'cal	5000 (as palmitate)	400	15	90	2.25	2.6	niacinamide, 30

** New listing

See Chapter 19, "Nutritional Products," for more information about these products.

Pyridoxine HCl (B6) (mg)	Cyanocobalamin (B12) (mcg)	Folic Acid (mcg)	Pantothenic Acid (mg)	Iron (elemental) (mg)	Calcium (elemental) (mg)	Phosphorus (mg)	Magnesium (mg)	Other Ingredients
5/5ml	25/5ml			100/5ml (as pyrophosphate), equivalent to 22mg (elemental)				l-lysine monohydrochloride, 100mg/5ml · methylparaben · propylparaben · cherry-strawberry flavor · potassium benzoate · glycerin
2	6	400	10	27	450			zinc, 15mg · tartrazine
10	6		25					zinc (elemental), 22.5mg · microcrystalline cellulose · hydroxypropyl methylcellulose · stearic acid · propylene glycol · titanium dioxide · FD&C blue#1 · aluminium lake · methylparaben · propylparaben · xanthan gum · sodium citrate · potassium sorbate · silicon dioxide · polysorbate 20 · magnesium stearate · polyvinyl pyrrolidone · vanillin
3	9	400	15					soybean oil · gelatin · glycerin · lecithin · corn oil · titanium dioxide · ethyl vanillin

CALCIUM PRODUCTS

	Product Manufacturer/Supplier	Dosage Form	Calcium (elemental)	Vitamin D	Other Ingredients
GL PU SO	**Calcet** Mission Pharmacal	tablet	153mg (as gluconate, lactate, and carbonate)	100 IU	sugar · polyethylene glycol · croscarmellose · color · povidone · magnesium stearate · carnauba wax · beeswax · sodium benzoate
** DY GL PU	**Calci-Caps** Nion Labs	tablet	125mg (as gluconate and dicalcium phosphate)	66.7 IU	lactose · starch · cellulose · magnesium silicate · hydrogenated vegetable oil · croscarmellose sodium · calcium carbonate sugar · titanium dioxide · wax · food shellac
** GL PU SO	**Calci-Caps with Iron** Nion Labs	tablet	125mg (as gluconate and dicalcium phosphate)	66.7 IU	ferrous gluconate, 7.4mg · starch · cellulose · magnesium silicate · calcium carbonate sugar · titanium dioxide · FD&C blue#1 · FD&C yellow#5 (tartrazine) · wax
GL PU SO	**Calci-Chew; Cherry, Lemon, or Orange** R & D Labs	chewable tablet	500mg (as carbonate)		sugar · citric acid · stearic acid · silica · magnesium stearate · flavoring
DY GL LA PU SO SU	**Calci-Mix** R & D Labs	capsule	500mg (as carbonate)		
GL PU SU	**Calciday-667** Hudson	tablet	667mg (as carbonate and oyster shell)		
** SU	**Calcium** Sundown	tablet	60mg (as gluconate)		
GL PU	**Calcium 600 + D3** Hudson	tablet	600mg (as oyster shell)	125 IU	
** SU	**Calcium and Magnesium** Sundown	tablet	158mg (as carbonate)		magnesium, 99mg
GL LA SU	**Calcium Carbonate** Roxane Labs	tablet	500mg; 1250mg (as carbonate)		colloidal silicon dioxide · crospovidone · magnesium stearate · povidone · titanium dioxide · cellulose · polyethylene glycol
DY	**Calcium Carbonate** Roxane Labs	suspension	100mg/ml (carbonate, 250mg/ml)		sorbitol solution, 40% · spearmint flavor · glycol · methylparaben · propylparaben · water · xanthan gum · sodium hypochlorite
	Calcium Carbonate 600 Republic Drug	tablet	1200mg (as carbonate)		
	Calcium Citrate Goldline Labs	caplet	200mg		
** DY GL LA PU SU	**Calcium Complex** Shaklee	tablet	1200mg		magnesium, 40mg · zinc, 1.5mg · manganese, 1.5mg · copper, 0.2mg · ground limestone · modified cellulose gum · carbohydrate gum
** DY GL PR PU	**Calcium Complex** Shaklee	chewable tablet	1000mg		magnesium, 40mg · zinc, 1.5mg · manganese, 1.5mg · copper, 0.2mg · corn syrup solids · non-fat dry milk · acacia gum · flavors

See Chapter 19, "Nutritional Products," for more information about these products.

CALCIUM PRODUCTS - continued

	Product Manufacturer/Supplier	Dosage Form	Calcium (elemental)	Vitamin D	Other Ingredients
** DY LA PU SU	**Calcium Magnesium** Shaklee	tablet	650mg	200 IU	phosphorus, 500mg · magnesium, 400mg · modified cellulose gum · dried yeast · ground limestone · modified food starch
** SU	**Calcium with Vitamin D** Sundown	tablet	600mg (as carbonate)	125 IU	
** SU	**Calcium, Magnesium, and Zinc** Sundown	tablet	167mg (as carbonate)		magnesium, 83.3mg (as oxide) · zinc, 8.3mg (as gluconate)
	Calcium-600 Vangard Labs	tablet	600mg; 1500mg (as carbonate)		
**	**Calel-D** Rhône-Poulenc Rorer Ph'cals	tablet	500mg	200 IU	corn starch · croscarmellose sodium · hydroxypropyl methylcellulose · polyethylene glycol · sodium lauryl stearate
** GL LA PU SO SU	**Caltrate 600** Lederle Consumer	tablet	600mg (as carbonate)		maltodextrin · cellulose · mineral oil · hydroxypropyl methylcellulose · titanium dioxide · sodium lauryl sulfate · gelatin · crospovidone · stearic acid · magnesium stearate
** GL LA PU SO SU	**Caltrate 600 + D** Lederle Consumer	tablet	600mg (as carbonate)	200 IU	maltodextrin · cellulose · mineral oil · hydroxypropyl methylcellulose · titanium dioxide · sodium lauryl sulfate · FD&C yellow#6 · gelatin · crospovidone · stearic acid · magnesium stearate
** GL LA PU SO SU	**Caltrate Plus** Lederle Consumer	tablet	600mg	200 IU	magnesium, 40mg · zinc, 7.5mg · manganese, 1.8mg · copper, 1mg · boron, 250mcg · maltodextrin · cellulose · mineral oil · hydroxypropyl methylcellulose · titanium dioxide · sodium lauryl sulfate · FD&C red#40 · FD&C yellow#6 · FD&C blue#1 · gelatin · crospovidone · stearic acid · magnesium stearate
**	**Caltrate Plus, Asst. Fruit or Spearmint** Lederle Consumer	chewable tablet	600mg	200 IU	magnesium, 40mg · zinc, 7.5mg · manganese, 1.8mg · copper, 1mg · boron, 250mcg
DY GL LA PU SO SU	**Citracal** Mission Pharmacal	tablet	200mg (as citrate)		polyethylene glycol · croscarmellose · povidone · magnesium stearate · carnauba wax · beeswax
** DY GL LA PU SO SU	**Citracal + D** Mission Pharmacal	caplet	315mg (as citrate)	200 IU	polyethylene glycol · croscarmellose · povidone · carnauba wax · magnesium stearate · beeswax
DY GL LA PU SU	**Citracal Liquitabs** Mission Pharmacal	effervescent tablet	500mg (as citrate)		citric acid · calcium carbonate · adipic acid · saccharin sodium · orange flavor · cellulose gum · aspartame

See Chapter 19, "Nutritional Products," for more information about these products.

CALCIUM PRODUCTS - continued

	Product Manufacturer/Supplier	Dosage Form	Calcium (elemental)	Vitamin D	Other Ingredients
GL PU SO	**Citron** Legere Ph'cals	caplet	1000mg (as citrate carbonate)		boron, 3mg (as chelate aspartate)
	Dical-D Abbott Labs	wafer	232mg	200 IU	phosphorus, 0.18g · sucrose · dextrose · talc · stearic acid · mineral oil · salt · natural and artificial flavorings
	Dical-D Abbott Labs	tablet	117mg	133 IU	phosphorus, 90mg · microcrystalline cellulose · sodium starch glycolate · corn starch · hydrogenated vegetable oil wax · magnesium stearate · talc
DY GL LA PU SO SU	**Fem Cal** Freeda Vitamins	tablet	100mg	100 IU	magnesium, 100mg · silicon, 2.5mg · manganese, 5mg · boron, 0.5mg
GL PU SU	**Florical** Mericon	capsule	145.6mg (as carbonate and oyster shell, 364mg)		fluoride, 3.75mg (as sodium fluoride, 8.3mg)
	Florical Mericon	tablet	145.6mg (as carbonate, 364mg)		fluoride, 3.75mg (as sodium fluoride, 8.3mg)
	Gencalc 600 Goldline Labs	tablet	600mg (as carbonate)		
** SU	**Liquid Calcium + D** Sundown	softgel	300mg (as carbonate)	100 IU	
** DY GL LA PU SO SU	**Mag/Cal Mega** Freeda Vitamins	tablet	133.3mg		magnesium, 266.6mg
SU	**Monocal** Mericon	tablet	250mg (as carbonate, 625mg)		fluoride, 3mg (as sodium mono-fluorophosphate, 22.75mg)
	Neo-Calglucon Sandoz Consumer	syrup	115mg/5ml (as gluconate)		sucrose · saccharin · citric acid · benzoic acid · sorbitol · flavors
DY GL PU SU	**Nephro-Calci** R & D Labs	tablet	600mg (as carbonate)		magnesium stearate · cellulose, <0.2mg
** GL SO SU	**NutraVescent Calcium** Northampton Medical	effervescent tablet	1000mg (as citrate)	400 IU	beta carotene, 1000 IU · citric acid · natural orange flavor · aspartame
**	**One-A-Day Calcium Plus** Bayer Consumer	chewable tablet	500mg	100 IU	magnesium, 50mg · sorbitol · maltodextrin · xylitol · starch · stearic acid · aspartame · flavors · polyethylene glycol · gelatin · polydextrose · poloxamer 407 · docusate sodium · vitamin D3

See Chapter 19, "Nutritional Products," for more information about these products.

CALCIUM PRODUCTS - continued

	Product Manufacturer/Supplier	Dosage Form	Calcium (elemental)	Vitamin D	Other Ingredients
GL LA PU SO SU	**Os-Cal 250 + D** SmithKline Beecham	tablet	250mg (as oyster shell)	125 IU	oyster shell powder · talc · corn syrup solids · hydroxypropyl methylcellulose · corn starch · polysorbate 80 · titanium dioxide · polyethylene glycol · propylparaben · methylparaben · simethicone · yellow#10 lake · blue#1 lake · carnauba wax · edetate sodium
DY GL LA PU SU	**Os-Cal 500** SmithKline Beecham	chewable tablet	500mg (as carbonate)		dextrose monohydrate · maltodextrin · microcrystalline cellulose · magnesium stearate · artificial flavors · sodium chloride
** GL LA PU SO	**Os-Cal 500** SmithKline Beecham	tablet	500mg (as oyster shell)		oyster shell powder · talc · corn syrup solids · hydroxypropyl methylcellulose · corn starch · polysorbate 80 · titanium dioxide · polyethylene glycol · propylparaben · methylparaben · polydextrose · triacetin · yellow#10 lake · blue#1 lake · carnauba wax
GL LA PU SO	**Os-Cal 500 + D** SmithKline Beecham	tablet	500mg	125 IU	oyster shell powder · talc · corn syrup solids · hydroxypropyl methylcellulose · corn starch · polysorbate 80 · titanium dioxide · polyethylene glycol · propylparaben · methylparaben · polydextrose · triacetin · yellow#10 lake · blue#1 lake · carnauba wax
	Oyst-Cal 500 Goldline Labs	tablet	500mg (as carbonate)		
	Oyst-Cal-D Goldline Labs	tablet	250mg	125 IU	tartrazine
GL PU SO SU	**Oyster Calcium** Hudson	tablet	375mg (as carbonate and oyster shell)	200 IU	vitamin A, 800 IU (as acetate)
GL PU SO SU	**Oyster Calcium 500 + D** Hudson	tablet	500mg (as oyster shell)	125 IU	
	Oyster Shell Calcium Schein Ph'cal	tablet	500mg (as carbonate and oyster shell, 1250mg)		oyster shell · cellulose · hydroxypropyl methylcellulose · hydroxypropyl cellulose · crospovidone · silica · polyethylene glycol · stearic acid · magnesium stearate · pharmaceutical glaze
** SU	**Oyster Shell Calcium** Sundown	tablet	500mg (as carbonate)		tartrazine
** SU	**Oyster Shell Calcium with Vitamin D** Sundown	tablet	250mg; 500mg (as carbonate)	125 IU	tartrazine (500mg tablet)
SO	**Oyster Shell Calcium-250 and Vitamin D** Vangard Labs	tablet	750mg (as oyster shell)	375 IU	
SO	**Oyster Shell Calcium-500** Vangard Labs	tablet	500mg; 1250mg (as carbonate)		
GL PU SU	**Oystercal 500** Hudson	tablet	500mg (as oyster shell)		

See Chapter 19, "Nutritional Products," for more information about these products.

CALCIUM PRODUCTS - continued

	Product Manufacturer/Supplier	Dosage Form	Calcium (elemental)	Vitamin D	Other Ingredients
GL PU SO SU	**Oystercal-D 250** Hudson	tablet	250mg (as oyster shell powder)	125 IU	
** DY GL LA PU SO SU	**Parvacal** Freeda Vitamins	tablet	500mg	200 IU	
GL	**Posture** Whitehall-Robins Healthcare	tablet	600mg (as tribasic phosphate)		croscarmellose sodium · ethylcellulose · magnesium stearate · microcrystalline cellulose · polyethylene glycol · povidone · sodium lauryl sulfate
GL	**Posture-D** Whitehall-Robins Healthcare	tablet	600mg (as tribasic phosphate)	125 IU	croscarmellose sodium · ethylcellulose · magnesium stearate · microcrystalline cellulose · polyethylene glycol · povidone · sodium lauryl sulfate
DY GL LA PU SO SU	**Super Cal/Mag** Freeda Vitamins	tablet	333.3mg		magnesium, 166.6mg
** DY GL LA PU SU	**Super Calci-Caps** Nion Labs	tablet	400mg (as oyster shell, bone meal, gluconate, and dicalcium phosphate)	400 IU	croscarmellose sodium · hydrogenated vegetable oil · stearic acid · titanium dioxide · magnesium silicate · wax · hydroxypropyl methylcellulose
GL LA PU SO	**Tums 500; Asst. Fruit or Peppermint** SmithKline Beecham	chewable tablet	500mg (as carbonate)		sucrose · starch · talc · mineral oil · flavors · sodium polyphosphate · adipic acid (Fruit) · yellow#6 lake (Fruit) · yellow#10 lake (Fruit) · blue#1 lake (Fruit) · red#27 lake · red#30 lake
** DY GL LA PU	**Vita-Cal** Shaklee	chewable tablet	750mg	200 IU	phosphorus, 500mg · thiamin, 3mg · riboflavin, 3mg · ground limestone · fructose · mannitol · sorbitol · primary grown yeast · spearmint oil · peppermint oil

** New listing

See Chapter 19, "Nutritional Products," for more information about these products.

IRON PRODUCTS

	Product Manufacturer/Supplier	Dosage Form	Iron (elemental)	Vitamins & Nutrients	Other Ingredients
**	**Fe-50 Extended Release** Northampton Medical	caplet	50mg (as sulfate)		corn starch · glyceryl monostearate · polyethylene glycol · titanium dioxide
**	**Femiron Daily Iron Supplement** Menley & James Labs	tablet	20mg (as fumarate)		alginic acid · calcium phosphate · FD&C red#40 · starch · magnesium stearate · stearic acid · silicon dioxide · polyethylene glycol · white wax · carnauba wax
	Feosol SmithKline Beecham	capsule	50mg (as sulfate)		sugar spheres · glycerin · confectioners sugar · starch · povidone · white wax · gelatin · D&C red#7 · polyethylene glycol · glyceryl distearate · ferric oxide · FD&C red#40 · FD&C blue#1 · D&C red#33 · D&C yellow#10
	Feosol SmithKline Beecham	elixir	44mg/5ml (as sulfate)		alcohol, 5% · purified water · sucrose · glucose · citric acid · saccharin sodium · FD&C yellow#6 · flavors
	Feosol SmithKline Beecham	tablet	65mg (as sulfate)		calcium sulfate · starch · glucose · hydroxypropyl methylcellulose · talc · stearic acid · polyethylene glycol · sodium lauryl sulfate · mineral oil · titanium dioxide · D&C yellow#10 · FD&C blue#2
AL DY GL LA SL	**Feostat** Forest Ph'cals	suspension	33mg/5ml (as fumarate)		sucrose, 1917.5mg/5ml · sorbitol solution · methylparaben · veegum · flavor
AL DY GL LA SL	**Feostat** Forest Ph'cals	drops	15mg/0.6ml (as fumarate)		sucrose · sorbitol · methylparaben · veegum · isoascorbic acid · flavor
GL LA PU SU	**Feostat** Forest Ph'cals	chewable tablet	33mg (as fumarate)		magnesium stearate · stearic acid hystrene · saccharin sodium · flavor
GL LA PU SO SU	**Fer-In-Sol** Mead Johnson Nutritionals	capsule	60mg (as sulfate)		gelatin · vegetable oil · glycerin · water · lecithin · yellow wax · artificial flavor and color · methylparaben · propylparaben
DY GL LA SL PE	**Fer-In-Sol** Mead Johnson Nutritionals	syrup	18mg/5ml (as sulfate)		alcohol, 5% · sugar · water · sorbitol · citric acid · salt · artificial flavor · sodium bisulfite
DY GL LA SL PE	**Fer-In-Sol** Mead Johnson Nutritionals	drops	15mg/0.6ml (as sulfate)		alcohol, 0.2% · sugar · sorbitol · water · citric acid · sodium bisulfite · natural flavors
GL PU SO	**Feratab** Upsher-Smith Labs	tablet	60mg; 300mg (as sulfate)		
GL SO	**Fergon** Bayer Consumer	tablet	36mg (as gluconate)		

See Chapter 19, "Nutritional Products," for more information about these products.

IRON PRODUCTS - continued

	Product Manufacturer/Supplier	Dosage Form	Iron (elemental)	Vitamins & Nutrients	Other Ingredients
	Fero-Grad-500 Filmtabs Abbott Labs	tablet	105mg (as sulfate)	sodium ascorbate, 500mg	cellulosic polymers · D&C red#7 · castor oil · magnesium stearate · methyl acrylate-methyl methacrylate copolymers · polyethylene glycol · povidone · pregelatinized starch (contains corn starch) · propylene glycol · talc · titanium dioxide · vanillin
	Fero-Gradumet Filmtabs Abbott Labs	tablet	105mg (as sulfate)		castor oil · cellulosic polymers · FD&C red#40 · FD&C yellow#6 · magnesium stearate · methyl acrylate-methyl methacrylate copolymers · polyethylene glycol · povidone · propylene glycol · titanium dioxide · vanillin
	Ferra-TD Goldline Labs	capsule	50mg (as sulfate)		
GL PU SU	**Ferro-Sequels** Lederle Consumer	timed-release tablet	50mg (as fumarate)		lactose · microcrystalline cellulose · hydroxypropyl methylcellulose · docusate sodium · magnesium stearate · sodium benzoate · silicon dioxide · mineral oil · titanium dioxide · yellow#10 · blue#1 · sodium lauryl sulfate
	Ferrous Fumarate Multisource	tablet	106mg (as fumarate)		
	Ferrous Gluconate Multisource	capsule	38mg (as gluconate)		
** GL PU SO	**Ferrous Gluconate** Upsher-Smith Labs	tablet	34mg; 300mg (as gluconate)		
** SU	**Ferrous Gluconate** Sundown	tablet	36mg (as gluconate)		
AL	**Ferrous Sulfate** Pharmaceutical Assoc.	liquid	60mg/5ml		
	Ferrous Sulfate Multisource	capsule	30mg (as sulfate)		
** SU	**Ferrous Sulfate** Sundown	tablet	65mg (as sulfate)		
**	**Ferrous Sulfate** Sundown	timed-release capsule	50mg (as sulfate)		sucrose
	Ferrous Sulfate Hematinic Schein Ph'cal	elixir	220mg/5ml (as sulfate)		alcohol, 5% · FD&C yellow#6
PE	**Ferrous Sulfate Pediatric Formula** Schein Ph'cal	drops	25mg/ml (as sulfate)		alcohol, 0.2% · sugar · sorbitol · water · citric acid · potassium sorbate · sodium bisulfite · flavors
	Ferrous-S.Q.L. Goldline Labs	capsule	50mg (as fumarate)		docusate sodium, 100mg
**	**Hemaspan** Bock Pharmacal	tablet	110mg	ascorbic acid, 200mg	docusate sodium, 20mg · shellac · povidone · NU-Tab Sugar · magnesium stearate · Eudragit E100 · FD&C blue#1 · FD&C red#40 · FD&C yellow#6 · titanium dioxide · talc · Opaspray beige · polyethylene glycol 8000 · artificial French vanilla

See Chapter 19, "Nutritional Products," for more information about these products.

IRON PRODUCTS - continued

	Product Manufacturer/Supplier	Dosage Form	Iron (elemental)	Vitamins & Nutrients	Other Ingredients
GL PU	**Hytinic** Hyrex Ph'cals	capsule	150mg (as polysaccharide-iron complex)		sodium, 0.2mEq
**	**I.L.X.** Kenwood Labs	elixir	70mg	nicotinamide, 10mg · B1, 5mg · B2, 2mg	liver concentrate, 98mg
**	**I.L.X. B12** Kenwood Labs	elixir	102mg	nicotinamide, 10mg · B1, 5mg · B2, 2mg · B12, 10mcg	liver fraction, 98mg
** SU	**I.L.X. B12 Sugar Free** Kenwood Labs	elixir	102mg	nicotinamide, 10mg · B1, 5mg · B2, 2mg · B12, 10mcg	liver fraction, 98mg
**	**Ircon** Kenwood Labs	tablet	200mg (as fumarate)		
**	**Ircon FA** Kenwood Labs	tablet	250mg (as fumarate)	folic acid, 800mcg	
	Iron Plus Vitaline	tablet	50mg (as gluconate and amino acid chelate)	ascorbic acid, 50mg · folic acid, 400mcg · B12, 5mcg	liver concentrate, 50mg
	Iron Plus Goldline Labs	caplet	50mg (as fumarate)		docusate sodium, 100mg
** DY GL LA PU SU	**Iron Plus Vitamin C** Shaklee	tablet	18mg	calcium, 136mg · phosphorus, 97mg · ascorbic acid, 60mg	maltodextrin · modified cellulose gum · beet powder · acacia gum · spinach powder · barley flour · locust bean gum · agar-agar
SU	**Irospan** Fielding	tablet	65mg	ascorbic acid, 150mg	
	Irospan Fielding	capsule	65mg	ascorbic acid, 150mg	
	Mol-Iron Schering-Plough HealthCare	tablet	39mg (as sulfate)		
GL PU SO	**Nephro-Fer** R & D Labs	tablet	115mg (as fumarate)		whey · stearic acid · hydrogenated vegetable oil · cellulose · silicon dioxide
DY GL LA SU	**Niferex** Central Ph'cals	elixir	20mg/ml (as polysaccharide-iron complex)		alcohol, 10%
	Niferex Central Ph'cals	tablet	50mg (as polysaccharide-iron complex)		
GL LA	**Niferex with Vitamin C** Central Ph'cals	tablet	50mg (as polysaccharide-iron complex)	sodium ascorbate, 168.75mg · ascorbic acid, 100mg	
LA	**Niferex-150** Central Ph'cals	capsule	150mg (as polysaccharide-iron complex)		
** SU	**Perfect Iron** Sundown	tablet	65mg (as carbonyl)		
	Simron SmithKline Beecham	capsule	10mg (as gluconate)		polysorbate 20 · FD&C red#40 · flavor · gelatin · glycerin · methylparaben · polyethylene glycol · propylparaben · simethicone · titanium dioxide · water

See Chapter 19, "Nutritional Products," for more information about these products.

IRON PRODUCTS - continued

	Product Manufacturer/Supplier	Dosage Form	Iron (elemental)	Vitamins & Nutrients	Other Ingredients
GL PU SO	**Slow Fe** Ciba Self-Medication	tablet	50mg (as sulfate)		cetostearyl alcohol · hydroxypropyl methylcellulose · lactose · magnesium stearate · polysorbate 80 · talc · titanium dioxide · yellow iron oxide · blue#2
	Slow Fe + Folic Acid Ciba Self-Medication	tablet	50mg (as sulfate)	folic acid, 400mcg	cetostearyl alcohol · hydroxypropyl methylcellulose · lactose · magnesium stearate · polysorbate 80 · talc · titanium dioxide · yellow iron oxide
	Vitron-C Ciba Self-Medication	tablet	66mg (as fumarate)	ascorbic acid, 125mg	colloidal silicon dioxide · flavor · glycine · hydroxypropyl methylcellulose · iron oxides · magnesium stearate · microcrystalline cellulose · polyethylene glycol · polysorbate 80 · povidone · saccharin sodium · talc · titanium dioxide

** New listing

See Chapter 19, "Nutritional Products," for more information about these products.

MISCELLANEOUS MINERAL PRODUCTS

	Product Manufacturer/Supplier	Dosage Form	Mineral(s)	Other Ingredients
** SU	**Chromium Picolinate** Sundown	tablet	chromium, 200mcg (as picolinate)	
**	**Chromium Picolinate** Mericon	tablet	chromium, 200mcg (as picolinate, 1.6mg)	
** DY GL LA PU SO SU	**Chromium, Organic** Freeda Vitamins	tablet	chromium, 200mcg; 400mcg	
** SU	**Manganese** Sundown	tablet	manganese, 50mg (as gluconate)	
** DY GL LA PU SO SU	**Manganese** Freeda Vitamins	tablet	manganese, 50mg (as gluconate)	
DY GL LA PU SO SU	**Maxi-Minerals** Freeda Vitamins	tablet	calcium, 300mg (as carbonate) · magnesium, 175mg (as oxide) · zinc, 50mg (as gluconate) · manganese, 20mg (as gluconate) · ferrous fumarate, 19.8mg · potassium gluconate, 10mg · copper gluconate, 8mg · iodide, 0.1mg · selenium, 10mcg	
** SU	**Mega Mineral** Sundown	tablet	calcium, 333.3mg (as carbonate) · magnesium, 133.3mg (as oxide) · potassium, 16.6mg · iron, 5mg (as carbonyl) · zinc, 5mg (as sulfate) · manganese, 0.83mg · copper, 0.66mg · chromium, 66.6mcg (from picolinate) · iodine, 50mcg · boron, 33.3mcg · molybdenum, 33.3mcg · selenium, 16.6 mcg · tin, 6.6mcg · nickel, 1.6mcg · vanadium, 3.3mcg	
**	**Orazinc 110** Mericon	tablet	zinc, 25mg (as sulfate)	
**	**Orazinc 220** Mericon	capsule	zinc, 50mg (as sulfate)	
**	**Permathene Maximum Strength Chromium Picolinate** CCA Industries	softgel	chromium, 200mcg (as chromium picolinate) · zinc oxide	phenylpropanolamine HCl, 75mg · beeswax · gelatin · glycerin · lecithin · soybean oil · vegetable oil · water
** SU	**Selenium** Sundown	tablet	selenium, 50mcg; 100mcg	brewers yeast
** DY GL LA PU SO SU	**Selenium, Oceanic** Freeda Vitamins	tablet	oceanic selenium, 50mcg; 100mcg; 200mcg	

See Chapter 19, "Nutritional Products," for more information about these products.

MISCELLANEOUS MINERAL PRODUCTS - continued

	Product Manufacturer/Supplier	Dosage Form	Mineral(s)	Other Ingredients
** DY LA PU SU	**Zinc** Goldline Labs	tablet	zinc, 50mg (as gluconate, 385mg)	
** DY GL LA PU SO SU	**Zinc** Freeda Vitamins	tablet	zinc, 8.5mg (as gluconate, 60mg)	
** DY GL LA PU SO SU	**Zinc** Goldline Labs	lozenge	zinc, 23mg (as citrate and gluconate)	
** DY GL LA PU SO SU	**Zinc** Goldline Labs	tablet	zinc, 25mg (as gluconate, 193mg)	
**	**Zinc 15** Mericon	tablet	zinc, 15mg (as sulfate)	
** DY GL LA PU SO SU	**Zinc, Elemental** Freeda Vitamins	tablet	zinc, 30mg (as gluconate, 235mg)	

** New listing

See Chapter 19, "Nutritional Products," for more information about these products.

ENTERAL FOOD SUPPLEMENT PRODUCTS

	Product Manufacturer/Supplier	Dosage Form	Calories (per mL)	Protein [a] (g)	Carbohydrate [a] (g)	Fat [a] (g)	Vitamins & Minerals	Comments
	Advera Ross Products/Abbott Labs	liquid	1.28	14.2/8fl oz	51.1/8fl oz	5.4/8fl oz	taurine, 0.05g/8fl oz · l-carnitine, 0.03g/8fl oz	for dietary management of patients with HIV infection or AIDS
	Alitra Q Ross Products/Abbott Labs	individual packet	1	15.8/packet	49.5/packet	4.65/packet	various [b,c,d] · glutamine, 21.3/1500calories · arginine · carnitine · taurine	elemental nutrition with glutamine · 300 calories/packet · 5 servings = 100% vitamin USRDA
**	**Amin-Aid Instant Drink** R & D Labs	individual packet	665kcal/packet	6.6/packet (as amino acids)	124.3/packet	15.7/packet		low protein formula for patients with acute or chronic renal failure
** GL LA	**Boost** Mead Johnson Nutritionals	liquid	1.01	43	174	17.5	various [b,c]	volume to meet 100% USRDA is 1180ml
	Carnation Instant Breakfast Carnation Nutritional	liquid	0.73	12.5/10fl oz	36/10fl oz	3.25/10fl oz	various [b,c,d]	
	Carnation Instant Breakfast Carnation Nutritional	individual packet	0.92	12.5	39	1.3	various [b,c,d]	prepare with skim milk
	Carnation Instant Breakfast Carnation Nutritional	individual packet	1.2	12.5	39	12	various [b,c,d]	prepare with whole milk
DY GL LA PU SU	**Casec** Mead Johnson Nutritionals	powder	380/100g	90/100g		2/100g		calcium caseinate
** DY GL LA	**Choice dm** Mead Johnson Nutritionals	liquid	1.06	45	106	51	various [b,c,d]	vanilla flavor · volume to meet 100% USRDA is 1000ml
CO GL LA	**Citrotein** Sandoz Nutrition	powder	0.66	41	122	1.6	various [b,c,d]	orange and punch flavors
LA	**Compleat Modified Formula** Sandoz Nutrition	liquid	1.07	43	140	37	various [b,c,d]	
	Compleat Regular Formula Sandoz Nutrition	liquid	1.07	43	130	43	various [b,c,d]	milk base
DY GL LA SU	**Criticare HN** Mead Johnson Nutritionals	liquid	1.06	38	220	5.3	various [b,c]	volume to meet 100% USRDA is 1890ml

See Chapter 19, "Nutritional Products," for more information about these products.

ENTERAL FOOD SUPPLEMENT PRODUCTS - continued

	Product Manufacturer/Supplier	Dosage Form	Calories (per mL)	Protein [a] (g)	Carbohy-drate [a] (g)	Fat [a] (g)	Vitamins & Minerals	Comments
CO DY GL LA SU	**Deliver 2.0** Mead Johnson Nutritionals	liquid	2	75	200	102	various [b,c]	volume to meet 100% USRDA is 1000ml
** LA SU	**DiabetiSource** Sandoz Nutrition	liquid	1	50	90	49	various [b,c,d]	fructose sweetened · includes traditional food ingredients · fiber content: fruits and vegetables
	Egg Nog Sandoz Nutrition	powder	1.2	62.3	154	37.5	various [b]	prepare with whole milk
LA	**Ensure** Ross Products/Abbott Labs	liquid	1.06	9/8fl oz	40/8fl oz	6/8fl oz	various [b,c,d]	
GL	**Ensure** Ross Products/Abbott Labs	pudding	250	6.8/5oz	34.0/5oz	9.7/5oz	various [b,c,d]	
GL LA	**Ensure** Ross Products/Abbott Labs	powder	1.06	8.8/8fl oz	34.3/8fl oz	8.8/8fl oz	various [b,c,d]	
**	**Ensure High Protein** Ross Products/Abbott Labs	liquid	0.95	12/8fl oz	31/8fl oz	6/8fl oz	various [b,c,d]	
LA	**Ensure HN** Ross Products/Abbott Labs	liquid	1.06	10.5/8fl oz	33.4/8fl oz	8.4/8fl oz	various [b,c,d]	high nitrogen
**	**Ensure Light** Ross Products/Abbott Labs	liquid	0.84	10/8fl oz	33/8fl oz	3/8fl oz	various [b,c,d]	chocolate, strawberry, and vanilla flavors
LA	**Ensure Plus** Ross Products/Abbott Labs	liquid	1.5	13/8fl oz	47.3/8fl oz	12.6/8fl oz	various [b,c,d]	high calorie
LA	**Ensure Plus HN** Ross Products/Abbott Labs	liquid	1.5	14.8/8fl oz	47.3/8fl oz	11.8/8fl oz	various [b,c,d] · l-carnitine, 0.038g/8fl oz · taurine, 0.038g/8fl oz	high nitrogen · high calorie
LA	**Ensure with Fiber** Ross Products/Abbott Labs	liquid	1.1	9.4/8fl oz	38.3/8fl oz	8.8/8fl oz	various [b,c,d]	dietary fiber, 3.4g/8oz
LA	**Fibersource** Sandoz Nutrition	liquid	1.2	43	170	41	various [b,c,d]	contains fiber
LA	**Fibersource HN** Sandoz Nutrition	liquid	1.2	53	160	41	various [b,c,d]	contains fiber
LA	**Forta Drink** Ross Products/Abbott Labs	powder	85/0.8oz mix	5/0.8oz mix	15/0.8oz mix	<1/0.8oz mix	various [b,c,d]	
	Forta Shake Ross Products/Abbott Labs	powder	140/1.4oz mix	9/1.4oz mix	26/1.4oz mix	<1/1.4oz mix	various [b,c,d]	milk base

See Chapter 19, "Nutritional Products," for more information about these products.

ENTERAL FOOD SUPPLEMENT PRODUCTS - continued

	Product Manufacturer/Supplier	Dosage Form	Calories (per mL)	Protein [a] (g)	Carbohy-drate [a] (g)	Fat [a] (g)	Vitamins & Minerals	Comments
	Glucerna Ross Products/Abbott Labs	liquid	1	9.9/8fl oz	22.2/8fl oz	13.2/8fl oz	various [b,c,d] · l-carnitine · taurine · m-inositol	for patients with abnormal glucose tolerance · high fiber (dietary fiber, 3.4g/8oz)
	Health Shake (Frozen) Sandoz Nutrition	liquid	1.58	50.9	271	33.9	various [b,c]	
	Health Shake, No Sugar Added (Frozen) Sandoz Nutrition	liquid	1.4	67.8	197.7	39.6	various [b,c]	soluble dietary fiber, 3g/serving
LA	**High Protein Broth** Sandoz Nutrition	powder	0.67	39	122	2.3		prepare with water
LA	**High Protein Gelatin** Sandoz Nutrition	powder	1.2	99.6	215.8	3.32		prepare with water
GL LA SU	**Impact** Sandoz Nutrition	liquid	1	56	130	28	various [b,c,d]	contains arginine, dietary nucleotides, and fish oil
** GL LA SU	**Impact 1.5** Sandoz Nutrition	liquid	1.5	80	140	69	various [b,c,d]	calorically dense · contains arginine, dietary nucleotides, and fish oil
GL LA SU	**Impact with Fiber** Sandoz Nutrition	liquid	1	56	140	28	various [b,c,d]	contains RNA, arginine, and fish oil · fiber content: soy fiber and partially hydrolyzed guar gum
	Instant Breakfast Sandoz Nutrition	liquid	1.04	50	137.6	33.4	various [b]	
	Instant Breakfast Sandoz Nutrition	powder	1.2	63	156	38	various [b]	prepare with whole milk
	Introlite Ross Products/Abbott Labs	liquid	0.53	22.2	70.5	18.4	various [b,c,d]	for introductory tube feeding · 700 calories = 100% USRDA
CO DY GL LA SU	**Isocal** Mead Johnson Nutritionals	liquid	1.06	34	135	44	various [b,c]	volume to meet 100% USRDA is 1890ml
CO DY GL LA SU	**Isocal HN** Mead Johnson Nutritionals	liquid	1.06	44	124	45	various [b,c]	volume to meet 100% USRDA is 1180ml

See Chapter 19, "Nutritional Products," for more information about these products.

ENTERAL FOOD SUPPLEMENT PRODUCTS - continued

	Product Manufacturer/Supplier	Dosage Form	Calories (per mL)	Protein [a] (g)	Carbohy-drate [a] (g)	Fat [a] (g)	Vitamins & Minerals	Comments
LA	**IsoSource** Sandoz Nutrition	liquid	1.2	43	170	41	various [b,c,d]	
** GL LA	**IsoSource 1.5** Sandoz Nutrition	liquid	1.5	68	170	65	various [b,c,d]	fiber content: soy fiber and partially hydrolyzed guar gum
LA	**IsoSource HN** Sandoz Nutrition	liquid	1.2	53	160	41	various [b,c,d]	
** GL LA SU	**IsoSource VHN** Sandoz Nutrition	liquid	1	62	130	29	various [b,c,d]	fiber content: soy fiber and partially hydrolyzed guar gum
GL LA	**Isotein HN** Sandoz Nutrition	powder	1.19	68	160	34	various [b,c,d]	
LA	**Jevity** Ross Products/Abbott Labs	liquid	1.06	10.5/8oz	35.9/8oz	8.7/8oz	various [b,c,d] · l-carnitine, 0.027g/8oz · taurine, 0.027g/8oz	high nitrogen · added fiber (dietary fiber, 3.4g/8oz)
CO DY GL LA	**Lipisorb** Mead Johnson Nutritionals	liquid	1.35	57	161	57	various [b,c]	volume to meet 100% USRDA is 1180ml
DY GL LA PU	**Lipisorb** Mead Johnson Nutritionals	powder	4.7/g	16.5/100g	54/100g	23/100g	various [b]	volume to meet 100% USRDA is 1180ml prepared
CO DY GL LA SO SU	**MCT Oil** Mead Johnson Nutritionals	oil	8.3/g			1/g		
GL	**Meritene** Sandoz Nutrition	powder	1.06	69	120	34	various [b,c,d]	milk base · chocolate, milk chocolate, strawberry, and vanilla flavors
	Milk Shake Sandoz Nutrition	powder	1.58	50.9	271	33.9	various [b]	prepare with whole milk
	Milk Shake Plus Sandoz Nutrition	powder	1.2	63	156	38	various [b]	prepare with whole milk
CO DY GL LA PU SU	**Modulcal** Mead Johnson Nutritionals	powder	3.8/g		0.95/g			maltodextrin

See Chapter 19, "Nutritional Products," for more information about these products.

ENTERAL FOOD SUPPLEMENT PRODUCTS - continued

	Product Manufacturer/Supplier	Dosage Form	Calories (per mL)	Protein [a] (g)	Carbohy-drate [a] (g)	Fat [a] (g)	Vitamins & Minerals	Comments
LA	**Nepro** Ross Products/Abbott Labs	liquid	2	16.6/8fl oz	51.1/8fl oz	22.7/8fl oz	various [b,c,d] · l-carnitine, 0.062g/8fl oz · taurine, 0.038g/8fl oz	for dialyzed patients with renal failure
**	**Nutra Start** Advanced Nutrition Foods	liquid	0.89	10/8fl oz	40/8fl oz	2.5/8fl oz	various [b,c,d]	chocolate and vanilla flavors
CO LA	**NutrAssist** Chronimed	liquid	1.5	60	180	61	various [b,c,d]	high calorie · high protein
	Nutritious Pudding Sandoz Nutrition	powder	1.67	60	233	53.4	various [b]	prepare with whole milk
	Nutritious Pudding (Frozen) Sandoz Nutrition	pudding	1.67	60	233	53	various [b]	
LA	**Osmolite** Ross Products/Abbott Labs	liquid	1.06	8.8/8fl oz	34.3/8fl oz	8.9/8fl oz	various [b,c,d] · l-carnitine, 0.019g/8fl oz · taurine, 0.019g/8fl oz	isotonic
LA	**Osmolite HN** Ross Products/Abbott Labs	liquid	1.06	10.5/8fl oz	33.4/8fl oz	8.5/8fl oz	various [b,c,d] · l-carnitine, 0.027g/8fl oz · taurine, 0.027g/8fl oz	high nitrogen · isotonic
	Perative Ross Products/Abbott Labs	liquid	1.3	15.8/8fl oz	42.0/8fl oz	8.8/8fl oz	various [b,c,d] · l-carnitine, 0.031g/8fl oz · taurine, 0.031g/8fl oz	for management of metabolically stressed patients · 1500 calories=100% USRDA
LA	**Polycose** Ross Products/Abbott Labs	liquid	2		500			glucose polymers to supply carbohydrate calories
LA	**Polycose** Ross Products/Abbott Labs	powder	380/100g		940			glucose polymers to supply carbohydrate calories
	Pro Mod Ross Products/Abbott Labs	powder	28/6.6g (scoop)	5/6.6g (scoop)	<0.67/6.6g (scoop)	<0.6/6.6g (scoop)		protein supplement
LA	**Promote** Ross Products/Abbott Labs	liquid	1	14.8/8fl oz	30.8/8fl oz	6.2/8fl oz	various [b,c,d] · l-carnitine, 0.029g/8fl oz · taurine, 0.029g/8fl oz	high protein

See Chapter 19, "Nutritional Products," for more information about these products.

ENTERAL FOOD SUPPLEMENT PRODUCTS - continued

	Product Manufacturer/Supplier	Dosage Form	Calories (per mL)	Protein [a] (g)	Carbohy-drate [a] (g)	Fat [a] (g)	Vitamins & Minerals	Comments
LA	**Pulmocare** Ross Products/Abbott Labs	liquid	1.5	14.8/8fl oz	25/8fl oz	22.1/8fl oz	various [b,c,d] · l-carnitine, 0.036g/8fl oz · taurine, 0.036g/8fl oz	for pulmonary patients
CO LA	**ReSource** Sandoz Nutrition	liquid	1.06	37	140	37	various [b,c,d]	chocolate, strawberry, and vanilla flavors
CO GL LA	**ReSource Crystals** Sandoz Nutrition	powder	1.06	37	140	37	various [b,c,d]	vanilla flavor
** GL LA SU	**ReSource Fructose Sweetened / ReSource Diabetic** Sandoz Nutrition	liquid	1.06	63	99	47	various [b,c,d]	fructose sweetened · fiber content: partially hydrolyzed guar gum · chocolate, strawberry, and vanilla flavors
** CO LA	**ReSource Fruit Beverage** Sandoz Nutrition	liquid	0.76	37	150	0	various [b,c,d]	orange, peach, and wild berry flavors
** GL LA PE	**ReSource Just for Kids** Sandoz Nutrition	liquid	1	30	110	50	various [b,c,d]	renal solute load: 190mOsm/1000ml · chocolate, strawberry, and vanilla flavors
	ReSource Nutritious Juice Drink (Frozen) Sandoz Nutrition	liquid	1	33.9	231	1	various [b,c]	
CO LA	**ReSource Plus** Sandoz Nutrition	liquid	1.5	55	200	53	various [b,c,d]	chocolate, strawberry, and vanilla flavors
	ReSource Shake Sandoz Nutrition	liquid	1.5	50.9	254	33.9	various [b]	<1g of lactose/serving
**	**ReSource Shake Plus (Frozen)** Sandoz Nutrition	liquid	1.7	63	244	50.6	various [b]	
**	**ReSource Shake Thickened (Frozen)** Sandoz Nutrition	liquid	1.5	50.9	254	33.9	various [b]	
DY GL LA	**Respalor** Mead Johnson Nutritionals	liquid	1.52	76	148	71	various [b,c]	volume to meet 100% USRDA is 1420ml
** GL LA SU	**SandoSource Peptide** Sandoz Nutrition	liquid	1	50	160	17	various [b,c,d]	semi-elemental peptide-based diet with supplemental arginine

See Chapter 19, "Nutritional Products," for more information about these products.

ENTERAL FOOD SUPPLEMENT PRODUCTS - continued

	Product Manufacturer/Supplier	Dosage Form	Calories (per mL)	Protein [a] (g)	Carbohy-drate [a] (g)	Fat [a] (g)	Vitamins & Minerals	Comments
	Suplena Ross Products/Abbott Labs	liquid	2	7.1/8fl oz	60.6/8fl oz	22.7/8fl oz	various [b,c,d] · l-carnitine, 0.038g/8fl oz · taurine, 0.038g/8fl oz	for dietary management of renal patients prone to uremia · 1900 calories=100% USRDA
GL LA	**Sustacal** Mead Johnson Nutritionals	liquid	1.01	61	140	23	various [b]	chocolate, egg nog, strawberry, and vanilla flavors · volume to meet 100% USRDA is 1060ml
** DY GL PU	**Sustacal** Mead Johnson Nutritionals	individual packet	0.74	47	135	1.1	various [b]	mix with water · vanilla flavor · volume to meet 100% USRDA is 3200ml
GL PU	**Sustacal** Mead Johnson Nutritionals	pudding	1.7/g	6.8/5oz	32/5oz	9.5/5oz	various [b]	milk base · butterscotch, chocolate, and vanilla flavors
DY GL PU	**Sustacal** Mead Johnson Nutritionals	powder	1.08	79	180	2.6	various [b]	mix with skim milk · vanilla flavor · volume to meet 100% USRDA is 810ml
CO GL LA	**Sustacal Basic** Mead Johnson Nutritionals	liquid	1.06	38	146	38	various [b,c]	chocolate, strawberry, and vanilla flavors · volume to meet 100% USRDA is 1890ml
CO GL LA PU	**Sustacal Plus** Mead Johnson Nutritionals	liquid	1.52	61	190	58	various [b,c]	chocolate, egg nog, strawberry, and vanilla flavors · volume to meet 100% USRDA is 1180ml
CO GL LA	**Sustacal with Fiber** Mead Johnson Nutritionals	liquid	1.06	46	139	35	various [b]	chocolate, strawberry, and vanilla flavors · volume to meet 100% USRDA is 1420ml
CO GL LA	**Tolerex** Sandoz Nutrition	powder	1	21	230	1.5	various [b,c,d]	elemental diet · contains 100% free amino acids
DY GL LA PU	**TraumaCal** Mead Johnson Nutritionals	liquid	1.5	82	142	68	various [b,c]	vanilla flavor · volume to meet 100% USRDA is 2000ml

See Chapter 19, "Nutritional Products," for more information about these products.

ENTERAL FOOD SUPPLEMENT PRODUCTS - continued

	Product Manufacturer/Supplier	Dosage Form	Calories (per mL)	Protein [a] (g)	Carbohy-drate [a] (g)	Fat [a] (g)	Vitamins & Minerals	Comments
LA	**Two Cal HN** Ross Products/Abbott Labs	liquid	2	19.8/8fl oz	51.4/8fl oz	21.5/8fl oz	various [b,c,d]	high calorie · high nitrogen
CO DY LA PU	**Ultracal** Mead Johnson Nutritionals	liquid	1.06	44	123	45	various [b,c]	vanilla flavor · volume to meet 100% USRDA is 1180ml
LA	**Vital High Nitrogen** Ross Products/Abbott Labs	individual packet	1	12.5/packet	55.4/packet	3.25/packet	various [b,c,d]	for patients with limited digestion, absorption · 300 calories/packet
** CO GL LA SU PE	**Vivonex Pediatric** Sandoz Nutrition	powder	0.8	24	130	24	various [b,c,d]	100% elemental diet for children ages 1-10 · contains 100% free amino acids and free glutamine
CO GL LA SU	**Vivonex Plus** Sandoz Nutrition	powder	1	45	190	6.7	various [b,c,d]	100% elemental high nitrogen diet · contains 100% free amino acids and free glutamine
CO GL LA SU	**Vivonex T.E.N.** Sandoz Nutrition	powder	1	38	210	2.8	various [b,c,d]	high nitrogen elemental diet · contains 100% free amino acids and free glutamine

** New listing
[a] Unless otherwise specified, content given in grams per liter. Powder products must be added to liquid according to package directions.
[b] Includes vitamins A, D, E, ascorbic acid, thiamine, riboflavin, niacin, pyridoxine HCl, cyanocobalamin, and/or various other substances having vitamin acitvity
[c] Includes iron, calcium, phosophorus, iodine, magnesium, copper, zinc, potassium, sodium, manganese, chromium, selenium, and/or molybdenum
[d] Includes choline, biotin, inositol, and/or folic acid

See Chapter 19, "Nutritional Products," for more information about these products.

This page intentionally left blank.

INFANTS' AND CHILDREN'S FORMULA PRODUCTS

	Product Manufacturer/Supplier	Dosage Form	Kcal (per oz) [b]	Protein Type	Protein (g/L)	Carbo-hydrate Type	Carbo-hydrate (g/L)	Fat Type
	Natural Milks							
	Cow Milk, Whole Cows	liquid	20	casein, 80% · whey, 20%	31	lactose	49	cow milk fat
	Human Breast Milk, Mature Mother	liquid	21	casein, 40% · whey, 60%	9	lactose	68	human milk fat
	Milk-based Formulas							
PE	**Carnation Follow-Up** Carnation Nutritional	concentrate · powder · ready-to-feed	20	nonfat milk	18	lactose · corn syrup	89.2	palm olein · soy oil · coconut oil · high-oleic safflower oil
DY GL PU SU PE	**Enfamil** Mead Johnson Nutritionals	concentrate · powder · ready-to-feed	20	nonfat milk, whey-predominant	14.5	lactose	73	palm olein · soy oil · coconut oil · high-oleic sunflower oil
** GL PU SU PE	**Enfamil Next Step** Mead Johnson Nutritionals	concentrate · powder · ready-to-feed	20	nonfat milk	17.6	corn syrup solids · lactose	75	palm olein · soy oil · coconut oil · high oleic sunflower oil
DY GL PU SU PE	**Enfamil with Iron** Mead Johnson Nutritionals	concentrate · powder · ready-to-feed	20	nonfat milk, whey-predominant	14.5	lactose	73	palm olein · soy oil · coconut oil · high-oleic sunflower oil
DY GL PU SU PE	**Gerber Baby Formula Low Iron** Gerber Products	powder	20	nonfat milk, casein-predominant	14.3	lactose	74	palm olein · soy oil · coconut oil · high-oleic sunflower oil
DY GL PU SU PE	**Gerber Baby Formula with Iron** Gerber Products	concentrate · powder	20	nonfat milk, casein-predominant	14.3	lactose	74	palm olein · soy oil · coconut oil · high-oleic sunflower oil
** DY GL LA PU PE	**Kindercal** Mead Johnson Nutritionals	ready-to-feed	31.3	calcium caseinate · sodium caseinate · milk protein concentrate	34	maltodextrin · sucrose	135	canola oil · MCT oil · high oleic sunflower oil
DY GL LA PU SU PE	**Lactofree** Mead Johnson Nutritionals	concentrate · powder · ready-to-feed	20	nonfat milk, casein-predominant	14.3	corn syrup solids	74	palm olein · soy oil · coconut oil · high-oleic sunflower oil
PE	**Similac** Ross Products/Abbott Labs	concentrate · powder · ready-to-feed	20	nonfat milk, casein-predominant	14.5	lactose	72.3	soy oil · coconut oil

See Chapter 20, "Infant Formula Products," for more information about these products.

Fat (g/L)	Sodium (mEq/L)	Potassium (mEq/L)	Calcium (mg/L)	Phosphorus (mg/L)	Ca:P Ratio	Iron (mg/L)	Osmolality (mOsm/kg)	Renal Solute Load	Comments [c]
38	21	39	1200	920	1.3:1	0.5	288	308	
40	7	13	340	150	2.3:1	0.5	300	93	
27.7	11.5	23.4	912.6	609	1.5:1	13	326	122	for babies 4-12 months and older eating cereal and other baby foods
36	8	18.7	530	360	1.47:1	4.7	300	132	
34	12.2	23	810	570	1.43:1	12.2	270	168	alternative to cow milk for toddlers
36	8	18.7	530	360	1.47:1	12.2	300	132	
36	8.7	18.7	530	360	1.47:1	4.7	320	132	
36	8.7	18.7	530	360	1.47:1	12.2	320	132	
44	16.1	34	850	850	1:1	10.6	310	290	volume to meet 100% USRDA for 1-10 yr. olds is 946mL (1.06 Kcal/mL)
36	8.7	18.9	550	370	1.49:1	12.2	200	132	milk-based
36.5	8	18.1	493	380	1.3:1	1.5	300	96.3	

INFANTS' AND CHILDREN'S FORMULA PRODUCTS - continued

	Product Manufacturer/Supplier	Dosage Form	Kcal (per oz) [b]	Protein Type	Protein (g/L)	Carbo-hydrate Type	Carbo-hydrate (g/L)	Fat Type
PE	**Similac Toddler's Best; Berry, Chocolate, or Vanilla** Ross Products/Abbott Labs	ready-to-feed	20	nonfat milk, casein-predominant	23.3	sucrose · lactose	73.4	high-oleic safflower oil · coconut oil · soy oil
PE	**Similac with Iron** Ross Products/Abbott Labs	concentrate · powder · ready-to-feed	20	nonfat milk, casein-predominant	14.5	lactose	72.3	soy oil · coconut oil
	Soy-based Therapeutic Formulas							
** PE	**Carnation Alsoy** Carnation Nutritional	concentrate · powder · ready-to-feed	20	soy protein isolate	19	corn maltodextrin · sucrose	75	palm olein · soy oil · coconut oil · high oleic safflower oil
** PE	**Carnation Follow-Up Soy** Carnation Nutritional	powder	20	soy protein isolate	21	corn maltodextrin · sucrose	75	palm olein · soy oil · coconut oil · high oleic safflower oil
** GL LA PE	**Enfamil Next Step Soy** Mead Johnson Nutritionals	powder	20	soy protein isolate · L-methionine	22	corn syrup solids · sucrose	80	palm olein · soy oil · coconut oil · high-oleic sunflower oil
** DY GL LA PE	**Enfamil Next Step Soy** Mead Johnson Nutritionals	concentrate	20	soy protein isolate · L-methionine	20	corn syrup · sucrose	68	palm olein · soy oil · coconut oil · high-oleic sunflower oil
DY GL PE	**Gerber Soy Baby Formula** Gerber Products	concentrate · powder	20	soy protein isolate	20	corn syrup · sucrose	68	palm olein · soy oil · coconut oil · high-oleic sunflower oil
LA PE	**Isomil** Ross Products/Abbott Labs	concentrate · powder · ready-to-feed	20	soy protein isolate · L-methionine	18	corn syrup · sucrose	68.3	soy oil · coconut oil
LA PE	**Isomil DF** Ross Products/Abbott Labs	ready-to-feed	20	soy protein isolate · L-methionine	18	corn syrup solids · sucrose · soy fiber	68.3	soy oil · coconut oil
LA PE	**Isomil SF** Ross Products/Abbott Labs	concentrate	20	soy protein isolate · L-methionine	18	glucose polymers	68.3	soy oil · coconut oil
DY GL LA SU PE	**ProSobee** Mead Johnson Nutritionals	concentrate · powder · ready-to-feed	20	soy protein isolate · L-methionine	20	corn syrup solids	68	palm olein · soy oil · coconut oil · high-oleic sunflower oil

See Chapter 20, "Infant Formula Products," for more information about these products.

Fat (g/L)	Sodium (mEq/L)	Potassium (mEq/L)	Calcium (mg/L)	Phosphorus (mg/L)	Ca:P Ratio	Iron (mg/L)	Osmolality (mOsm/kg)	Renal Solute Load	Comments [c]
31.3	12.6	25.6 (Berry, Vanilla); 38.7 (Chocolate)	1040	747	1.4:1	12	[d]	175	for toddlers over 12 months
36.5	8	18.1	493	380	1.3:1	12	300	96.3	
33.5	9.7	20.1	710	412	1.72:1	12.17	270	118	for milk-free feeding during baby's first year
30	12.3	20.4	912.6	608.4	1.5:1	12.17	270	130	for babies 4-12 months and older eating cereal and other baby foods, and who require milk-free or lactose-free feeding
30	13	26	780	610	1.28:1	12.2	260	200	alternative to cow milk for toddlers
36	10.4	21	710	560	1.27:1	12.2	230	179	alternative to cow milk for toddlers
36	10.4	21	710	560	1.27:1	12.2	230	179	
36.9	13	18.7	710	510	1.4:1	12	280	115.6	
36.9	13	18.7	710	510	1.4:1	12	240	115.3	for dietary management of diarrhea in infants and toddlers · total dietary fiber, 6g/L
36.9	13	18.7	710	510	1.4:1	12	180	115.6	
36	10.4	21	710	560	1.27:1	12.2	200	179	

INFANTS' AND CHILDREN'S FORMULA PRODUCTS - continued

	Product Manufacturer/Supplier	Dosage Form	Kcal (per oz) [b]	Protein Type	Protein (g/L)	Carbo-hydrate Type	Carbo-hydrate (g/L)	Fat Type
LA PE	**RCF (Ross Carbohydrate Free)** Ross Products/Abbott Labs	concentrate	12 (diluted 1:1 with water, no carbohydrates added)	soy protein isolate · L-methionine	20	selected by physician	0.04	soy oil · coconut oil
	Other Therapeutic Formulas							
DY GL LA PU SU PE	**3232A Formula** Mead Johnson Nutritionals	powder	20	casein hydrolysate	19	modified tapioca starch	91 (includes 62g added according to label directions)	medium chain triglyceride oil · corn oil
LA PE	**Alimentum** Ross Products/Abbott Labs	ready-to-feed	20	casein hydrolysate supplemented with L-cystine, L-tyrosine, and L-tryptophan	18.6	sucrose · modified tapioca starch	68.9	medium chain triglycerides · safflower oil · soy oil
PE	**Carnation Good Start** Carnation Nutritional	concentrate · powder · ready-to-feed	20	enzymatically hydrolyzed reduced minerals · whey	16	lactose · maltodextrin	74.4	palm olein · soy oil · coconut oil · high-oleic safflower oil
DY GL LA PU SU PE	**Lofenalac** Mead Johnson Nutritionals	powder	20	casein hydrolysate with L-tyrosine, L-tryptophan, L-histidine HCl, L-methionine (see comments)	22	corn syrup solids · modified tapioca starch	88	corn oil
DY GL LA PU SU PE	**Nutramigen** Mead Johnson Nutritionals	concentrate · powder · ready-to-feed	20	casein hydrolysate supplemented with L-cystine, L-tyrosine, and L-tryptophan	19	corn syrup solids · modified cornstarch	74	palm olein · soy oil · coconut oil · high oleic sunflower oil

See Chapter 20, "Infant Formula Products," for more information about these products.

Fat (g/L)	Sodium (mEq/L)	Potassium (mEq/L)	Calcium (mg/L)	Phosphorus (mg/L)	Ca:P Ratio	Iron (mg/L)	Osmolality (mOsm/kg)	Renal Solute Load	Comments [c]
36	13	18.7	700	500	1.4:1	1.5	74	123.6	carbohydrate-free base · carbohydrate must be added before feeding
29	12.6	18.9	640	430	1.5:1	12.8	varies with preparation	170	for disaccharidase deficiencies, impaired glucose transport and intractable diarrhea · carbohydrate must be added before feeding
37.5	13	20.5	710	510	1.4:1	12	370	123.2	for protein sensitivity or allergy, protein maldigestion, or fat malabsorption
34.5	7	17	433	243	1.8:1	10	265	99.3	whey hydrolyzed formula intended for routine feeding of healthy full-term infants
26	13.9	17.6	640	470	1.34:1	12.7	360	186	protein is incomplete; it contains inadequate levels of phenyloclanine needed for normal growth
34	13.9	18.9	640	430	1.49:1	12.2	320	171	for protein sensitivity, food allergies, and severe diarrhea

INFANTS' AND CHILDREN'S FORMULA PRODUCTS - continued

	Product / Manufacturer/Supplier	Dosage Form	Kcal (per oz) [b]	Protein Type	Protein (g/L)	Carbo-hydrate Type	Carbo-hydrate (g/L)	Fat Type
DY GL LA PU PE	**Portagen** Mead Johnson Nutritionals	powder	20	sodium caseinate	24	corn syrup solids · sucrose	78	medium chain triglyceride oil · corn oil
** DY GL LA PU SU PE	**Pregestimil** Mead Johnson Nutritionals	nursette bottle · ready-to-feed	24	casein hydrolysate supplemented with L-cystine, L-tyrosine, and L-tryptophan	23	corn syrup solids · modified corn starch	83	medium chain triglycerides · corn oil · soy oil · high-oleic safflower oil
** DY GL LA PU SU PE	**Pregestimil** Mead Johnson Nutritionals	nursette bottle · ready-to-feed	20	casein hydrolysate supplemented with L-cystine, L-tyrosine, and L-tryptophan	19	corn syrup solids · modified corn starch	69	medium chain triglycerides · corn oil · soy oil · high-oleic safflower oil
DY GL LA PU SU PE	**Pregestimil** Mead Johnson Nutritionals	powder	20	casein hydrolysate supplemented with L-cystine, L-tyrosine, and L-tryptophan	19	corn syrup solids · modified corn starch · dextrose	69	medium chain triglycerides · corn oil · soy oil · high-oleic safflower oil
PE	**Similac PM 60/40** Ross Products/Abbott Labs	powder	20	whey protein · sodium caseinate	15.8	lactose	69	soy oil · coconut oil
	Formulas for Premature Infants							
DY GL PU SU PE	**Enfamil Premature Formula** Mead Johnson Nutritionals	nursette bottle · ready-to-feed	20	nonfat milk, whey-predominant	20	corn syrup solids · lactose	75	medium chain triglycerides · soy oil · coconut oil
DY GL PU SU PE	**Enfamil Premature Formula** Mead Johnson Nutritionals	nursette bottle · ready-to-feed	24	nonfat milk, whey-predominant	24	corn syrup solids · lactose	90	medium chain triglycerides · soy oil · coconut oil
DY GL PU SU PE	**Enfamil Premature Formula with Iron** Mead Johnson Nutritionals	nursette bottle · ready-to-feed	24	nonfat milk, whey-predominant	24	corn syrup solids · lactose	90	medium chain triglycerides · soy oil · coconut oil

See Chapter 20, "Infant Formula Products," for more information about these products.

Fat (g/L)	Sodium (mEq/L)	Potassium (mEq/L)	Calcium (mg/L)	Phosphorus (mg/L)	Ca:P Ratio	Iron (mg/L)	Osmolality (mOsm/kg)	Renal Solute Load	Comments [c]
32	16.1	22	640	470	1.34:1	12.7	230	200	for malabsorption problems and pancreatic insufficiency · higher amounts of vitamins added · infants with cholestatic disease may require supplementation of linoleic acid if Portagen is used as the sole or major food
45	16.5	23	930	610	1.53:1	15.2	320	210	for fat malabsorption, severe diarrhea, GI immaturity, and protein intolerance
38	13.9	18.9	780	510	1.53:1	12.7	280	174	for fat malabsorption, severe diarrhea, GI immaturity, and protein intolerance
38	11.7	18.9	640	430	1.49:1	12.7	320	169	for fat malabsorption, severe diarrhea, GI immaturity, and protein intolerance
37.6	7	14.8	380	190	2:1	1.5	280	96.3	low in sodium, potassium, and minerals
35	11.7	17.9	1120	560	2:1	1.7	260	176	
41	13.9	21	1340	670	2:1	2	310	210	
41	13.9	21	1340	670	2:1	14.6	310	210	

INFANTS' AND CHILDREN'S FORMULA PRODUCTS - continued

	Product Manufacturer/Supplier	Dosage Form	Kcal (per oz) [b]	Protein Type	Protein (g/L)	Carbo-hydrate Type	Carbo-hydrate (g/L)	Fat Type
DY GL PU SU PE	**Enfamil Premature Formula with Iron** Mead Johnson Nutritionals	nursette bottle · ready-to-feed	20	nonfat milk, whey-predominant	20	corn syrup solids · lactose	75	medium chain triglycerides · soy oil · coconut oil
PE	**Similac Special Care 24 with Iron** Ross Products/Abbott Labs	ready-to-feed	24	nonfat milk, whey-predominant	22	lactose · glucose polymer	86.1	medium chain triglycerides · soy oil · coconut oil
	Miscellaneous Products							
DY GL PU SU PE	**Enfamil Human Milk Fortifier** Mead Johnson Nutritionals	powder	14	whey protein · sodium caseinate	0.7	corn syrup solids · lactose	2.7	
DY GL LA PU SU PE	**MSUD Diet** Mead Johnson Nutritionals	powder	20	amino acids (see comments)	11.5	corn syrup solids · modified tapioca starch	91	corn oil
PE	**PediaSure** Ross Products/Abbott Labs	ready-to-feed	30	low lactose whey protein · sodium caseinate	30	hydrolyzed corn starch · sucrose	110	high-oleic safflower and soy oils · medium chain triglycerides
GL PE	**PediaSure with Fiber** Ross Products/Abbott Labs	ready-to-feed	30	low lactose whey protein · sodium caseinate	30	hydrolyzed corn starch · sucrose · soy fiber	114	high-oleic safflower and soy oils · medium chain triglycerides
DY GL LA PU PE	**Phenyl-Free** Mead Johnson Nutritionals	powder	25	amino acids (see comments)	42	sucrose · corn syrup solids · modified tapioca starch	137	corn oil · coconut oil

** New listing
[a] Refer to the text of Chapter 13, "Antidiarrheal Products," for information about fluid and electrolyte replacement products.
[b] Unless otherwise noted, calorie content and other nutritional information pertain to ready-to-feed formula.
[c] Formulas contain appropriate range of vitamins, minerals, and trace elements unless noted otherwise in "Comments" section.
[d] Osmolality not determined by manufacturer/supplier.

See Chapter 20, "Infant Formula Products," for more information about these products.

Fat (g/L)	Sodium (mEq/L)	Potassium (mEq/L)	Calcium (mg/L)	Phosphorus (mg/L)	Ca:P Ratio	Iron (mg/L)	Osmolality (mOsm/kg)	Renal Solute Load	Comments [c]
35	11.7	17.9	1120	560	2:1	12.2	260	176	
44.1	15.2	26.9	1460	730	2:1	15	280	148.7	
<0.1	0.3	0.4	90	45	2:1		120		values are listed for 4 packets of fortifier only, before mixing with breast milk · adequate nutrients only when added to breast milk
28	11.3	17.9	700	380	1.84:1	12.7	300	122	protein is incomplete; it contains inadequate levels of leucine, isoleucine, and valine needed for normal growth
50	16.5	33.5	970	800	1.2:1	14	310	198.5	liquid nutrition for children 1-6 years of age · tube or oral feeding
50	16.5	33.5	970	800	1.2:1	14	345	198.5	liquid nutrition for children 1-6 years of age · tube or oral feeding · total dietary fiber, 1.2g/8fl oz
14.2	37	74	1690	1690	1:1	25	790	460	not recommended for use with infants · protein is incomplete; it contains no phenylalanine

APPETITE SUPPRESSANT PRODUCTS

	Product Manufacturer/Supplier	Dosage Form	Phenylpropa- nolamine HCl	Other Ingredients
GL PU SO	**Acutrim 16 Hour Steady Control** Ciba Self-Medication	timed-release tablet	75mg	cellulose acetate · hydroxypropyl methylcellulose · stearic acid
GL PU SO	**Acutrim Late Day Strength** Ciba Self-Medication	timed-release tablet	75mg	cellulose acetate · FD&C yellow#6 · hydroxypropyl methylcellulose · isopropyl alcohol · propylene glycol · riboflavin · stearic acid · titanium dioxide
GL PU SO	**Acutrim Maximum Strength** Ciba Self-Medication	timed-release tablet	75mg	cellulose acetate · FD&C yellow#10 · FD&C blue#1 · FD&C yellow#6 · hydroxypropyl methylcellulose · povidone · propylene glycol · stearic acid · titanium dioxide
GL PU SO	**Amfed T.D.** Legere Ph'cals	capsule	75mg	
GL PU SO	**Control** Thompson Medical	timed-release caplet	75mg	hydroxypropyl methylcellulose · magnesium stearate · red iron oxide · stearic acid · titanium dioxide · microcrystalline cellulose · povidone · silicon dioxide · carnauba wax
GL PU SO	**Dexatrim Caffeine Free Extended Duration** Thompson Medical	timed-release tablet	75mg	calcium sulfate · D&C yellow#10 aluminum lake · ethylcellulose · FD&C yellow#6 aluminum lake · hydroxypropyl methylcellulose · iron oxide · magnesium stearate · propylene glycol · povidone · stearic acid · titanium dioxide · triacetin · carnauba wax
GL PU SO	**Dexatrim Caffeine Free Maximum Strength** Thompson Medical	timed-release caplet	75mg	stearic acid · magnesium stearate · D&C yellow#10 aluminum lake · FD&C yellow#6 aluminum lake · hydroxypropyl methylcellulose · iron oxide · polyethylene glycol · titanium dioxide · carnauba wax · microcrystalline cellulose · polysorbate 80 · povidone · silicon dioxide
	Dexatrim Caffeine Free Plus Vitamins Thompson Medical	caplet · timed-release caplet	timed-release caplet, 75mg	caplet: vitamins A, D, E, C, B6, B2, B1, B12 · dibasic calcium phosphate · magnesium oxide · niacinamide · ferrous fumarate · zinc · calcium pantothenate · copper · folic acid · potassium iodide timed-release caplet: ascorbic acid, 180mg · croscarmellose sodium · ethylcellulose · FD&C red#40 aluminum lake · FD&C yellow#6 aluminum lake · hydroxypropyl methylcellulose · magnesium stearate · polyethylene glycol · polysorbate 80 · stearic acid · titanium dioxide · may also contain: calcium sulfate dihydrate · carnauba wax · FD&C blue#1 aluminum lake · lactose · microcrystalline cellulose · povidone · silicon dioxide
GL PU SO	**Dexatrim Caffeine Free with Vitamin C** Thompson Medical	timed-release caplet	75mg	ascorbic acid, 180mg · FD&C blue#1 aluminum lake · FD&C red#40 aluminum lake · FD&C yellow#6 aluminum lake · hydroxypropyl methylcellulose · magnesium stearate · microcrystalline cellulose · povidone · stearic acid · silicon dioxide · carnauba wax
GL PU SO	**Dieutrim** Legere Ph'cals	capsule	75mg	benzocaine, 9mg
	Mini Slims BDI Ph'cals	timed-release capsule	75mg	

See Chapter 21, "Weight Control Products," for more information about these products.

APPETITE SUPPRESSANT PRODUCTS - continued

	Product Manufacturer/Supplier	Dosage Form	Phenylpropa-nolamine HCl	Other Ingredients
**	**Permathene Maximum Strength Chromium Picolinate** CCA Industries	softgel	75mg	chromium, 200mcg (as chromium picolinate) · beeswax · gelatin · glycerin · lecithin · soybean oil · vegetable oil · water · zinc oxide
**	**Permathene with Calcium** CCA Industries	tablet	25mg	calcium · croscarmellose · lactose ANH · magnesium stearate · microcrystalline cellulose · stearic acid
	Permathene-12 CCA Industries	timed-release caplet	75mg	dicalcium phosphate · FD&C red#40 · FD&C yellow#6 · lactose D/C · magnesium stearate · microcrystalline cellulose · primellose · stearic acid
	Permathene-12 Maximum Strength with Vitamin C CCA Industries	timed-release caplet	75mg	ascorbic acid · dicalcium phosphate · FD&C yellow#10 · lactose D/C · magnesium stearate · microcrystalline cellulose · primellose · stearic acid
	Permathene-16 CCA Industries	timed-release caplet	75mg	D&C yellow#10 · dicalcium phosphate · FD&C blue#1 · lactose D/C · magnesium stearate · microcrystalline cellulose · primellose · stearic acid
	Protrim Legere Ph'cals	caplet	37.5mg	benzocaine, 9mg
GL PU SO	**Protrim S.R.** Legere Ph'cals	caplet	75mg	
	Super Odrinex Fox Pharmacal	tablet	25mg	cellulose · dicalcium phosphate · magnesium stearate · stearic acid · yellow#6
LA SO	**Thinz Back-To-Nature** Alva-Amco Pharmacal	timed-release tablet	75mg	dicalcium phosphate · natural oat bran · wheat bran · apple fiber · fillers · coating
GL LA SO	**Thinz-Span** Alva-Amco Pharmacal	timed-release capsule	75mg	

** New listing

See Chapter 21, "Weight Control Products," for more information about these products.

ARTIFICIAL TEAR PRODUCTS

	Product Manufacturer/Supplier	Dosage Form	Viscosity Agent	Preservative	pH	Other Ingredients
	20/20 Tears S.S.S. Company	drops	polyvinyl alcohol, 1.4%	disodium edetate, 0.05% · benzalkonium chloride, 0.01%	4.5-5.8	sodium chloride · potassium chloride
	Adsorbotear Alcon Labs	drops	povidone, 1.67% · hydroxyethyl cellulose, 0.41%	thimerosal, 0.004%	7.1-7.6	
PR PU	**Akwa Tears** Akorn	ointment	white petrolatum · mineral oil · lanolin		5.21	
PU	**Akwa Tears** Akorn	drops	polyvinyl alcohol, 1.4%	benzalkonium chloride, 0.01% · disodium edetate	5.21	sodium chloride · dibasic sodium phosphate · monobasic sodium phosphate · purified water
	AquaSite CIBA Vision Ophthalmics	drops	Dextran 70, 0.1%	sorbic acid, 0.2% · disodium edetate	6.5-7	PEG-400, 0.2% · polycarbophil · purified water · sodium chloride · sodium hydroxide
	Artificial Tears Schein Ph'cal	drops	polyvinyl alcohol, 1.4%	disodium edetate · benzalkonium chloride		sodium chloride · may contain hydrochloric acid and/or sodium hydroxide
PR	**Bion Tears** Alcon Labs	drops	hydroxypropyl methylcellulose, 0.3% · Dextran 70, 0.1%		6-9	sodium chloride · potassium chloride · sodium bicarbonate · magnesium chloride · calcium chloride · zinc chloride
PR	**Celluvisc** Allergan	drops	carboxymethylcellulose sodium, 1%		6.2-6.8	calcium chloride · potassium chloride · purified water · sodium chloride · sodium lactate
	Comfort Tears Allergan	liquid	hydroxyethyl cellulose	disodium edetate, 0.02% · benzalkonium chloride, 0.005%	6.7-7.2	sodium chloride
	Dry Eye Therapy Bausch & Lomb	drops	glycerin, 0.3%			calcium chloride · magnesium chloride · potassium chloride · sodium chloride · sodium citrate · sodium phosphate · zinc chloride
	Duolube Bausch & Lomb	ointment	white petrolatum, 80% · mineral oil, 20%			
	DuraTears Naturale Alcon Labs	ointment	petrolatum · mineral oil · lanolin			
**	**GenTeal Lubricant** CIBA Vision Ophthalmics	drops	hydroxypropyl methylcellulose	sodium perborate		boric acid · sodium chloride · potassium chloride · phosphoric acid · purified water
	Hypotears CIBA Vision Ophthalmics	drops	polyvinyl alcohol, 1% · polyethylene glycol 400	benzalkonium chloride, 0.01%	6.6	dextrose · purified water
PR	**Hypotears** CIBA Vision Ophthalmics	ointment	white petrolatum · light mineral oil			
PR	**Hypotears PF** CIBA Vision Ophthalmics	drops	polyvinyl alcohol, 1% · polyethylene glycol 400	disodium edetate	5-7.5	dextrose · purified water
	Isopto Alkaline Alcon Labs	drops	hydroxypropyl methylcellulose, 1%	benzalkonium chloride, 0.01%	6.0-7.8	
	Isopto Tears Alcon Labs	drops	hydroxypropyl methylcellulose, 0.5%	benzalkonium chloride, 0.01%	6.0-7.8	

See Chapter 22, "Ophthalmic Products," for more information about these products.

ARTIFICIAL TEAR PRODUCTS - continued

	Product Manufacturer/Supplier	Dosage Form	Viscosity Agent	Preservative	pH	Other Ingredients
** PR	**Lacri-Lube N.P.** Allergan	ointment	white petrolatum, 57.3% · mineral oil, 42.5% · lanolin alcohol			
**	**Lacri-Lube S.O.P.** Allergan	ointment	white petrolatum, 56.8% · mineral oil, 42.5% · lanolin alcohol	chlorobutanol		
PU	**Liquifilm Tears** Allergan	drops	polyvinyl alcohol, 1.4%	chlorobutanol, 0.5%	3.3-7	sodium chloride · purified water · may contain hydrochloric acid or sodium hydroxide
	Moisture Drops Bausch & Lomb	drops	hydroxypropyl methylcellulose, 0.5% · glycerin, 0.2% · povidone, 0.1%	benzalkonium chloride, 0.01% · disodium edetate		sodium chloride · potassium chloride · sodium borate · boric acid
PU	**Murine Tears Lubricant** Ross Products/Abbott Labs	drops	povidone, 0.6% · polyvinyl alcohol, 0.5%	benzalkonium chloride · disodium edetate	6-7.3	dextrose · potassium chloride · sodium bicarbonate · sodium chloride · sodium citrate · sodium phosphate · purified water
	Murocel Lubricant Ophthalmic Bausch & Lomb	solution	methylcellulose, 1% · propylene glycol	methylparaben, 0.023% · propylparaben, 0.01%		sodium chloride · boric acid · sodium borate
	Ocucoat Lubricating Storz Ophthalmics	drops	hydroxypropyl methylcellulose, 0.8% · Dextran 70, 0.1%	benzalkonium chloride, 0.01%	5.5-7.8	monobasic sodium phosphate · disbasic sodium phosphate · potassium chloride · dextrose · purified water · may also contain hydrochloric acid and/or sodium hydroxide
PR	**Ocucoat PF Lubricating** Storz Ophthalmics	drops	hydroxypropyl methylcellulose, 0.8% · Dextran 70, 0.1%		5.5-7.8	monobasic sodium phosphate · disbasic sodium phosphate · potassium chloride · dextrose · purified water · may also contain hydrochloric acid and/or sodium hydroxide
	Puralube Tears E. Fougera	drops	polyvinyl alcohol, 1% · polyethylene glycol 400, 1%	benzalkonium chloride · disodium edetate		dextrose · purified water
PR PU	**Refresh** Allergan	drops	polyvinyl alcohol, 1.4% · povidone, 0.6%		5.5-6.5	sodium chloride · purified water · may contain hydrochloric acid or sodium hydroxide
** PR	**Refresh P.M.** Allergan	ointment	white petrolatum, 56.8% · mineral oil, 41.5% · lanolin alcohols			purified water · sodium chloride
PR PU	**Refresh Plus CelluFresh Formula** Allergan	drops	carboxymethylcellulose sodium, 0.5%		6-7	calcium chloride · magnesium chloride · potassium chloride · purified water · sodium chloride · sodium lactate · may contain hydrochloric acid or sodium hydroxide
**	**Stye Sterile Lubricant** Del Ph'cals	ointment	petrolatum, 55% · mineral oil, 32%			
	Teargen II Goldline Labs	drops	hydroxypropyl methylcellulose, 0.3% · Dextran, 0.1%	benzalkonium chloride, 0.01%		

See Chapter 22, "Ophthalmic Products," for more information about these products.

ARTIFICIAL TEAR PRODUCTS - continued

	Product Manufacturer/Supplier	Dosage Form	Viscosity Agent	Preservative	pH	Other Ingredients
	Tearisol CIBA Vision Ophthalmics	drops	hydroxypropyl methylcellulose, 0.5%	benzalkonium chloride, 0.01%	7.5	boric acid · potassium chloride · sodium carbonate
	Tears Naturale Alcon Labs	drops	hydroxypropyl methylcellulose, 0.3% · Dextran 70, 0.1%	benzalkonium chloride, 0.01% · disodium EDTA	6.6-7.8	potassium chloride · sodium chloride · sodium hydroxide · purified water
PR	**Tears Naturale Free** Alcon Labs	drops	hydroxypropyl methylcellulose, 0.3% · Dextran 70, 0.1%		6.0-8.0	sodium chloride · potassium chloride · sodium borate · sodium HCl and/or sodium hydroxide · purified water
	Tears Naturale II Alcon Labs	drops	hydroxypropyl methylcellulose, 0.3% · Dextran 70, 0.1%	polyquad, 0.001%	6.5-8.0	potassium chloride · sodium chloride · sodium borate · hydrochloric acid and/or sodium hydroxide · purified water
PU	**Tears Plus** Allergan	drops	polyvinyl alcohol, 1.4% · povidone, 0.6%	chlorobutanol, 0.5%	3.5-7	purified water · sodium chloride · may contain hydrochloric acid or sodium hydroxide
PU	**Tears Renewed** Akorn	drops	hydroxypropyl methylcellulose 2906, 0.3% · Dextran 70, 0.1%	benzalkonium chloride, 0.01% · disodium edetate	6.7-7.3	sodium chloride · potassium chloride · hydrochloric acid and/or sodium hydroxide · purified water
PR	**Tears Renewed** Akorn	ointment	white petrolatum · light mineral oil			
	Ultra Tears Alcon Labs	drops	hydroxypropyl methylcellulose, 1%	benzalkonium chloride, 0.01%	6.0-7.8	
**	**Visine Lubricating** Pfizer Consumer	drops	hydroxypropyl methylcellulose, 0.2% · glycerin, 0.2%	sodium borate · boric acid · disodium edetate	6.3-6.5	

** New listing

See Chapter 22, "Ophthalmic Products," for more information about these products.

OPHTHALMIC DECONGESTANT PRODUCTS

	Product Manufacturer/Supplier	Dosage Form	Viscosity Agent	Vasoconstrictor	Preservative	Buffer	pH	Other Ingredients
	20/20 Drops S.S.S. Company	drops	glycerin, 0.4%	naphazoline HCl, 0.012%	benzalkonium chloride, 0.01%	boric acid, 1.25% · sodium carbonate, 0.004%	6	potassium chloride · zinc sulfate · camphor
PU	**AK-Nefrin** Akorn	drops	polyvinyl alcohol, 1.4%	phenylephrine HCl, 0.12%	benzalkonium chloride, 0.005%	monobasic sodium phosphate · dibasic sodium phosphate · hydrochloric acid and/or sodium hydroxide	6.2-6.8	sodium chloride · purified water · disodium edetate
	Allerest Eye Drops Ciba Self-Medication	drops		naphazoline HCl, 0.012%	benzalkonium chloride · EDTA	boric acid · sodium borate	5.5-6.3	water
PU	**Clear eyes ACR Astringent/Lubricant Eye Redness Reliever** Ross Products/Abbott Labs	drops	glycerin, 0.2%	naphazoline HCl, 0.012%	benzalkonium chloride · disodium edetate	boric acid · sodium citrate	5.5-6.3	zinc sulfate, 0.25% · sodium chloride · purified water
PU	**Clear eyes Lubricant Eye Redness Reliever** Ross Products/Abbott Labs	drops	glycerin, 0.2%	naphazoline HCl, 0.012%	benzalkonium chloride · disodium edetate	boric acid · sodium borate	5.5-6.3	purified water
	Collyrium Fresh Wyeth-Ayerst Labs	drops	glycerin, 1%	tetrahydrozoline HCl, 0.05%	benzalkonium chloride, 0.01% · disodium edetate, 0.01%	boric acid · sodium borate · hydrochloric acid		
	Comfort Eye Drops Akorn	drops		naphazoline HCl, 0.03%	disodium edetate, 0.02% · benzalkonium chloride, 0.005%			
	Degest 2 Akorn	drops	hydroxyethyl cellulose · povidone	naphazoline HCl, 0.012%	disodium edetate, 0.02% · benzalkonium chloride, 0.0067%			
	Estivin II Alcon Labs	drops	hydroxypropyl methylcellulose, 0.3% · Dextran 70, 0.1%	naphazoline HCl, 0.012%	benzalkonium chloride, 0.01%		5.5-6.5	
**	**Eye-Sed** Scherer Labs	drops		tetrahydrozoline HCl, 0.05%	disodium edetate · benzalkonium chloride	sodium borate · boric acid	5.8-7	zinc sulfate, 0.25% · sodium chloride

See Chapter 22, "Ophthalmic Products," for more information about these products.

OPHTHALMIC DECONGESTANT PRODUCTS - continued

	Product Manufacturer/Supplier	Dosage Form	Viscosity Agent	Vasoconstrictor	Preservative	Buffer	pH	Other Ingredients
**	**EyeSine** Akorn	drops		tetrahydrozoline HCl, 0.05%	benzalkonium chloride, 0.01% · disodium edetate	boric acid · sodium borate	5.8-6.5	sodium chloride · purified water
	Geneye Goldline Labs	drops		tetrahydrozoline HCl, 0.05%				
	Isopto-Frin Alcon Labs	drops	hydroxypropyl methylcellulose, 0.5%	phenylephrine HCl, 0.12%	benzalkonium chloride, 0.01%	sodium citrate · sodium phosphate · sodium biphosphate	4.0-7.5	
PU	**Murine Plus Lubricant Eye Redness Reliever** Ross Products/Abbott Labs	drops	povidone, 0.6% · polyvinyl alcohol, 0.5%	tetrahydrozoline HCl, 0.05%	benzalkonium chloride · disodium edetate	sodium phosphate	6-7.3	dextrose · potassium chloride · purified water · sodium bicarbonate · sodium chloride
	Naphcon Alcon Labs	drops		naphazoline HCl, 0.012%	benzalkonium chloride, 0.01% · disodium EDTA	boric acid	5.5-7.0	sodium chloride · potassium chloride
	Naphcon-A Alcon Labs	solution		naphazoline HCl, 0.025%	benzalkonium chloride, 0.01% · disodium edetate	boric acid · sodium borate · hydrochloric acid and/or sodium hydroxide	5-7	pheniramine maleate, 0.3% · sodium chloride · purified water
	Ocu Clear Schering-Plough HealthCare	drops		oxymetazoline HCl, 0.025%	benzalkonium chloride, 0.01% · EDTA	sodium hydroxide	6.4	
**	**OcuHist** Pfizer Consumer	drops		naphazoline HCl, 0.025%	disodium edetate, 0.1% · benzalkonium chloride, 0.01%	boric acid · sodium borate · hydrochloric acid and/or sodium hydroxide	5.5-6.5	pheniramine maleate, 0.3% · purified water
	Opcon-A Bausch & Lomb	drops	hydroxypropyl methylcellulose 0.5%	naphazoline HCl, 0.027%	disodium edetate, 0.1% · benzalkonium chloride, 0.01%	boric acid · sodium borate	5.5-6.3	pheniramine maleate, 0.315% · sodium chloride · purified water
	Optigene Pfeiffer Ph'cals	drops		tetrahydrozoline HCl, 0.05%	EDTA, 0.1% · benzalkonium chloride, 0.01%		6-7	

See Chapter 22, "Ophthalmic Products," for more information about these products.

OPHTHALMIC DECONGESTANT PRODUCTS - continued

	Product Manufacturer/Supplier	Dosage Form	Viscosity Agent	Vasoconstrictor	Preservative	Buffer	pH	Other Ingredients
PU	**Prefrin Liquifilm** Allergan	drops	polyvinyl alcohol, 1.4%	phenylephrine HCl, 0.12%	benzalkonium chloride, 0.005%	monobasic sodium phosphate · dibasic sodium phosphate · may contain hydrochloric acid or sodium hydroxide	6.3-7.1	disodium edetate · purified water · sodium acetate · sodium thiosulfate
PR PU	**Relief** Allergan	drops	polyvinyl alcohol, 1.4%	phenylephrine HCl, 0.12%		monobasic sodium phosphate · dibasic sodium phosphate · may contain hydrochloric acid and/or sodium chloride	6.3-7.1	disodium edetate · purified water · sodium acetate · sodium thiosulfate
**	**Sensitive Eyes Redness Reliever Lubricant** Bausch & Lomb	drops	polyethylene glycol 300, 0.2%	naphazoline HCl, 0.012%	benzalkonium chloride, 0.01% · disodium edetate	boric acid · sodium borate		sodium chloride
**	**Sensitive Eyes Redness Reliever Lubricant Maximum Strength** Bausch & Lomb	drops	hydroxypropyl methylcellulose, 0.5%	naphazoline HCl, 0.03%	benzalkonium chloride, 0.01% · disodium edetate	boric acid · sodium borate		sodium chloride
	Soothe Alcon Labs	drops	povidone, 1.67% · polyethylene glycol	tetrahydrozoline HCl, 0.05% · disodium edetate	benzalkonium chloride, 0.004%	boric acid · sodium borate · hydrochloric acid and/or sodium hydroxide	5.8-6.5	sodium chloride
	Vaso Clear CIBA Vision Ophthalmics	drops	polyvinyl alcohol	naphazoline HCl, 0.02%	benzalkonium chloride, 0.01% · EDTA		5.5-7	PEG-8000
	Vaso Clear A CIBA Vision Ophthalmics	drops	polyvinyl alcohol, 0.25%	naphazoline HCl, 0.02%	benzalkonium chloride, 0.005% · EDTA		5.5-6.6	zinc sulfate, 0.25% · PEG-8000
**	**Vasocon-A** CIBA Vision Ophthalmics	drops		naphazoline HCl, 0.05%	benzalkonium chloride		5.5-6.3	antazoline phosphate, 0.5%
PU	**Visine Allergy Relief** Pfizer Consumer	drops		tetrahydrozoline HCl, 0.05%	EDTA, 0.1% · benzalkonium chloride, 0.01%	boric acid · sodium citrate	6.3-6.5	zinc sulfate, 0.25% · sodium chloride
PU	**Visine L.R.** Pfizer Consumer	drops		oxymetazoline HCl, 0.025%	EDTA, 0.1% · benzalkonium chloride, 0.01%	boric acid · sodium borate	6.3-6.5	sodium chloride

See Chapter 22, "Ophthalmic Products," for more information about these products.

OPHTHALMIC DECONGESTANT PRODUCTS - continued

	Product Manufacturer/Supplier	Dosage Form	Viscosity Agent	Vasoconstrictor	Preservative	Buffer	pH	Other Ingredients
PU	**Visine Moisturizing** Pfizer Consumer	drops	polyethylene glycol 400, 1%	tetrahydrozoline HCl, 0.05%	EDTA, 0.1% · benzalkonium chloride, 0.013%	boric acid · sodium borate	6.3-6.5	sodium chloride
PU	**Visine Original Formula** Pfizer Consumer	drops		tetrahydrozoline HCl, 0.05%	EDTA, 0.1% benzalkonium chloride, 0.01%	boric acid · sodium borate	6.3-6.5	sodium chloride
	Zincfrin Alcon Labs	drops		phenylephrine HCl, 0.12%	benzalkonium chloride, 0.01%	citric acid · sodium citrate	7.0-7.8	zinc sulfate, 0.25%

** New listing

See Chapter 22, "Ophthalmic Products," for more information about these products.

MISCELLANEOUS OPHTHALMIC PRODUCTS

	Product Manufacturer/Supplier	Dosage Form	Buffer	pH	Preservative	Other Ingredients
	Irrigants					
	Blinx Akorn	solution	sodium phosphate		disodium edetate, 0.02% · benzalkonium chloride, 0.005%	sodium chloride · potassium chloride
	Collyrium for Fresh Eyes Wyeth-Ayerst Labs	solution	boric acid · sodium borate		benzalkonium chloride	water
	Dacriose CIBA Vision Ophthalmics	liquid	sodium phosphate		disodium edetate, 0.3% · benzalkonium chloride, 0.01%	sodium hydroxide, 0.01% · sodium chloride · potassium chloride
	Eye Wash Bausch & Lomb	liquid	borate		sorbic acid, 0.1% · EDTA, 0.025%	sodium chloride
	Eye-Stream Alcon Labs	liquid	sodium acetate, 0.39% · sodium citrate, 0.17%	6.5-7.5	benzalkonium chloride, 0.013%	potassium chloride, 0.075% · sodium chloride, 0.64% · calcium chloride, 0.048% · magnesium chloride, 0.03% · sodium hydroxide and/or hydrochloric acid
	Lavoptik Eye Wash Lavoptik	liquid	sodium phosphate	7	benzalkonium chloride, 0.005% · sodium edetate	sodium chloride, 0.49%
	Optigene Pfeiffer Ph'cals	solution	monobasic sodium phosphate · dibasic sodium phosphate	6-7	benzalkonium chloride · disodium edetate	sodium chloride
	Hyperosmotics					
**	**Adsorbonac** Alcon Labs	solution	sodium phosphate		thimerosal 0.04% · disodium edetate	sodium chloride, 2%; 5% · polyethylene glycol · hydroxythethyl cellulose · povidone · hydrochloric acid and/or sodium hydroxide
** PR	**AK-NaCl** Akorn	ointment		6-8		sodium chloride, 5% · lanolin oil · mineral oil · white petrolatum · purified water
**	**AK-NaCl** Akorn	solution	boric acid · sodium borate · hydrochloric acid and/or sodium hydroxide	6-8	methylparaben, 0.023% · propylparaben, 0.017%	sodium chloride, 5% · hydroxypropyl methylcellulose 2906 · propylene glycol · purified water
**	**Muro 128** Bausch & Lomb	ointment				sodium chloride, 5%
**	**Muro 128** Bausch & Lomb	solution				sodium chloride, 2%
	Eye Lid Scrubs					
	Eye-Scrub CIBA Vision Ophthalmics	liquid			EDTA · benzyl alcohol	PEG-200 glyceryl monotallowate · disodium laureth sulfosuccinate · cocoamido propyl amine oxide · PEG-78 glyceryl monococoate

See Chapter 22, "Ophthalmic Products," for more information about these products.

MISCELLANEOUS OPHTHALMIC PRODUCTS - continued

	Product Manufacturer/Supplier	Dosage Form	Buffer	pH	Preservative	Other Ingredients
PR PU	**Lid Wipes-SPF** Akorn	pad	sodium phosphate · monobasic sodium hydroxide · phosphoric acid	6-7.6		PEG-200 glyceryl tallowate · PEG-80 glyceryl cocoate · laureth-23 · cocoamido propyl amine oxide · sodium chloride · glycerin · water
	Prosthesis Lubricant/Cleanser					
	Enuclene Alcon Labs	solution		6.1-6.8	benzalkonium chloride, 0.02%	hydroxypropyl methylcellulose, 0.85% · tyloxapol, 0.25%

** New listing

See Chapter 22, "Ophthalmic Products," for more information about these products.

HARD LENS PRODUCTS

	Product Manufacturer/Supplier	Product Form	Use	Viscosity Agent	Preservative	Other Ingredients
**	**20/20 Lubricating & Rewetting Solution** S.S.S. Company	drops	rewetting · lubricating	polyvinyl alcohol, 1.4%	sodium edetate, 0.05% · benzalkonium chloride, 0.01%	sodium chloride · potassium chloride
	Adapettes for Sensitive Eyes Alcon Labs	liquid	lubricating · rewetting		sorbic acid, 0.2% · disodium edetate, 0.1%	boric acid · sodium borate · sodium chloride
	Adapt Alcon Labs	liquid	wetting · rewetting	hydroxyethyl cellulose	thimerosal, 0.004% · disodium edetate	poloxamer · povidone · sodium phosphate · sodium chloride
PU	**Blairex Hard Contact Lens Cleaner** Blairex Labs	liquid	cleaning			miracare 2MCA, 20% · water
**	**Blairex Sterile Contact Lens Cleaner** Blairex Labs	liquid	cleaning		disodium edetate, 0.1% · benzalkonium chloride, 0.01%	cocoamphodiacetate · glycols
**	**Blairex Sterile Contact Lens Conditioning Solution** Blairex Labs	liquid	wetting · soaking · disinfecting		disodium edetate, 0.1% · benzalkonium chloride, 0.01%	
	Clean-N-Soak Allergan	liquid	cleaning · soaking		phenylmercuric nitrate, 0.004%	cleaning agent
	Clerz 2 Alcon Labs	drops	lubricating · rewetting	hydroxyethyl cellulose	sorbic acid, 0.2% · disodium edetate, 0.1%	sodium chloride · potassium chloride · sodium borate
	LC-65 Daily Contact Lens Cleaner Allergan	liquid	cleaning	cocoamphocarboxyglycinate	EDTA	sodium lauryl sulfate · hexylene glycol · sodium chloride · sodium phosphate
	Lens Fresh Allergan	drops	rewetting · lubricating	hydroxyethyl cellulose	EDTA, 0.2% · sorbic acid, 0.1%	sodium chloride · boric acid · sodium borate
	Lens Lubricant Bausch & Lomb	liquid	rewetting · lubricating	povidone	EDTA, 0.1% · thimerosal, 0.004%	polyoxyethylene
	Liquifilm Allergan	solution	wetting	hydroxypropyl methylcellulose · polyvinyl alcohol	benzalkonium chloride, 0.004% · EDTA	sodium chloride · potassium chloride
	Opti-Clean Daily Cleaner Alcon Labs	liquid	cleaning	hydroxyethyl cellulose	disodium edetate, 0.1% · thimerosal, 0.004%	nylon 11 · polysorbate 21 · boric acid · sodium borate · sodium chloride
	Opti-Clean II Daily Cleaner for Sensitive Eyes Alcon Labs	liquid	cleaning	hydroxyethyl cellulose	polyquaternium-1 · disodium edetate	nylon 11 · polysorbate 21 · boric acid · sodium borate · sodium chloride
	Opti-Zyme Enzymatic Cleaner Alcon Labs	tablet	weekly protein cleaning			pancreatin
	Soaclens Alcon Labs	liquid	soaking · wetting	hydroxyethyl cellulose · polyvinyl alcohol	disodium edetate, 0.1% · thimerosal, 0.004%	sodium chloride · sodium phosphate · polyvinyl alcohol

See Chapter 23, "Contact Lens Products," for more information about these products.

HARD LENS PRODUCTS - continued

Product Manufacturer/Supplier	**Product Form**	**Use**	**Viscosity Agent**	**Preservative**	**Other Ingredients**
Total All-In-One Contact Lens Allergan	solution	wetting · cleaning · soaking	polyvinyl alcohol	benzalkonium chloride · EDTA	

** New listing

See Chapter 23, "Contact Lens Products," for more information about these products.

RIGID GAS-PERMEABLE LENS PRODUCTS

	Product Manufacturer/Supplier	Product Form	Use	Viscosity Agent	Preservative	Other Ingredients
**	**Blairex Sterile Contact Lens Cleaner** Blairex Labs	liquid	cleaning		disodium edetate, 0.1% · benzalkonium chloride, 0.01%	cocoamphodiacetate · glycols
**	**Blairex Sterile Contact Lens Conditioning Solution** Blairex Labs	liquid	wetting · soaking · disinfecting		disodium edetate, 0.1% · benzalkonium chloride, 0.01%	
PR	**Boston Advance Cleaner** Polymer Technology	liquid	cleaning			alkyl ether sulfate · ethoxylated alkyl phenol · triquaternary cocoa-based phospholipid · silica gel
**	**Boston Advance Comfort Formula Conditioning Solution** Polymer Technology	solution	wetting · soaking · disinfecting	cellulosic viscosifier	disodium edetate, 0.05% · chlorhexidine gluconate, 0.003% · polyaminopropyl biguanide, 0.0005%	cationic cellulose derivative polymer · derivatized polyethylene glycol · polyvinyl alcohol
PR	**Boston Cleaner** Polymer Technology	liquid	cleaning			alkyl ether sulfate · silica gel · titanium dioxide · fragrance
	Boston Conditioning Solution Polymer Technology	solution	wetting · soaking · disinfecting	hydroxyethyl cellulose	disodium edetate, 0.05% · chlorhexidine gluconate, 0.006%	polyvinyl alcohol · cationic cellulose derivatives
	Boston Rewetting Drops Polymer Technology	drops	lubricating · rewetting	hydroxyethyl cellulose	disodium edetate, 0.05% · chlorhexidine gluconate, 0.006%	polyvinyl alcohol · cationic cellulose derivatives
**	**Boston Simplicity** Polymer Technology	solution	cleaning · rinsing · disinfecting · conditioning	cellulosic viscosifier	disodium edetate, 0.05% · chlorhexidine gluconate, 0.003% · polyaminopropyl biguanide, 0.0005%	PEO sorbitan monolaurate · betaine surfactant · silicone glycol copolymer · derivatized polyethylene glycol
	Concentrated Cleaner Bausch & Lomb	liquid	cleaning			sodium chloride · sulfate surfactant
	Opti-Clean II Daily Cleaner for Sensitive Eyes Alcon Labs	liquid	cleaning	hydroxyethyl cellulose	EDTA, 0.1% · thimerosal, 0.004%	polysorbate 21 · cleaning agent · boric acid · sodium borate · sodium chloride · sodium hydroxide · purified water
	Opti-Zyme Enzymatic Cleaner Alcon Labs	tablet	weekly protein cleaning			pancreatin
	Pro Free/GP Weekly Enzymatic Cleaner [a] Allergan	tablet	weekly protein cleaning		disodium edetate	sodium chloride · sodium carbonate · sodium borate · papain
	Resolve/GP Daily Cleaner Allergan	liquid	cleaning	cocoamphocarboxyglycinate		fatty acid amide · surfactants · sodium lauryl sulfate · hexylene glycol · alkyl ether sulfate

See Chapter 23, "Contact Lens Products," for more information about these products.

RIGID GAS-PERMEABLE LENS PRODUCTS - continued

Product Manufacturer/Supplier	**Product Form**	**Use**	**Viscosity Agent**	**Preservative**	**Other Ingredients**
Wet & Soak Allergan	drops	rewetting · lubricating	hydroxyethyl cellulose	WSCP, 0.0060%	borate
Wet-N-Soak Plus Allergan	solution	wetting · soaking	polyvinyl alcohol	benzalkonium chloride, 0.003% · EDTA	
Wetting & Soaking Solution Bausch & Lomb	solution	rinsing · disinfecting · storage	polyvinyl alcohol · hydroxyethyl cellulose	EDTA, 0.05% · chlorhexidine gluconate, 0.006%	

** New listing
[a] Tablet must be dissolved in water.

See Chapter 23, "Contact Lens Products," for more information about these products.

SOFT LENS PRODUCTS

	Product Manufacturer/Supplier	Product Form	Use	Viscosity Agent	Preservative	Other Ingredients
	Multipurpose Solutions					
	Complete Multi-Purpose Allergan	solution	cleaning · rinsing · disinfecting · storing		polyhexamethylene biguanide · EDTA	sodium chloride · tromethamine · tyloxapol
**	**Opti-Free Express** Alcon Labs	solution	cleaning · rinsing · disinfecting · storing		polyquaternium-1 · disodium edetate	sodium citrate · sodium chloride · citric acid
	Opti-One Multi-Purpose Alcon Labs	solution	rinsing · chemical disinfecting · storing		disodium EDTA, 0.05% · polyquaternium-1, 0.001%	citric acid · sodium citrate · sodium chloride · sodium hydroxide and/or hydrochloric acid · purified water
	ReNu Multi-Purpose Bausch & Lomb	solution	cleaning · rinsing · chemical disinfecting · storing · enzyme diluent		EDTA · polyaminopropyl biguanide	sodium chloride · sodium borate · boric acid · poloxamine
	Surface Active Cleaners					
	Ciba Vision Cleaner Ciba Vision	liquid	cleaning	cocoamphocarboxyglycinate	EDTA, 0.2% · sorbic acid, 0.1%	sodium lauryl sulfate · hexylene glycol
	Daily Cleaner Bausch & Lomb	liquid	cleaning	hydroxyethyl cellulose · polyvinyl alcohol	EDTA, 0.2% · thimerosal, 0.004%	tyloxapol · sodium phosphate · sodium chloride
	DURAcare II Blairex Labs	liquid	cleaning		disodium edetate, 0.25% · sorbic acid, 0.1%	block copolymers of ethylene and propylene oxide · octylphenoxy polyethoxyethanol
	LC-65 Daily Contact Lens Cleaner Allergan	liquid	cleaning	cocoamphocarboxyglycinate	EDTA	sodium lauryl sulfate · hexylene glycol · sodium chloride · sodium phosphate
	Lens Clear Cleaner Allergan	liquid	cleaning	cocoamphocarboxyglycinate	EDTA, 0.2% · sorbic acid, 0.1%	sodium lauryl sulfate · hexylene glycol
	Lens Plus Daily Cleaner Allergan	liquid	cleaning	cocoamphocarboxyglycinate		sodium lauryl sulfate · hexylene glycol · sodium chloride · sodium phosphate
	MiraFlow Extra Strength Ciba Vision	liquid	cleaning			isopropyl alcohol, 20% · poloxamer 407 · amphoteric 10
	Opti-Clean Daily Cleaner Alcon Labs	liquid	cleaning	hydroxyethyl cellulose	disodium edetate, 0.1% · thimerosal, 0.004%	nylon 11 · polysorbate 21 · boric acid · sodium borate · sodium chloride
	Opti-Clean II Daily Cleaner for Sensitive Eyes Alcon Labs	liquid	cleaning	hydroxyethyl cellulose	polyquaternium-1 · disodium edetate	nylon 11 · polysorbate 21 · boric acid · sodium borate · sodium chloride
	Opti-Free Daily Cleaner Alcon Labs	liquid	cleaning	hydroxyethyl cellulose	polyquaternium-1 · disodium EDTA	nylon II · polysorbate 21 · sodium borate · boric acid · hydrochloric acid and/or sodium hydroxide · purified water
**	**Opti-Soak Conditioning** Alcon Labs	solution	cleaning	hydroxyethyl cellulose · polyvinyl alcohol	polyquaternium-1 · disodium edetate	sodium phosphate · sodium chloride · polysorbate 80
**	**Opti-Soak Daily Cleaner** Alcon Labs	liquid	cleaning	hydroxyethyl cellulose	polyquaternium-1 · disodium edetate	nylon 11 · polysorbate 21 · sodium borate · boric acid · sodium chloride

See Chapter 23, "Contact Lens Products," for more information about these products.

SOFT LENS PRODUCTS - continued

	Product Manufacturer/Supplier	Product Form	Use	Viscosity Agent	Preservative	Other Ingredients
**	**Pliagel** Alcon Labs	solution	cleaning		sorbic acid, 0.25% · trisodium edetate, 0.5%	poloxamer 407 · potassium chloride · sodium chloride
	Preflex for Sensitive Eyes Alcon Labs	liquid	cleaning	hydroxyethyl cellulose · polyvinyl alcohol	EDTA, 0.2% · sorbic acid, 0.2%	sodium chloride · sodium phosphate · tyloxapol · sodium chloride
**	**Pure Eyes 1 Cleaner/Rinse** Ciba Vision	liquid	cleaning · rinsing			boric acid · sodium borate · sodium perborate · phosphoric acid · pluronic surfactant
	Sensitive Eyes Daily Cleaner Bausch & Lomb	liquid	cleaning	hydroxypropyl methylcellulose	EDTA, 0.5% · sorbic acid, 0.25%	sodium chloride · borate buffer · surfactant
	Enzymatic Cleaners					
**	**Alcon Enzymatic Cleaner** Alcon Labs	tablet	weekly protein cleaning			citric acid · sodium bicarbonate · sucrose
	Complete Weekly Enzymatic Cleaner Allergan	tablet	weekly protein cleaning			subtilisin A
	Enzymatic Contact Lens Cleaner Allergan	tablet	weekly protein cleaning		EDTA	sodium chloride · papain · sodium carbonate · sodium borate
	Opti-Free Enzymatic Cleaner for Sensitive Eyes Alcon Labs	tablet	weekly protein cleaning	povidone		pancreatin · citric acid · sodium bicarbonate · polyethylene glycol · dehydrated alcohol · compressible sugar
	Opti-Zyme Enzymatic Cleaner Alcon Labs	tablet	weekly protein cleaning			pancreatin
	ReNu 1 Step Enzymatic Cleaner Bausch & Lomb	tablet	weekly protein cleaning			subtilisin · sodium carbonate · sodium chloride · boric acid
	ReNu Effervescent Enzymatic Bausch & Lomb	tablet	weekly protein cleaning			subtilisin PEG · sodium carbonate · sodium chloride · tartaric acid
	ReNu Thermal Enzymatic Bausch & Lomb	tablet	weekly protein cleaning			subtilisin PEG · sodium carbonate · sodium chloride · boric acid
	Sensitive Eyes Effervescent Enzymatic Bausch & Lomb	tablet	weekly protein cleaning			subtilisin PEG · sodium carbonate · sodium chloride · tartaric acid
	Ultrazyme Enzymatic Cleaner Allergan	tablet	weekly protein cleaning			subtilisin A · effervescing agents · buffers
	Chemical Disinfecting Products					
	Disinfecting Solution Bausch & Lomb	solution	rinsing · chemical disinfecting · storing		EDTA, 0.1% · chlorhexidine gluconate, 0.005% · thimerosal, 0.001%	sodium chloride · sodium borate · boric acid

See Chapter 23, "Contact Lens Products," for more information about these products.

SOFT LENS PRODUCTS - continued

	Product Manufacturer/Supplier	Product Form	Use	Viscosity Agent	Preservative	Other Ingredients
	Flex-Care for Sensitive Eyes Alcon Labs	liquid	rinsing · chemical disinfecting		EDTA, 0.1% · chlorhexidine gluconate, 0.005%	sodium chloride · sodium borate · boric acid
	Hydrocare Cleaning & Disinfecting Allergan	solution	chemical disinfecting	propylene glycol	tris (2-hydroxyethyl) tallow ammonium chloride, 0.013% · thimerosal, 0.002% · hydrochloric acid · bis (2-hydroxyethyl) tallow ammonium chloride	sodium bicarbonate · sodium phosphate · soluble polyhema · polysorbate 80
	Opti-Free for Disinfection Alcon Labs	solution	rinsing · chemical disinfecting · storing		EDTA, 0.05% · polyquaternium-1, 0.001%	citrate buffer · sodium chloride
	Hydrogen Peroxide Disinfecting Products and Rinsing/Neutralizing Products					
	AO SEPT Ciba Vision	liquid	disinfecting			hydrogen peroxide, 3% · sodium chloride, 0.85% · sodium stannate · phosphate buffers · phosphoric acid
**	**Mirasept Step 1** Alcon Labs	solution	disinfecting			hydrogen peroxide · sodium stannate · sodium nitrate
**	**Mirasept Step 2** Alcon Labs	solution	rinsing · neutralizing		sorbic acid · disodium edetate	boric acid · sodium borate · sodium pyruvate
	Oxysept 1 Disinfecting Allergan	solution	disinfecting			hydrogen peroxide, 3% · sodium stannate · sodium nitrate · phosphate buffers
	Oxysept 2 Neutralizing Allergan	tablet	neutralizing			catalase · buffering agents · tableting agents
	Oxysept 2 Rinse and Neutralizer Allergan	liquid	rinsing · neutralizing			catalase · sodium chloride · monobasic sodium phosphate · dibasic sodium phosphate
**	**Pure Eyes 2 Disinfectant/Soaking** Ciba Vision	solution	disinfecting · soaking · neutralizing			hydrogen peroxide, 3% · sodium chloride, 0.85% · sodium stannate · phosphate buffers · phosphoric acid · packaged with a plastic lens case with built-in neutralizer
	Quick CARE System, Finishing Ciba Vision	solution	rinsing · soaking · storing			hydrogen peroxide, 0.006% · sodium borate · boric acid · phosphoric acid
	Quick CARE System, Starting Ciba Vision	solution	cleaning · disinfecting · neutralizing			purified water · polyoxypropylene · polyoxyethylene block copolymer · disodium lauroamphodiacetate · isopropanol · sodium chloride

See Chapter 23, "Contact Lens Products," for more information about these products.

SOFT LENS PRODUCTS - continued

	Product Manufacturer/Supplier	Product Form	Use	Viscosity Agent	Preservative	Other Ingredients
	Ultracare Disinfecting Solution/Neutralizer [a] Allergan	solution · tablet	disinfecting · neutralizing	tablet: hydroxypropyl methylcellulose		solution: hydrogen peroxide, 3% · sodium stannate · sodium nitrate · phosphates · purified water · tablet: catalase
	Rewetting Products					
	20/20 Solution S.S.S. Company	solution	lubricating · rewetting	polyvinyl alcohol, 1.4%	disodium edetate, 0.05% · benzalkonium chloride, 0.01%	sodium chloride · potassium chloride
	Adapettes for Sensitive Eyes Alcon Labs	liquid	lubricating · rewetting		sorbic acid, 0.2% · disodium edetate, 0.1%	boric acid · sodium borate · sodium chloride
	Clerz 2 Alcon Labs	drops	lubricating · rewetting	hydroxyethyl cellulose	boric acid, 0.2% · disodium edetate, 0.1%	sodium chloride · potassium chloride · sodium borate
	Lens Drops Ciba Vision	drops	lubricating · rewetting		EDTA, 0.2% · sorbic acid, 0.15%	sodium chloride · borate buffer · carbamide · poloxamer 407
	Lens Fresh Allergan	drops	lubricating · rewetting	hydroxyethyl cellulose	EDTA, 0.2% · sorbic acid, 0.1%	sodium chloride · boric acid · sodium borate
	Lens Lubricant Bausch & Lomb	liquid	lubricating · rewetting	povidone	EDTA, 0.1% · thimerosal, 0.004%	polyoxyethylene
	Lens Plus Allergan	drops	rewetting			sodium chloride · boric acid
	Opti-Free Alcon Labs	drops	rewetting		polyquaternium-1, 0.001%	citric acid · sodium citrate · sodium chloride
**	**Opti-Soak Soothing** Alcon Labs	drops	rewetting	hydroxypropyl methylcellulose · Dextran	polyquaternium-1 · disodium edetate	sodium chloride · potassium chloride
	Opti-Tears Soothing Alcon Labs	drops	lubricating · rewetting	hydroxypropyl methylcellulose · Dextran 70	EDTA, 0.1% · polyquaternium-1, 0.001%	sodium chloride · potassium chloride · sodium hydroxide and/or HCl · purified water
	ReNu Rewetting Bausch & Lomb	drops	rewetting		sorbic acid, 0.15% · EDTA	borate buffer
**	**Sensitive Eyes Plus Lubricating** Bausch & Lomb	drops	lubricating	hydroxypropyl methylcellulose	sorbic acid · disodium edetate	poloxamine · sodium chloride
	Sensitive Eyes Rewetting Bausch & Lomb	drops	rewetting		sorbic acid, 0.1% · EDTA	borate buffer
	Saline Products					
	Alcon Saline for Sensitive Eyes Alcon Labs	liquid	thermal disinfecting · storing		sorbic acid, 0.125% · edetate disodium, 0.1%	sodium borate · boric acid · sodium chloride
PR	**Blairex Sterile Saline** Blairex Labs	solution	rinsing · thermal disinfecting · storing			sodium chloride, 0.7% · boric acid · sodium borate
	Ciba Vision Saline Ciba Vision	liquid	rinsing · storing			sodium chloride · boric acid

See Chapter 23, "Contact Lens Products," for more information about these products.

SOFT LENS PRODUCTS - continued

	Product Manufacturer/Supplier	Product Form	Use	Viscosity Agent	Preservative	Other Ingredients
	Hydrocare Preserved Saline Allergan	solution	rinsing · thermal disinfecting · storing		disodium edetate, 0.01% · thimerosal, 0.001%	sodium hexametaphosphate · sodium chloride · boric acid · sodium borate · sodium hydroxide
	Lens Plus Sterile Saline Allergan	solution	rinsing · thermal disinfecting · storing			sodium chloride · boric acid
	Opti-Soft Alcon Labs	solution	rinsing · thermal disinfecting · storing		EDTA, 0.1% · polyquaternium-1, 0.001%	sodium chloride · borate buffer
	Preserved Saline Bausch & Lomb	solution	rinsing · thermal disinfecting · storing		thimerosal, 0.001% · EDTA	boric acid · sodium chloride
	Purisol 4 Nomax	liquid	rinsing · storing			sodium chloride · boric acid · sodium borate
	ReNu Saline Bausch & Lomb	liquid	rinsing · thermal disinfecting · storing · enzyme diluent		EDTA · polyaminopropyl biguanide	sodium chloride · boric acid
	Sensitive Eyes Plus Saline Bausch & Lomb	solution	rinsing · thermal disinfecting · storing · enzyme diluent		polyaminopropyl biguanide	sodium chloride · potassium chloride
	Sensitive Eyes Saline Bausch & Lomb	aerosol spray	rinsing · thermal disinfecting · storing · enzyme diluent			sodium chloride · boric acid · sodium borate
	Sensitive Eyes Saline Bausch & Lomb	solution	rinsing · thermal disinfecting · storing · enzyme diluent		sorbic acid, 0.1% · EDTA	sodium chloride · borate buffer
	Sensitive Eyes Saline/Cleaning Bausch & Lomb	solution	cleaning · rinsing · thermal disinfecting · storing		sorbic acid · EDTA	sodium chloride · borate buffer · surfactant
	SoftWear Saline Ciba Vision	liquid	rinsing · storing			sodium chloride · sodium borate · boric acid · sodium perborate
	Sterile Preserved Saline Blairex Labs	solution	rinsing · chemical disinfecting · storing		sorbic acid, 0.1% · disodium edetate	sodium chloride
	Sterile Saline Bausch & Lomb	liquid	rinsing · thermal disinfecting · storing		EDTA	sodium chloride · borate buffer
PR	**Unisol 4 Saline** Alcon Labs	solution	rinsing · thermal disinfecting · storing			sodium chloride · sodium borate · boric acid · purified water
** PR	**Unisol Plus** Alcon Labs	solution	rinsing · thermal disinfecting			sodium chloride · sodium borate · boric acid

** New listing
[a] Disinfects and neutralizes in one step

See Chapter 23, "Contact Lens Products," for more information about these products.

OTIC PRODUCTS

	Product Manufacturer/Supplier	Dosage Form	Anti-infective	Other Ingredients
	Auro Del Ph'cals	drops	carbamide peroxide, 6.5%	
	Auro-Dri Del Ph'cals	drops	isopropyl alcohol, 97.25%	
	Aurocaine Republic Drug	drops	carbamide peroxide	chlorobutanol, 0.5% · glycerin · propylene glycol
	Aurocaine 2 Republic Drug	drops	boric acid, 2.75% · isopropyl alcohol	
	Debrox SmithKline Beecham	drops	carbamide peroxide, 6.5%	citric acid · glycerin · propylene glycol · sodium stannate · water
	Dent's Ear Wax Drops C. S. Dent	drops	carbamide peroxide	glycerin
**	**Dri-Ear** Pfeiffer Ph'cals	drops	isopropyl alcohol, 95%	glycerin, 5%
	E.R.O. Scherer Labs	drops	carbamide peroxide, 6.5%	anhydrous glycerin
	E.R.O. Ear Wax Removal System Scherer Labs	drops	carbamide peroxide, 6.5%	anhydrous glycerin · packaged with syringe
	Ear Drops Goldline Labs	drops	carbamide peroxide, 6.5%	
	Ear Wax Removal System Bausch & Lomb	drops	carbamide peroxide, 6.5%	anhydrous glycerin base
	Ear-Dry Scherer Labs	drops	isopropyl alcohol, 95%	anhydrous glycerin, 5%
	Earsol-HC Parnell Ph'cals	drops	alcohol	hydrocortisone, 1% · propylene glycol · benzyl benzoate · water · yerba santa · fragrance
	Mollifene Pfeiffer Ph'cals	drops	carbamide peroxide, 6.5%	anhydrous glycerin · propylene glycol · sodium stannate · citric acid
	Murine Ear Wax Removal System Ross Products/Abbott Labs	drops	carbamide peroxide, 6.5% · alcohol, 6.3%	glycerin · polysorbate 20
	Swim-Ear E. Fougera	drops	isopropyl alcohol, 95%	anhydrous glycerin, 5%

** New listing

See Chapter 24, "Otic Products," for more information about these products.

ORAL DISCOMFORT PRODUCTS

	Product Manufacturer/Supplier	Dosage Form	Anesthetic/ Analgesic	Debriding Agent/ Wound Cleanser	Other Ingredients
AL	**Amosan** Oral-B Labs	powder		sodium peroxyborate monohydrate	sodium bitartrate · saccharin · peppermint, menthol, and vanilla flavors
	Anbesol Whitehall-Robins Healthcare	liquid	benzocaine, 6.4% · phenol, 0.5%		alcohol, 70% · camphor · glycerin · menthol · potassium iodide · povidone iodine
	Anbesol Whitehall-Robins Healthcare	gel	benzocaine, 6.3% · phenol, 0.5%		alcohol, 70% · camphor · carbomer 934P · D&C red#33 · D&C yellow#10 · FD&C blue#1 · FD&C yellow#6 · flavor · glycerin
AL PE	**Anbesol Baby, Grape** Whitehall-Robins Healthcare	gel	benzocaine, 7.5%		benzoic acid · carbomer 934P · D&C red#33 · disodium edetate · FD&C blue#1 · flavor · glycerin · methylparaben · polyethylene glycol · propylparaben · purified water · saccharin
AL PE	**Anbesol Baby, Original** Whitehall-Robins Healthcare	gel	benzocaine, 7.5%		carbomer 934P · clove oil · D&C red#33 · disodium edetate · glycerin · glycerin · polyethylene glycol · purified water · saccharin
	Anbesol Maximum Strength Whitehall-Robins Healthcare	gel · liquid	benzocaine, 20%		alcohol, 60% · carbomer 934P (gel) · D&C yellow#10 · FD&C blue#1 · FD&C red#40 · flavor · polyethylene glycol · saccharin
PE	**Babee Teething** S.S.S. Company	lotion	benzocaine, 2.5% · menthol · camphor		alcohol, 20% · witch hazel
	Benzodent Denture Analgesic [a] Chattem	ointment	benzocaine, 20%		8-hydroxyquinoline sulfate · petrolatum · sodium CMC · eugenol · color
	Blistex Lip Medex Blistex	ointment	camphor, 1% · menthol, 1% · phenol, 0.5%		petrolatum · cocoa butter · flavor · lanolin · mixed waxes · oil of cloves
	Blistex Medicated Blistex	ointment	menthol, 0.6% · camphor, 0.5% · phenol, 0.5%		allantoin, 1%
AL	**Campho-phenique [b]** Bayer Consumer	gel	camphor, 10.8% · phenol, 4.7%		eucalyptus oil
	Cankaid E. E. Dickinson	liquid		carbamide peroxide, 10%	citric acid · monohydrate · sodium citrate dihydrate · disodium edetate
**	**Carmex Lip Balm** Carma Labs	ointment	menthol · camphor · salicylic acid · phenol		alum · fragrance · petrolatum · lanolin · cocoa butter · wax
	ChapStick Medicated Lip Balm Whitehall-Robins Healthcare	stick	camphor, 1% · menthol, 0.6% · phenol, 0.5%		petrolatum 41% · paraffin wax · mineral oil · cocoa butter · 2-octyl dodecanol · arachidyl propionate · polyphenylmethylsiloxane 556 · white wax · isopropyl lanolate · carnauba wax · isopropyl myristate · lanolin · fragrance · methylparaben · propylparaben · oleyl alcohol · cetyl alcohol
	ChapStick Medicated Lip Balm, Jar or Squeeze Tube Whitehall-Robins Healthcare	ointment	camphor, 1% · menthol, 0.6% · phenol, 0.5%		petrolatum 60% (Jar) · petrolatum, 67% (Squeeze Tube) · microcrystalline wax · mineral oil · cocoa butter · lanolin · paraffin wax (Jar) · fragrance · methylparaben · propylparaben
	Cold Sore Lotion [b] Pfeiffer Ph'cals	lotion	camphor · menthol		alcohol, 85% · gum benzoin, 7% · thymol · eucalyptol

See Chapter 25, "Oral Health Products," for more information about these products.

ORAL DISCOMFORT PRODUCTS - continued

	Product Manufacturer/Supplier	Dosage Form	Anesthetic/ Analgesic	Debriding Agent/ Wound Cleanser	Other Ingredients
	Curasore S.S.S. Company	liquid	pramoxine HCl, 1%		ethyl ether · ethyl alcohol
	Dent's 3 In 1 Toothache Relief C. S. Dent	drops · gel · gum	benzocaine, 20% (drops · gum); 5% (gel)		drops: denatured alcohol, 74% · chlorobutanol anhydrous, 0.09% · propylene glycol · FD&C red#40 · eugenol · gel: distilled water · methylparaben · propylparaben · propylene glycol · carbopol 934-P · methyl salicylate · FD&C red#40 · 2.2' iminodiethanol · gum: petrolatum · cotton and wax base · beeswax · FD&C red#40 aluminum lake · eugenol
	Dent's Double-Action Kit C. S. Dent	drops · tablet	benzocaine, 20% (drops) · acetaminophen, 325mg (tablet)		drops: denatured alcohol, 74% · chlorobutanol anhydrous, 0.09% · propylene glycol · FD&C red#40 · eugenol
	Dent's Extra Strength Toothache Gum C. S. Dent	gum	benzocaine, 20%		petrolatum · cotton and wax base · beeswax · FD&C red#40 aluminum lake · eugenol
	Dent's Maxi-Strength Toothache Treatment C. S. Dent	drops	benzocaine, 20%		denatured alcohol, 74% · chlorobutanol anhydrous, 0.09% · propylene glycol · FD&C red#40 · eugenol
DY	**Dent-Zel-Ite Oral Mucosal Analgesic** Alvin Last	liquid	benzocaine, 5% · camphor		alcohol, 81% · wintergreen · glycerin
	Dent-Zel-Ite Temporary Dental Filling Alvin Last	liquid	camphor		alcohol, 55% · sandarac gum · methyl salicylate
	Dent-Zel-Ite Toothache Relief Alvin Last	drops	eugenol, 85% · camphor		alcohol, 13.5% · wintergreen
	Gly-Oxide SmithKline Beecham	liquid		carbamide peroxide, 10%	citric acid · flavor · glycerin · propylene glycol · sodium stannate · water
	HDA Toothache Gel S.S.S. Company	gel	benzocaine, 6.5%		clove oil
AL	**Herpecin-L Cold Sore Lip Balm** Campbell Labs	stick			allantoin · padimate O · titanium dioxide
DY GL SL	**Hurricaine, Wild Cherry [a]** Beutlich, L.P. Ph'cals	aerosol spray	benzocaine, 20%		polyethylene glycol · saccharin · flavoring · alcohol
AL DY GL SL	**Hurricaine, Wild Cherry or Pina Colada [a]** Beutlich, L.P. Ph'cals	liquid	benzocaine, 20%		polyethylene glycol · saccharin · flavoring
AL DY GL SL	**Hurricaine; Wild Cherry, Pina Colada, or Watermelon [a]** Beutlich, L.P. Ph'cals	gel	benzocaine, 20%		polyethylene glycol · saccharin · flavoring

See Chapter 25, "Oral Health Products," for more information about these products.

ORAL DISCOMFORT PRODUCTS - continued

	Product Manufacturer/Supplier	Dosage Form	Anesthetic/ Analgesic	Debriding Agent/ Wound Cleanser	Other Ingredients
	Kank-A Professional Strength [a] Blistex	liquid	benzocaine, 20% · benzyl alcohol		benzoin tincture compound · cetylpyridinium chloride · ethylcellulose · SD alcohol, 24% · dimethyl isosorbide · castor oil · flavor · tannic acid · propylene glycol · saccharin
** AL AF DY SO SU PE	**Little Teethers Oral Pain Relief** Vetco	gel	benzocaine, 7.5%		carbomer · glycerin · flavor · potassium sorbate · acesulfame K · PEGs
	Lotion-Jel C. S. Dent	gel	benzocaine, 5%		distilled water · methylparaben · propylparaben · propylene glycol · carbopol 934-P · methyl salicylate · FD&C red#40 · 2.2' iminodiethanol
	Medadyne Vetco	liquid	benzocaine, 10% · benzyl alcohol · menthol · camphor		benzalkonium chloride · tannic acid · flavors · SD alcohol · thymol
	Numzident Adult Strength Goody's Ph'cals	gel	benzocaine, 10%		PEG 400, 47.86% · glycerin, 30% · PEG 3350, 10% · saccharin sodium, 1% · purified water, 0.75% · cherry vanilla flavor, 0.4%
	Numzit Teething Goody's Ph'cals	gel	benzocaine, 7.5%		PEG-400, 66.2% · PEG-3350, 26.1% · saccharin sodium, 0.036% · clove oil, 0.09% · peppermint oil, 0.018% · purified water, 0.056%
	Numzit Teething Goody's Ph'cals	lotion	benzocaine, 0.2%		alcohol, 12.1% · glycerin, 2% · kelgin MV, 0.5% · saccharin sodium, 0.02% · methylparaben, 0.1% · FD&C red#40, 0.1% · FD&C blue#1, 0.009%
	Orabase Colgate-Palmolive	gel	benzocaine, 15%		ethanol · propylene glycol · hydroxypropyl cellulose · tannic acid · salicylic acid · flavor · saccharin sodium
AL PE	**Orabase Baby [a]** Colgate-Palmolive	gel	benzocaine, 7.5%		glycerin · PEG · carbopol · preservative · sweetener · flavor
AL	**Orabase Lip Cream** Colgate-Palmolive	cream	benzocaine, 5% · menthol, 0.5% · camphor · phenol		allantoin, 1% · sodium carboxymethylcellulose · veegum · Tween 80 · phenonip · PEG · biopure · talc · kaolin · lanolin · petrolatum · oil of clove · hydrated silica
AL	**Orabase Plain [a]** Colgate-Palmolive	paste			pectin · gelatin · carboxymethylcellulose sodium · polyethylene · mineral oil · flavors · preservative · guar · tragacanth
AL	**Orabase-B with Benzocaine [a]** Colgate-Palmolive	paste	benzocaine, 20%		plasticized hydrocarbon gel · guar · carboxymethylcellulose · tragacanth · pectin · preservatives · flavors
**	**Oragesic** Parnell Ph'cals	solution	benzyl alcohol, 2% · menthol		water · sorbitol · sodium chloride · yerba santa · poloxamer 407 · saccharin · cetylpyridinium chloride · disodium EDTA
AL PE	**Orajel Baby** Del Ph'cals	gel	benzocaine, 7.5%		FD&C red#40 · flavor · glycerin · polyethylene glycols · saccharin sodium · sorbic acid · sorbitol

See Chapter 25, "Oral Health Products," for more information about these products.

ORAL DISCOMFORT PRODUCTS - continued

	Product Manufacturer/Supplier	Dosage Form	Anesthetic/ Analgesic	Debriding Agent/ Wound Cleanser	Other Ingredients
AL PE	**Orajel Baby Nighttime Formula** Del Ph'cals	gel	benzocaine, 10%		FD&C red#40 · flavor · glycerin · polyethylene glycols · saccharin sodium · sorbic acid · sorbitol
**	**Orajel CoverMed, Tinted Light or Medium** Del Ph'cals	cream	dyclonine HCl, 1.0%		
	Orajel Denture Del Ph'cals	gel	benzocaine, 10%		chlorothymol · FD&C red#40 · flavor · polyethylene glycols · purified water · saccharin sodium · sorbic acid · eugenol
	Orajel Maximum Strength Del Ph'cals	gel	benzocaine, 20%		clove oil · flavor · polyethylene glycols · saccharin sodium · sorbic acid
	Orajel Mouth-Aid Del Ph'cals	gel	benzocaine, 20%		zinc chloride, 0.1% · benzalkonium chloride, 0.02% · allantoin · carbomer · disodium edetate · peppermint oil · polyethylene glycol · polysorbate 60 · propyl gallate · propylene · polysorbate 60 · glycol · purified water · povidone · saccharin sodium · sorbic acid · stearyl alcohol
	Orajel Mouth-Aid Del Ph'cals	liquid	benzocaine, 20% · phenol, 0.5%		cetylpyridinium chloride, 0.1% · ethylcellulose
	Orajel Perioseptic Del Ph'cals	liquid		carbamide peroxide, 15%	citric acid · disodium edetate · flavor · methylparaben · propylene glycol · purified water · sodium chloride · saccharin sodium
	Orajel Regular Strength Del Ph'cals	gel	benzocaine, 10%		clove oil · flavor · polyethylene glycols · saccharin sodium · sorbic acid
	Orasol Goldline Labs	liquid	benzocaine, 6.3% · phenol, 0.5%		alcohol, 70%
GL SL	**Peroxyl Hygienic Dental Rinse** Colgate-Palmolive	liquid		hydrogen peroxide, 1.5%	alcohol, 5% · pluronic F108 · sorbitol · saccharin sodium · dye · polysorbate 20 · mint flavor
GL SU	**Peroxyl Oral Spot Treatment** Colgate-Palmolive	gel		hydrogen peroxide, 1.5%	ethyl alcohol, 5% · mint flavor · pluronic F108 · polysorbate 20 · sorbitol · saccharin sodium · dye · pluronic F127
DY GL SU PE	**Probax [b]** Fischer Ph'cals	ointment			propolis, 2% · petrolatum · mineral oil
**	**Red Cross Canker Sore Medication [b]** Mentholatum	ointment	benzocaine, 20% · phenol		carbomer 974P · mineral oil · petrolatum · propylparaben
	Red Cross Toothache Medication Mentholatum	drops	eugenol, 85%		sesame oil
**	**Rid-a-Pain Dental Drops** Pfeiffer Ph'cals	liquid	benzocaine, 6.3% · phenol, 0.5%		alcohol, 70%
AL	**SensoGARD [b]** Dentco	gel	benzocaine, 20%		methylparaben · polycarbophil · polyethylene glycol · propylparaben · sorbitan monooleate

See Chapter 25, "Oral Health Products," for more information about these products.

ORAL DISCOMFORT PRODUCTS - continued

	Product Manufacturer/Supplier	Dosage Form	Anesthetic/ Analgesic	Debriding Agent/ Wound Cleanser	Other Ingredients
	Tanac Del Ph'cals	liquid	benzocaine, 10%		benzalkonium chloride, 0.125% · saccharin
	Tanac Del Ph'cals	stick	benzocaine, 7.5%		benzalkonium chloride, 0.125%
	Tanac Medicated Del Ph'cals	gel	dyclonine HCl, 1.0%		allantoin, 0.5%
	Tanac Roll-On Del Ph'cals	lotion	benzocaine, 5%		benzalkonium chloride, 0.12% · saccharin sodium · glycerin · polyethylene glycol · tannic acid
	Vaseline Lip Therapy Chesebrough-Pond's	ointment	camphor, 0.8% · menthol, 0.8% · phenol, 0.5%		white petrolatum, 93.8% · borage seed oil · sunflower seed oil · tocopheryl acetate · bisabolol · retinyl palmitate · panthenol · aloe extract · kukui nut oil · lecithin · stearic acid · corn oil · soya sterol · salicylic acid · zinc sulfate · methyl salicylate · flavor
**	**Zilactin B** Zila Ph'cals	gel	benzocaine, 10%		
	Zilactin Medicated Zila Ph'cals	gel	benzyl alcohol, 10%		
	Zilactin-L Zila Ph'cals	liquid	lidocaine, 2.5%		

** New listing
[a] Carries American Dental Association (ADA) seal indicating safety and efficacy
[b] For cold sore treatment only

See Chapter 25, "Oral Health Products," for more information about these products.

ORAL HYGIENE PRODUCTS

	Product Manufacturer/Supplier	Dosage Form	Antiseptic	Other Ingredients
	Astring-O-Sol Mentholatum	liquid	SD alcohol 38-B, 75.6% · methyl salicylate	water · myrrh extract · zinc chloride · citric acid
	Betadine Mouthwash/Gargle Purdue Frederick	liquid	alcohol, 8.8%	povidone-iodine, 0.5%
	Cepacol Mouthwash/Gargle J. B. Williams	liquid	alcohol, 14% · cetylpyridinium chloride, 0.05%	disodium edetate · colors · flavors · glycerin · polysorbate 80 · saccharin · sodium B phosphate · sodium phosphate · water
	Cepacol Mouthwash/Gargle, Mint J. B. Williams	liquid	alcohol, 14.5% · cetylpyridinium chloride, 0.5%	colors · flavors · glucono delta-lactone · glycerin · poloxamer-407 · saccharin sodium · sodium gluconate · water
**	**DentSure Denture Rinse, Peppermint** Pfizer Consumer	liquid	alcohol, 14.4%	water · glycerin · tetrapotassium pyrophosphate · benzoic acid · poloxamer 407 · sodium benzoate · saccharin sodium
** DY GL	**Dr. Tichenor's Antiseptic** Dr. G. H. Tichenor	liquid	SDA alcohol 38-B, 70%	oil of peppermint · extract of arnica · water
	Listerine [a] Warner Wellcome Consumer	liquid	alcohol, 26.9% · eucalyptol, 0.092% · thymol, 0.064% · methyl salicylate, 0.06% · menthol, 0.042%	benzoic acid · poloxamer 407 · caramel
	Listerine, Cool Mint or FreshBurst [a] Warner Wellcome Consumer	liquid	alcohol, 21.6% · eucalyptol, 0.092% · thymol, 0.064% · methyl salicylate, 0.06% · menthol, 0.042%	water · sorbitol solution · poloxamer 407 · benzoic acid · flavoring · saccharin sodium · sodium citrate · citric acid · FD&C green#3 · D&C yellow#10 (Mint)
** AL	**Listermint Mouthrinse** Warner Wellcome Consumer	liquid		water · zinc chloride · glycerin · poloxamer 335 · sodium lauryl sulfate · flavor · saccharin sodium · D&C yellow#10 · FD&C green#3 · PEG 600 · sodium benzoate · benzoic acid
**	**Mentadent Mouthwash, Cool Mint or Fresh Mint** Chesebrough-Pond's	liquid	alcohol, 12%	water · sorbitol · sodium bicarbonate · hydrogen peroxide · poloxamer 407 · sodium lauryl sulfate · flavor · polysorbate 20 · methyl salicylate (Cool Mint) · saccharin sodium · phosphoric acid · blue#1 · yellow#5 (Cool Mint)
	Mouth Wash Antiseptic Goldline Labs	liquid	alcohol, 26.9% · eucalyptol, 0.09% · thymol, 0.06% · methyl salicylate, 0.06% · menthol, 0.04%	
	Oral-B Anti-Plaque Rinse Oral-B Labs	liquid	alcohol, 8% · cetylpyridinium chloride	water · glycerin · saccharin sodium · methylparaben · propylparaben · FD&C blue #1 · D&C yellow #10 · poloxamer 407
**	**Plax Advanced Formula, Mint Sensation** Pfizer Consumer	liquid	alcohol, 8.5%	water · glycerin · tetrasodium pyrophosphate · benzoic acid · flavor · poloxamer 407 · sodium benzoate · sodium lauryl sulfate · saccharin sodium · xanthan gum · FD&C blue#1
	Plax Advanced Formula, Original Flavor Pfizer Consumer	liquid	alcohol, 8.5%	sodium lauryl sulfate · water · glycerin · sodium benzoate · tetrasodium pyrophosphate · benzoic acid · poloxamer 407 · saccharin · flavor · xanthan gum

See Chapter 25, "Oral Health Products," for more information about these products.

ORAL HYGIENE PRODUCTS - continued

	Product Manufacturer/Supplier	Dosage Form	Antiseptic	Other Ingredients
	Plax Advanced Formula, Softmint Pfizer Consumer	liquid	alcohol, 8.5%	sodium lauryl sulfate · water · glycerin · sodium benzoate · tetrasodium pyrophosphate · benzoic acid · poloxamer 407 · saccharin sodium · flavor · xanthan gum · flavor enhancer · FD&C blue#1 · FD&C yellow#5
**	**Plus+White Anti-Stain Oral Rinse** CCA Industries	liquid	cetylpyridinium chloride · domiphen bromide	water · glycerin · poloxamer 338 · flavor · saccharin sodium · FD&C blue#1 · tetrasodium EDTA · disodium EDTA · methylparaben
** AL	**Rembrandt Mouth Refreshing Rinse** Den-Mat	liquid		methylparaben · water · sodium citrate · sodium lauryl sulfate · natural and artificial flavors · polysorbate 20 · citric acid · sodium benzoate · saccharin sodium
	Scope, Cool Peppermint Procter & Gamble	liquid	SD alcohol 38-F, 14% · cetylpyridinium chloride · domiphen bromide	purified water · glycerin · poloxamer 407 · saccharin sodium · sodium benzoate · N-ethylmethylcarboxamide · benzoic acid · FD&C blue#1
**	**Swish, Cool Mint** Unico	liquid	SD alcohol 38-F, 18.9% · cetylpyridinium chloride · domiphen bromide	purified water · glycerin · saccharin sodium · sodium benzoate · flavor · benzoic acid · FD&C blue#1 · FD&C yellow#5
**	**Swish, Peppermint** Unico	liquid	SD alcohol 38-F, 14% · cetylpyridinium chloride · domiphen bromide	purified water · glycerin · poloxamer 407 · saccharin sodium · sodium benzoate · flavor · benzoic acid · FD&C blue#1
AL	**Tech 2000** Care-Tech Labs	liquid	cetylpyridinium chloride	water · glycerin · poloxamer 407 · flavor · FD&C blue#1 · FD&C yellow#5 · nutritive dextrose or sucrose and/or calcium saccharin
AL	**Tom's Natural Mouthwash, Cinnamon or Spearmint** Tom's of Maine	liquid	menthol	water · glycerin · aloe vera juice · witch hazel · poloxamer 335 · spearmint oil · ascorbic acid
	Viadent Oral Rinse Colgate-Palmolive	liquid	alcohol, 10% · sanguinaria extract, 0.03%	zinc chloride, 0.2% · glycerin · polysorbate 80 · flavor · saccharin sodium · poloxamer 237 · citric acid

** New listing
[a] Carries American Dental Association (ADA) seal indicating safety and efficacy

See Chapter 25, "Oral Health Products," for more information about these products.

TOPICAL FLUORIDE PRODUCTS

	Product Manufacturer/Supplier	Dosage Form	Therapeutic Agent	Other Ingredients
DY GL	**Fluorigard Anti-Cavity [a]** Colgate-Palmolive	liquid	sodium fluoride, 0.05%	ethyl alcohol · pluronic F108, F127 · sweetener · flavor · glycerin · sorbitol · preservatives
	Oral-B Anti-Cavity [a] Oral-B Labs	liquid	sodium fluoride, 0.05%	water · sodium benzoate · potassium sorbate · saccharin sodium · glycerin · PEG-40 · FD&C blue#1 · phosphoric acid
AL	**Reach Act Adult Anti-Cavity Treatment, Cinnamon** Johnson & Johnson Consumer	liquid	sodium fluoride, 0.05%	cetylpyridinium chloride · D&C red#33 · edetate calcium disodium · FD&C yellow#5 · flavors · glycerin · monobasic sodium phosphate · dibasic sodium phosphate · poloxamer 407 · polysorbate 80 · propylene glycol · sodium benzoate · saccharin sodium · water
AL	**Reach Act Adult Anti-Cavity Treatment, Mint** Johnson & Johnson Consumer	liquid	sodium fluoride, 0.05%	cetylpyridinium chloride · edetate calcium disodium · FD&C green#3 · FD&C yellow#5 · flavor · glycerin · menthol · methyl salicylate · monobasic sodium phosphate · dibasic sodium phosphate · poloxamer 407 · polysorbate 20 · potassium sorbate · propylene glycol · sodium benzoate · saccharin sodium · water
AL PE	**Reach Act for Kids [a]** Johnson & Johnson Consumer	liquid	sodium fluoride, 0.05%	cetylpyridinium chloride · D&C red#33 · dibasic sodium phosphate · edetate calcium disodium · flavors · glycerin · monobasic sodium phosphate · poloxamer 407 · polysorbate 80 · propylene glycol · sodium benzoate · saccharin sodium · water

** New listing
[a] Carries American Dental Association (ADA) seal indicating safety and efficacy

See Chapter 25, "Oral Health Products," for more information about these products.

DENTIFRICE PRODUCTS

	Product Manufacturer/Supplier	Dosage Form	Abrasive Ingredient	Therapeutic Ingredient	Foaming Agent	Other Ingredients [b]
	Aim Anti Tartar Formula Chesebrough-Pond's	gel	hydrated silica	sodium fluoride, 0.23%	sodium lauryl sulfate	sorbitol and related polyols · water · glycerin · zinc citrate trihydrate · SD alcohol 38B · flavor · xanthan gum · saccharin sodium · sodium benzoate · blue#1 · yellow #10
	Aim Baking Soda Chesebrough-Pond's	gel	hydrated silica · sodium bicarbonate	sodium fluoride, 0.23%	sodium lauryl sulfate	sorbitol and related polyols · water · glycerin · SD alcohol 38B · flavor · xanthan gum · saccharin sodium · sodium benzoate · blue #1 · yellow #10
**	**Aim Extra Strength [a]** Chesebrough-Pond's	gel	hydrated silica	sodium monofluorophosphate, 1.2%	sodium lauryl sulfate	sorbitol and other related polyols · water · glycerin · SD alcohol 38B · flavor · xanthan gum · saccharin sodium · sodium benzoate · blue #1 · yellow #10
	Aim Regular Strength Chesebrough-Pond's	gel	hydrated silica	sodium fluoride, 0.23%	sodium lauryl sulfate	sorbitol and other related polyols · water · glycerin · SD alcohol 38B · flavor · xanthan gum · saccharin sodium · sodium benzoate · blue #1 · yellow #10
	Aquafresh Baking Soda SmithKline Beecham	paste	calcium carbonate · hydrated silica · sodium bicarbonate	sodium monofluorophosphate	sodium lauryl sulfate	calcium carrageenan · cellulose gum · colors · flavor · glycerin · PEG-8 · sodium benzoate · saccharin sodium · sorbitol · titanium dioxide · water
	Aquafresh Extra Fresh [a] SmithKline Beecham	paste	hydrated silica · calcium carbonate	sodium monofluorophosphate	sodium lauryl sulfate	sorbitol · water · glycerin · PEG-8 · titanium dioxide · cellulose gum · flavor · saccharin sodium · sodium benzoate · calcium carrageenan · colors
	Aquafresh for Kids [a] SmithKline Beecham	paste	hydrated silica · calcium carbonate	sodium monofluorophosphate	sodium lauryl sulfate	sorbitol · water · glycerin · PEG-8 · titanium dioxide · cellulose gum · flavor · saccharin sodium · calcium carrageenan · sodium benzoate · colors
	Aquafresh Sensitive SmithKline Beecham	paste	hydrated silica	potassium nitrate · sodium fluoride	sodium lauryl sulfate	colors · flavors · glycerin · sodium benzoate · saccharin sodium · sorbitol · titanium dioxide · water · xanthan gum
	Aquafresh Tartar Control [a] SmithKline Beecham	paste	hydrated silica	sodium fluoride	sodium lauryl sulfate	tetrapotassium pyrophosphate · tetrasodium pyrophosphate · sorbitol · glycerin · PEG-8 · flavor · xanthan gum · saccharin sodium · sodium benzoate · D&C red#30 lake · FD&C blue#1 · D&C yellow#10 · titanium dioxide · water

See Chapter 25, "Oral Health Products," for more information about these products.

DENTIFRICE PRODUCTS - continued

	Product Manufacturer/Supplier	Dosage Form	Abrasive Ingredient	Therapeutic Ingredient	Foaming Agent	Other Ingredients [b]
	Aquafresh Triple Protection [a] SmithKline Beecham	paste	hydrated silica · calcium carbonate	sodium monofluorophosphate	sodium lauryl sulfate	PEG-8 · sorbitol · cellulose gum · sodium benzoate · titanium dioxide · calcium carrageenan · flavor · saccharin sodium · colors · water
	Aquafresh Whitening SmithKline Beecham	paste	hydrated silica	sodium fluoride	sodium lauryl sulfate	D&C yellow#10 · FD&C blue#1 · flavor · glycerin · PEG-8 · sodium benzoate · sodium hydroxide · saccharin sodium · sodium tripolyphosphate · sorbitol · titanium dioxide · water · xanthan gum
DY	**Arm & Hammer Dental Care** Church & Dwight	paste	sodium bicarbonate	sodium fluoride	sodium lauryl sulfate	water · glycerin · saccharin sodium · PEG-8 · flavor blend · cellulose gum · sodium lauryl sarcosinate
	Arm & Hammer Dental Care Church & Dwight	gel	hydrated silica · sodium bicarbonate	sodium fluoride	sodium lauryl sulfate	sorbitol · glycerin · water · flavor blend · cellulose gum · sodium lauryl sarcosinate · saccharin sodium · FD&C blue#1 · FD&C yellow#5
	Arm & Hammer Dental Care Tartar Control Church & Dwight	paste	sodium bicarbonate	sodium fluoride	sodium lauryl sulfate	water · glycerin · sodium pyrophosphates · saccharin sodium · PEG-8 · flavor blend · sodium phosphates · cellulose gum · sodium lauryl sarcosinate
	Arm & Hammer Dental Care Tartar Control Church & Dwight	gel	sodium bicarbonate · hydrated silica	sodium fluoride	sodium lauryl sulfate	water · sorbitol · glycerin · sodium pyrophosphates · flavor · cellulose gum · saccharin sodium · sodium lauryl sarcosinate · FD&C blue#1 · FD&C yellow#5
DY	**Arm & Hammer Dental Care Toothpowder** Church & Dwight	powder	sodium bicarbonate	sodium fluoride		mint flavor · saccharin sodium · trisodium phosphate · magnesium oxide · PEG-8
DY SU	**Arm & Hammer PeroxiCare** Church & Dwight	paste	sodium bicarbonate · silica	sodium fluoride	sodium carbonate peroxide · sodium lauryl sulfate	PEG-8 · poloxamer 338 · flavor · water · saccharin sodium · sodium lauryl sarcosinate
	Caffree Anti-Stain [a] Block Drug	paste	diatomaceous earth · aluminum silicate	sodium monofluorophosphate	sodium lauryl sulfate	water · glycerin · sorbitol · titanium dioxide · hydroxyethyl cellulose · flavor · saccharin sodium · methylparaben · propylparaben

See Chapter 25, "Oral Health Products," for more information about these products.

DENTIFRICE PRODUCTS - continued

	Product Manufacturer/Supplier	Dosage Form	Abrasive Ingredient	Therapeutic Ingredient	Foaming Agent	Other Ingredients [b]
	Close-Up Anti-Plaque Chesebrough-Pond's	gel	hydrated silica	stannous fluoride, 0.41%	sodium lauryl sulfate	sorbitol · water · PEG-32 · SD alcohol 38B · flavor · zinc citrate trihydrate · cellulose gum · saccharin sodium · sodium benzoate · sodium hydroxide · blue #1
	Close-Up Baking Soda Chesebrough-Pond's	paste	hydrated silica · sodium bicarbonate	sodium monofluorophosphate, 0.79% (fluoride, 0.15%)	sodium lauryl sulfate	sorbitol and related polyols · water · glycerin · SD alcohol 38B · flavor · cellulose gum · saccharin sodium · sodium benzoate · red#33 · red#40 · titanium dioxide
	Close-Up Crystal Clear, Mint Chesebrough-Pond's	gel	hydrated silica	sodium monofluorophosphate, 0.79% (fluoride, 0.15%)	sodium lauryl sulfate	sorbitol · water · glycerin · SD alcohol 38B · flavor · cellulose gum · saccharin sodium · polysorbate 20 · sodium benzoate · sodium chloride · blue#1 · mica · red#33 · titanium dioxide
	Close-Up Original Chesebrough-Pond's	gel	hydrated silica	sodium fluoride, 0.23%	sodium lauryl sulfate	sorbitol and other related polyols · water · glycerin · SD alcohol 38B · flavor · xanthan gum · saccharin sodium · sodium benzoate · sodium chloride · red #33 · red #40
	Close-Up Tartar Control Chesebrough-Pond's	gel	hydrated silica	sodium monofluorophosphate, 0.79% (fluoride, 0.15%)	sodium lauryl sulfate	sorbitol and related polyols · water · glycerin · zinc citrate trihydrate · SD alcohol 38B · flavor · cellulose gum · saccharin sodium · sodium benzoate · sodium chloride · red#33 · red#40
	Colgate [a] Colgate-Palmolive	paste	dicalcium phosphate dihydrate	sodium monofluorophosphate, 0.76%	sodium lauryl sulfate	glycerin · cellulose gum · tetrasodium pyrophosphate · saccharin sodium · flavor
**	**Colgate Baking Soda & Peroxide Tartar Control** Colgate-Palmolive	paste	hydrated silica · sodium bicarbonate	sodium monofluorophosphate, 0.76%	sodium lauryl sulfate	glycerin · propylene glycol · water · PEG-12 · tetrasodium pyrophosphate · sodium carbonate · flavor · titanium dioxide · calcium peroxide · saccharin sodium · xanthan gum · cellulose gum
	Colgate Baking Soda [a] Colgate-Palmolive	gel	hydrated silica · sodium bicarbonate	sodium fluoride, 0.243%	sodium lauryl sulfate	glycerin · PEG-12 · cellulose gum · flavor · saccharin sodium · FD&C blue#1 · D&C yellow#10
	Colgate Baking Soda [a] Colgate-Palmolive	paste	hydrated silica · sodium bicarbonate	sodium fluoride, 0.243%	sodium lauryl sulfate	glycerin · cellulose gum · flavor · saccharin sodium · titanium dioxide

See Chapter 25, "Oral Health Products," for more information about these products.

DENTIFRICE PRODUCTS - continued

	Product Manufacturer/Supplier	Dosage Form	Abrasive Ingredient	Therapeutic Ingredient	Foaming Agent	Other Ingredients [b]
	Colgate Baking Soda Tartar Control Colgate-Palmolive	gel · paste	hydrated silica · sodium bicarbonate	sodium fluoride, 0.243%	sodium lauryl sulfate	glycerin · tetrasodium pyrophosphate · PVM/MA copolymer · cellulose gum · flavor · saccharin sodium · sodium hydroxide · titanium dioxide (paste) · FD&C blue#1 & D&C yellow#10 (gel)
PE	**Colgate Junior [a]** Colgate-Palmolive	gel	hydrated silica	sodium fluoride, 0.243%	sodium lauryl sulfate	sorbitol · PEG-12 · flavor · tetrasodium pyrophosphate · cellulose gum · saccharin sodium · mica · titanium dioxide · FD&C blue#1 · D&C yellow#10
	Colgate Peak Colgate-Palmolive	paste	sodium bicarbonate · hydrated silica · precipitated calcium carbonate		sodium lauryl sulfate	glycerin · cellulose gum · flavor · saccharin sodium · titanium dioxide · sodium benzoate
	Colgate Tartar Control Micro Cleansing Formula [a] Colgate-Palmolive	gel · paste	synthetic amorphous silica, 27% · hydrated amorphous silica, 3%	sodium fluoride, 0.243%	sodium lauryl sulfate	water · sorbitol · glycerin · PEG-12 · tetrasodium pyrophosphate · PVM/MA copolymer · cellulose gum · flavor · sodium hydroxide · titanium dioxide (paste) · saccharin sodium · carrageenan · FD&C blue#1 (gel)
	Colgate Winterfresh [a] Colgate-Palmolive	gel	hydrated silica	sodium fluoride, 0.243%	sodium lauryl sulfate	sorbitol · glycerin · PEG-12 · flavor · tetrasodium pyrophosphate · cellulose gum · saccharin sodium · FD&C blue#1
	Crest Baking Soda Tartar Control, Mint [a] Procter & Gamble	gel · paste	hydrated silica · sodium bicarbonate	sodium fluoride, 0.243%	sodium lauryl sulfate	water · glycerin · sorbitol · tetrasodium pyrophosphate · PEG-6 · sodium carbonate · flavor · cellulose gum · saccharin sodium · titanium dioxide (paste) · FD&C blue#1 (gel)
	Crest Baking Soda, Mint [a] Procter & Gamble	gel · paste	hydrated silica · sodium bicarbonate	sodium fluoride, 0.243%	sodium lauryl sulfate	sorbitol · water · glycerin · sodium carbonate · flavor · cellulose gum · saccharin sodium · titanium dioxide (paste) · FD&C blue#1 (gel)
	Crest Cavity Fighting, Cool Mint [a] Procter & Gamble	gel	hydrated silica	sodium fluoride, 0.243%	sodium lauryl sulfate	sorbitol · water · trisodium phosphate · flavor · sodium phosphate · xanthan gum · saccharin sodium · carbomer 956 · FD&C blue#1

See Chapter 25, "Oral Health Products," for more information about these products.

DENTIFRICE PRODUCTS - continued

	Product Manufacturer/Supplier	Dosage Form	Abrasive Ingredient	Therapeutic Ingredient	Foaming Agent	Other Ingredients [b]
	Crest Cavity Fighting, Icy Mint or Regular [a] Procter & Gamble	paste	hydrated silica	sodium fluoride, 0.243%	sodium lauryl sulfate	sorbitol · water · glycerin · Mint · trisodium phosphate · flavor · sodium phosphate · cellulose gum (Mint) · xanthan gum (Regular) · saccharin sodium · carbomer 956 · titanium dioxide · FD&C blue#1
PE	**Crest for Kids, Sparkle Fun [a]** Procter & Gamble	gel	hydrated silica	sodium fluoride, 0.243%	sodium lauryl sulfate	sorbitol · water · trisodium phosphate · sodium phosphate · xanthan gum · flavor · saccharin sodium · carbomer 956 · mica · titanium dioxide · FD&C blue#1
**	**Crest Gum Care** Procter & Gamble	gel · paste	hydrated silica	stannous fluoride, 0.454%	sodium lauryl sulfate	sorbitol · water · saccharin sodium · sodium gluconate · stannous chloride · titanium dioxide (paste) · sodium hydroxide · hydroxyethyl cellulose · carrageenan · flavor · FD&C blue#1 (gel)
DY	**Crest Sensitivity Protection, Mild Mint [a]** Procter & Gamble	paste	hydrated silica	potassium nitrate, 5% · sodium fluoride, 0.243%	sodium lauryl sulfate	water · glycerin · sorbitol · trisodium phosphate · cellulose gum · flavor · xanthan gum · saccharin sodium · titanium dioxide
	Crest Tartar Control, Fresh Mint or Smooth Mint [a] Procter & Gamble	gel	hydrated silica	sodium fluoride, 0.243%	sodium lauryl sulfate	water · sorbitol · glycerin · tetrapotassium pyrophosphate · PEG-6 · disodium pyrophosphate · tetrasodium pyrophosphate · flavor · xanthan gum · saccharin sodium · carbomer 956 · FD&C blue#1 · FD&C yellow#5 (Smooth Mint)
	Crest Tartar Control, Original Flavor [a] Procter & Gamble	paste	hydrated silica	sodium fluoride, 0.243%	sodium lauryl sulfate	water · sorbitol · glycerin · tetrapotassium pyrophosphate · PEG-6 · disodium pyrophosphate · tetrasodium pyrophosphate · flavor · xanthan gum · saccharin sodium · carbomer 956 · titanium dioxide · FD&C blue#1
** DY SU	**Dr. Tichenor's Toothpaste** Dr. G. H. Tichenor	paste	hydrated silica	sodium fluoride	sodium lauryl sulfate	sorbitol · water · glycerin · insoluble sodium metaphosphate · peppermint oil · cellulose gum · saccharin sodium · sodium phosphate · titanium dioxide · magnesium aluminum silicate

See Chapter 25, "Oral Health Products," for more information about these products.

DENTIFRICE PRODUCTS - continued

	Product Manufacturer/Supplier	Dosage Form	Abrasive Ingredient	Therapeutic Ingredient	Foaming Agent	Other Ingredients [b]
DY	**Gleem** Procter & Gamble	paste	hydrated silica	sodium fluoride, 0.243%	sodium lauryl sulfate	sorbitol · water · trisodium phosphate · flavor · sodium phosphate · xanthan gum · saccharin sodium · carbomer 956 · titanium dioxide
	Interplak Bausch & Lomb	paste	hydrated silica	sodium fluoride	sodium lauryl sulfate	purified water · poloxamer 407 · sorbitol · glycerin · flavor · dibasic sodium phosphate · saccharin sodium · monobasic sodium phosphate · sodium benzoate · D&C yellow#10
**	**Listerine Toothpaste, Cool Mint** Warner Wellcome Consumer	paste	hydrated silica	sodium monofluorophosphate	sodium lauryl phosphate	thymol · methyl salicylate · eucalyptol · menthol · sorbitol · water · glycerin · flavors · saccharin sodium · cellulose gum · xanthan gum · phosphoric acid · titanium dioxide · sodium phosphate · benzoic acid · FD&C blue#1 · D&C yellow#10
**	**Listerine Toothpaste, Cool Mint** Warner Wellcome Consumer	gel	hydrated silica	sodium monofluorophosphate	sodium lauryl sulfate	thymol · methyl salicylate · eucalyptol · menthol · sorbitol · glycerin · flavors · saccharin sodium · cellulose gum · xanthan gum · phosphoric acid · sodium phosphate · benzoic acid · FD&C blue#1 · D&C yellow#10
**	**Mentadent Gum Care** Chesebrough-Pond's	gel · paste	hydrated silica · sodium bicarbonate	sodium fluoride, 0.15%	sodium lauryl sulfate · hydrogen peroxide	zinc citrate trihydrate, 2% · water · glycerin · sorbitol · poloxamer 407 · PEG-32 · SD alcohol 38B · menthol · methyl salicylate · cellulose gum · saccharin sodium · phosphoric acid · green#3 · titanium dioxide
**	**Mentadent Tartar Control** Chesebrough-Pond's	gel · paste	hydrated silica · sodium bicarbonate	sodium fluoride, 0.24%	sodium lauryl sulfate · hydrogen peroxide	sorbitol syrup · water · glycerol · poloxamer 407 · PEG-32 · zinc citrate · SD alcohol 38B · flavor · cellulose gum · menthol · saccharin sodium · titanium dioxide · phosphoric acid · FD&C blue#1
	Mentadent with Baking Soda & Peroxide [a] Chesebrough-Pond's	paste	hydrated silica · sodium bicarbonate	sodium fluoride, 0.24% (fluoride, 0.15%)	sodium lauryl sulfate · hydrogen peroxide	water · sorbitol · glycerin · poloxamer 407 · PEG- 32 · SD alcohol 38B · flavor · cellulose gum · saccharin sodium · phosphoric acid · blue#1 · titanium dioxide
** SU	**Natural White** Natural White	paste	hydrated silica	sodium fluoride	sodium lauryl sulfate	sorbitol · water · glycerin · titanium dioxide · cellulose gum · flavor · sodium benzoate

See Chapter 25, "Oral Health Products," for more information about these products.

DENTIFRICE PRODUCTS - continued

	Product Manufacturer/Supplier	Dosage Form	Abrasive Ingredient	Therapeutic Ingredient	Foaming Agent	Other Ingredients [b]
** SU	**Natural White Tartar Control** Natural White	paste	hydrated silica	sodium fluoride	sodium lauryl sulfate	sorbitol · water · glycerin · tetrapotassium pyrophosphate · titanium dioxide · cellulose gum · flavor · sodium benzoate · FD&C blue#1 · D&C yellow#10
** PE	**Orajel Baby Tooth & Gum Cleanser** Del Ph'cals	gel	poloxamer 407, 2% · simethicone, 0.12% · Microdent			carboxymethylcellulose · sodium · citric acid · flavor · glycerin · methylparaben · potassium sorbate · propylene glycol · propylparaben · water · saccharin sodium · sorbitol
	Oral-B Sensitive Oral-B Labs	paste	hydrated silica	potassium nitrate, 5% · sodium fluoride, 0.243%	sodium lauryl sulfate	sorbitol · water · glycerin · PEG-8 · trisodium phosphate · flavor · cellulose gum · titanium dioxide · saccharin sodium
	Oral-B Sesame Street, Bubblegum or Fruity [a] Oral-B Labs	paste	hydrated silica	sodium fluoride, 0 248%	sodium lauryl sulfate	sorbitol · water · glycerin · acesulfame K · flavor · xanthan gum · carbomer · sodium hydroxide · FD&C red#3
	Oral-B Tooth and Gum Care Oral-B Labs	paste	calcium pyrophosphate	stannous fluoride, 0.454%	sodium lauryl sulfate	sorbitol · water · glycerin · flavor · xanthan gum · PVM/MA copolymer · PEG-8 · zinc citrate · carbomer · saccharin sodium · sodium hydroxide
DY SU	**Pearl Drops Whitening Baking Soda Tartar Control** Carter Products	paste	sodium bicarbonate · hydrated silica	sodium fluoride	sodium lauryl sulfate	water · sorbitol · glycerin · tetrapotassium pyrophosphate · tetrasodium pyrophosphate · PEG-12 · flavor · titanium dioxide · saccharin sodium · cellulose gum
DY SU	**Pearl Drops Whitening Extra Strength** Carter Products	paste	hydrated silica · calcium pyrophosphate · dicalcium phosphate	sodium monofluorophosphate	sodium lauryl sulfate	water · sorbitol · glycerin · PEG-12 · flavor · titanium dioxide · cellulose gum · trisodium phosphate · sodium phosphate · saccharin sodium
DY SU	**Pearl Drops Whitening Regular Tartar Control** Carter Products	paste	hydrated silica	sodium fluoride	sodium lauryl sulfate	water · sorbitol · glycerin · tetrapotassium pyrophosphate · tetrasodium pyrophosphate · PEG-12 · flavor · titanium dioxide · cellulose gum · saccharin sodium
DY SU	**Pearl Drops Whitening Toothpolish, Spearmint** Carter Products	paste	calcium pyrophosphate · hydrated silica · aluminum hydroxide · dicalcium phosphate	sodium monofluorophosphate	sodium lauryl sulfate	water · sorbitol · glycerin · flavor · PEG-12 · titanium dioxide · cellulose gum · trisodium phosphate · sodium phosphate · saccharin sodium

See Chapter 25, "Oral Health Products," for more information about these products.

DENTIFRICE PRODUCTS - continued

	Product Manufacturer/Supplier	Dosage Form	Abrasive Ingredient	Therapeutic Ingredient	Foaming Agent	Other Ingredients [b]
	Pepsodent Baking Soda Chesebrough-Pond's	paste	hydrated silica	sodium fluoride, 0.24%	sodium lauryl sulfate	sorbitol · water · sodium bicarbonate · PEG-32 · SD alcohol 38B · flavor · xanthan gum · saccharin sodium · titanium dioxide
	Pepsodent Original Chesebrough-Pond's	paste	hydrated silica	sodium fluoride, 0.23%	sodium lauryl sulfate	sorbitol and related polyols · water · glycerin · SD alcohol 38B · flavor · xanthan gum · saccharin sodium · sodium benzoate · titanium dioxide
	Platinum Whitening Colgate-Palmolive	paste		sodium monofluorophosphate, 0.76%	sodium lauryl sulfate	water · hydrated silica · sorbitol · aluminum oxide · glycerin · PEG-12 · tetrapotassium pyrophosphate · PVM/MA copolymer · flavor · sodium hydroxide · saccharin sodium · titanium dioxide
**	**Plus+White Plus Peroxide** CCA Industries	paste	dicalcium phosphate · hydrated silica	sodium monofluorophosphate	sodium lauryl sulfate · calcium peroxide	glycerin · propylene glycol · sorbitol · carbomer · saccharin sodium · sodium carbonate · urea · titanium dioxide · flavor · ethylcellulose
**	**Plus+White with Fluoride** CCA Industries	paste	dicalcium phosphate · alumina · hydrated silica	sodium monofluorophosphate	sodium lauryl sulfate	glycerin · cellulose gum · water · sodium benzoate · saccharin sodium · trisodium phosphate · titanium dioxide · flavor · FD&C blue#1
**	**Plus+White with Fluoride** CCA Industries	gel	alumina · hydrated silica	sodium monofluorophosphate	sodium lauryl sulfate	glycerin · cellulose gum · sorbitol · PEG-32 · water · sodium benzoate · saccharin sodium · FD&C blue#1 · sodium phosphate · trisodium phosphate · flavor
	Promise Block Drug	paste	dicalcium phosphate	potassium nitrate · sodium monofluorophosphate	sodium lauryl sulfate	water · hydroxyethyl cellulose · flavor · saccharin sodium · methylparaben · propylparaben · D&C yellow#10 · FD&C blue#1 · glycerin · sorbitol · silicon dioxide
	Pycopay Block Drug	powder	sodium bicarbonate · calcium carbonate · tricalcium phosphate · magnesium carbonate			sodium chloride · eugenol · methyl salicylate
**	**Rembrandt Whitening Baking Soda** Den-Mat	paste	sodium bicarbonate · silica	sodium monofluorophosphate (fluoride, 0.15%)	sodium lauryl sulfate	glycerin · sorbitol · alumina · water · sodium citrate · sodium carrageenan · papain · flavor · sodium hydroxide · FD&C blue#1 · saccharin sodium
**	**Rembrandt Whitening Natural** Den-Mat	paste	dicalcium phosphate · silica	sodium monofluorophosphate		glycerin · xylitol · water · sodium citrate · natural flavors · papain · sodium carrageenan · citric acid

See Chapter 25, "Oral Health Products," for more information about these products.

DENTIFRICE PRODUCTS - continued

	Product Manufacturer/Supplier	Dosage Form	Abrasive Ingredient	Therapeutic Ingredient	Foaming Agent	Other Ingredients [b]
	Rembrandt Whitening Sensitive Den-Mat	paste	dicalcium phosphate dihydrate	potassium nitrate, 5% · sodium monofluorophosphate, 0.76%	sodium lauryl sulfate	glycerin · sorbitol · water · alumina · papain · sodium citrate · flavor · sodium carboxymethylcellulose · saccharin sodium · methylparaben · citric acid · FD&C red#40
	Rembrandt Whitening, Mint or Regular Den-Mat	paste	dicalcium phosphate dihydrate	sodium monofluorophosphate, 0.76%	sodium lauryl sulfate	glycerin · sorbitol · water · alumina · sodium citrate · flavor · sodium carrageenan · papain · saccharin sodium · methylparaben · citric acid · FD&C blue#1 · FD&C yellow#5
	Rembrandt with Peroxide Den-Mat	gel		sodium monofluorophosphate	carbamide peroxide · sodium lauryl sulfate	glycerin · sodium citrate · carbomer · titanium dioxide · flavor · triethanolamine
DY	**Revelation** Alvin Last	powder	calcium carbonate		vegetable soap powder	methyl salicylate · menthol
DY	**Sensodyne Baking Soda** Dentco	paste	silica · sodium bicarbonate	potassium nitrate · sodium fluoride	sodium lauryl sulfate	water · glycerin · flavor · hydroxyethyl cellulose · titanium dioxide · saccharin sodium
	Sensodyne, Cool Gel Dentco	gel	silica	potassium nitrate · sodium fluoride	sodium methyl cocoyl taurate	water · sorbitol · glycerin · sodium carboxyethylcellulose · flavor · saccharin sodium · FD&C blue#1 · trisodium phosphate
	Sensodyne, Fresh Mint [a] Dentco	paste	dicalcium phosphate	potassium nitrate · sodium monofluorophosphate	sodium lauryl sulfate	water · glycerin · sorbitol · hydroxyethyl cellulose · flavor · saccharin sodium · methylparaben · propylparaben · D&C yellow#10 · FD&C blue#1 · silicon dioxide
** SU PE	**Slimer** Perio	paste	hydrated silica	sodium fluoride, 0.15%		sorbitol · water · glycerin · PEG-32 · flavor · ethyl alcohol · propylene glycol · glyceryl triacetate · cellulose gum · saccharin sodium · sodium benzoate · FD&C blue#1 · FD&C red#33
	Thermodent Mentholatum	paste	diatomaceous earth · silica	strontium chloride hexahydrate	sodium methyl cocoyl taurate	sorbitol · glycerin · titanium dioxide · guar gum · PEG-40 stearate · hydroxyethyl cellulose · flavor · preservative · water
** FL	**Tom's Natural Baking Soda with Propolis & Myrrh** Tom's of Maine	paste	calcium carbonate · sodium bicarbonate		sodium lauryl sulfate	glycerin · water · carrageenan · peppermint oil · myrrh · propolis
PE	**Tom's Natural for Children, with Calcium & Fluoride** Tom's of Maine	paste	calcium carbonate · hydrated silica	sodium monofluorophosphate	sodium lauryl sulfate	glycerin · water · fruit extracts · carrageenan

See Chapter 25, "Oral Health Products," for more information about these products.

DENTIFRICE PRODUCTS - continued

	Product Manufacturer/Supplier	Dosage Form	Abrasive Ingredient	Therapeutic Ingredient	Foaming Agent	Other Ingredients [b]
	Tom's Natural with Baking Soda, Calcium, & Fluoride Tom's of Maine	paste	calcium carbonate · sodium bicarbonate	sodium monofluorophosphate	sodium lauryl sulfate	glycerin · water · carrageenan · xylitol · peppermint oil
**	**Tom's Natural with Calcium & Fluoride** Tom's of Maine	paste	calcium carbonate · hydrated silica	sodium monofluorophosphate	sodium lauryl sulfate	glycerin · water · xylitol · carrageenan · natural wintergreen oil
	Tom's Natural with Calcium & Fluoride [a] Tom's of Maine	paste	calcium carbonate	sodium monofluorophosphate	sodium lauryl sulfate	glycerin · water · xylitol (spearmint) · carrageenan · either cinnamon, fennel oil or spearmint · peppermint oil (cinnamon, spearmint)
FL	**Tom's Natural with Propolis & Myrrh** Tom's of Maine	paste	calcium carbonate		sodium lauryl sulfate	glycerin · water · carrageenan · spearmint, peppermint, cassia, or fennel oil · myrrh · propolis
	Ultra Brite Colgate-Palmolive	paste	hydrated silica · alumina	sodium monofluorophosphate, 0.76%	sodium lauryl sulfate	glycerin · cellulose gum · carrageenan gum · sodium benzoate · titanium dioxide · saccharin sodium · flavor
	Ultra Brite [a] Colgate-Palmolive	gel	hydrated silica	sodium monofluorophosphate, 0.76%	sodium lauryl sulfate	sorbitol · PEG-12 · flavor · cellulose gum · saccharin sodium · glycerin · FD&C blue#1 · D&C red#33
	Ultra Brite Baking Soda Colgate-Palmolive	paste	hydrated silica · sodium bicarbonate · alumina	sodium monofluorophosphate, 0.76%	sodium lauryl sulfate	glycerin · tetrasodium pyrophosphate · cellulose gum · flavor · saccharin sodium · titanium dioxide
	Viadent Fluoride Colgate-Palmolive	paste	hydrated silica	sodium monofluorophosphate, 0.8% · sanguinaria extract, 0.075%	sodium lauryl sulfate	sorbitol · titanium dioxide · carboxymethylcellulose · flavor · saccharin sodium · citric acid · zinc chloride
	Viadent Fluoride Colgate-Palmolive	gel	hydrated silica	sodium monofluorophosphate, 0.8% · sanguinaria extract, 0.075%	sodium lauryl sulfate	saccharin sodium · zinc chloride · teaberry flavor · sodium carboxymethylcellulose · sorbitol
FL	**Viadent Original** Colgate-Palmolive	paste	dicalcium phosphate	sanguinaria extract, 0.075%	sodium lauryl sulfate	glycerin · sorbitol · titanium dioxide · zinc chloride · carrageenan · flavor · saccharin sodium · citric acid

** New listing
[a] Carries American Dental Association (ADA) seal indicating safety and efficacy
[b] Sodium bicarbonate can also be considered an abrasive.

See Chapter 25, "Oral Health Products," for more information about these products.

ARTIFICIAL SALIVA PRODUCTS

	Product Manufacturer/Supplier	Dosage Form	Viscosity Agent	Preservative	Other Ingredients
	Entertainer's Secret Throat Relief KLI Corp.	pump spray	sodium carboxymethylcellulose	methylparaben · propylparaben	potassium chloride · dibasic sodium phosphate
**	**Glandosane Mouth Moisturizer; Lemon, Mint, or Unflavored** Kenwood Labs	aerosol spray	sodium carboxymethylcellulose, 0.51g		sorbitol, 1.52g · sodium chloride, 0.043g · potassium chloride, 0.061g · calcium chloride dihydrate, 0.007g · magnesium chloride hexahydrate, 0.003g · dipotassium hydrogen phosphate, 0.017g · flavoring · carbon dioxide
	Moi-Stir Mouth Moistening Kingswood Labs	pump spray	carboxymethylcellulose		
	Moi-Stir Oral Swabsticks [a] Kingswood Labs	swab	carboxymethylcellulose		
	MouthKote Parnell Ph'cals	spray		sodium benzoate	water · xylitol · sorbitol · yerba santa · citric acid · flavor · ascorbic acid · saccharin sodium
	Optimoist Colgate-Palmolive	liquid	hydroxyethyl cellulose	sodium benzoate	citric acid · calcium phosphate · sodium monofluorophosphate · sweetener · xylitol · polysorbate 20 · flavor · sodium hydroxide
	Saliva Substitute [a] Roxane Labs	spray	sodium carboxymethylcellulose	methylparaben	sorbitol · flavoring
	Salivart Synthetic Saliva [a] Gebauer	aerosol spray	sodium carboxymethylcellulose, 1%		sorbitol, 3% · potassium chloride, 0.12% · sodium chloride, 0.084% · calcium chloride dihydrate · magnesium chloride hexahydrate · potassium phosphate dibasic · nitrogen (as propellant)

** New listing
[a] Carries American Dental Association (ADA) seal indicating safety and efficacy

See Chapter 25, "Oral Health Products," for more information about these products.

DENTURE CLEANSER PRODUCTS

	Product Manufacturer/Supplier	Dosage Form	Cleaning/Abrasive Agent	Other Ingredients
	Ban-A-Stain Brimms Labs	liquid	phosphoric acid, 25%	deionized water · imidurea · methylparaben · xanthan gum · alkyl phenoxy polyethoxy ethanol · oil of cassis · FD&C red#40
	Complete [a] Procter & Gamble	paste	calcium carbonate · silica	water · glycerin · sorbitol · cellulose gum · sodium lauryl sulfate · flavor · magnesium aluminum silicate · saccharin sodium · methylparaben · propylparaben
	Dentu-Creme Dentco	paste	dicalcium phosphate dihydrate · calcium carbonate · aluminum silicate	propylene glycol · sodium lauryl sulfate · glycerin · hydroxyethyl cellulose · flavor · magnesium aluminum silicate · saccharin sodium · methylparaben · propylparaben
	Efferdent Antibacterial [a] Warner Wellcome Consumer	tablet	sodium carbonate · sodium bicarbonate · potassium monopersulfate · sodium perborate	fragrance · colors
**	**Efferdent Plus** Warner Wellcome Consumer	tablet	sodium bicarbonate · sodium perborate · potassium monopersulfate · detergents	fragrance · colors (including FD&C yellow#5) · saccharin sodium · chelating agents
	Efferdent, 2 Layer Warner Wellcome Consumer	tablet	sodium bicarbonate · sodium carbonate · potassium monopersulfate · detergents	fragrance · colors · saccharin sodium · chelating agents
	Polident Block Drug	tablet · powder	sodium carbonate · sodium bicarbonate	potassium monopersulfate · sodium perborate monohydrate · surfactant · sodium acid pyrophosphate (powder) · citric acid (tablet) · fragrance
	Smokers' Polident Block Drug	tablet	sodium carbonate · sodium bicarbonate · potassium monopersulfate · sodium perborate monohydrate · surfactant	citric acid · chelating agents · proteolytic enzyme · fragrance

** New listing
[a] Carries American Dental Association (ADA) seal indicating safety and efficacy

See Chapter 25, "Oral Health Products," for more information about these products.

DENTURE ADHESIVE PRODUCTS

	Product Manufacturer/Supplier	Dosage Form	Adhesive Agent	Other Ingredients
	Confident Block Drug	cream	carboxymethylcellulose gum, 32%	ethylene oxide polymer, 13% · petrolatum · liquid petrolatum · propylparaben
	Corega Block Drug	powder	karaya gum, 94.6%	water-soluble ethylene oxide polymer, 5% · flavor
**	**Cushion Grip** Schering-Plough HealthCare	gel		alcohol, 26.2% · triacetin · polyvinyl acetate
	Dentrol Block Drug	liquid	carboxymethylcellulose sodium	ethylene oxide polymer · mineral oil · polyethylene · flavor · propylparaben
	Denturite Brimms Labs	liquid · powder		liquid: butyl phthalyl butyl glycolate · vinyl acetate · SDA alcohol · powder: polyethyl methacrylate polymer
	Effergrip [a] Warner Wellcome Consumer	cream	carboxymethylcellulose sodium · polyvinylmethylether maleic acid calcium sodium double salt	color · flavor · preservatives · vehicle
	Ezo Cushions Medtech Labs	pad		paraffin wax · cotton
	Fasteeth Procter & Gamble	powder	sodium carboxymethylcellulose	calcium/zinc poly (vinyl methyl ether maleate) · corn starch · silicon dioxide · peppermint oil, rectified
	Fasteeth Extra Hold Procter & Gamble	powder	sodium carboxymethylcellulose	calcium/zinc poly (vinyl methyl ether maleate) · silicon dioxide · peppermint oil, rectified
	Fixodent Procter & Gamble	cream	sodium carboxymethylcellulose	calcium/zinc poly (vinyl methyl ether maleate) · mineral oil · petrolatum · silicon dioxide · color
	Fixodent Fresh Procter & Gamble	cream	sodium carboxymethylcellulose	calcium/zinc poly (vinyl methyl ether maleate) · mineral oil · petrolatum · silicon dioxide · color · peppermint flavor · methyl lactate · menthol
	Plasti-Liner Brimms Labs	strip		polyethyl methacrylate polymer · butyl phthalyl butyl glycolate · triacetin
	Poli-Grip Block Drug	cream	karaya gum, 51%	petrolatum, 36.7% · liquid petrolatum · magnesium oxide · propylparaben · flavor
	Poli-Grip Super Block Drug	cream	carboxymethylcellulose sodium	calcium sodium methyl vinyl ether maleic acid salt · petrolatum · mineral oil · flavor · propylparaben
	Poli-Grip Super Block Drug	powder	carboxymethylcellulose sodium	calcium sodium methyl vinyl ether maleic acid salt copolymer · flavor
	Polident Dentu-Grip Block Drug	cream	carboxymethylcellulose gum, 49%	ethylene oxide polymer, 21% · flavor
	Quik-Fix Brimms Labs	liquid · powder		liquid: methyl methacrylate monomer · hydroxyethyl methacrylate monomer · colorsatable concentrate · triacetin · powder: polyethyl methacrylate polymer · polymethyl methacrylate polymer
	Sea-Bond Combe	pad		ethylene oxide polymer · sodium alginate
	Wernet's Block Drug	cream	carboxymethylcellulose gum, 32%	petrolatum · mineral oil · ethylene oxide polymer, 13% · propylparaben · flavor, 0.5%
	Wernet's Block Drug	powder	karaya gum, 94.6%	water-soluble ethylene oxide polymer, 5% · flavor, 0.4%

See Chapter 25, "Oral Health Products," for more information about these products.

DENTURE ADHESIVE PRODUCTS - continued

Product Manufacturer/Supplier	**Dosage Form**	**Adhesive Agent**	**Other Ingredients**
Wernet's Super Block Drug	powder	carboxymethylcellulose gum	ethylene oxide polymer · dicalcium phosphate · monosodium phosphate · flavor

** New listing
[a] Carries American Dental Association (ADA) seal indicating safety and efficacy

See Chapter 25, "Oral Health Products," for more information about these products.

DERMATITIS PRODUCTS

	Product Manufacturer/Supplier	Dosage Form	Hydro-cortisone	Astringent	Other Ingredients
**	**Aquanil HC** Person & Covey	lotion	1%	cetyl alcohol · stearyl alcohol	purified water · glycerin · benzyl alcohol · sodium laureth · sulfate · xanthan gum
	Bactine Hydrocortisone 1% Bayer Consumer	cream	1%	cetearyl alcohol · hydrocortisone alcohol · aluminum sulfate · calcium acetate	beeswax · dextrin · glycerin · light mineral oil · methylparaben · water · sodium lauryl sulfate · white petrolatum
	Caldecort Ciba Self-Medication	cream	1%		cetostearyl alcohol · sodium lauryl sulfate · white petrolatum · propylene glycol · purified water
**	**Cortaid FastStick** Pharmacia & Upjohn	stick	1%	alcohol, 55%	butylated hydroxytoluene · methylparaben · purified water
	Cortaid Maximum Strength Pharmacia & Upjohn	spray	1%	alcohol, 55%	glycerin · methylparaben · water
	Cortaid Maximum Strength Pharmacia & Upjohn	ointment	1%		butylparaben · cholesterol · methylparaben · microcrystalline wax · mineral oil · white petrolatum
	Cortaid Maximum Strength Pharmacia & Upjohn	cream	1%	cetyl alcohol	glycerin · methylparaben · water · aloe · ceteareth-20 · cetyl palmitate · isopropyl myristate · isopropyl pentanoate
	Cortaid Sensitive Skin Formula Pharmacia & Upjohn	cream	0.5%		aloe · butylparaben · cetyl palmitate · glyceryl stearate · methylparaben · propylethylene glycol · stearamidoethyl diethylamine · water
	Cortaid Sensitive Skin Formula Pharmacia & Upjohn	ointment	0.5%		aloe · butylparaben · cholesterol · methylparaben · mineral oil · white petrolatum · microcrystalline wax
	Corticaine UCB Pharma	cream	0.5%		
	Cortizone-10 Thompson Medical	ointment	1%		white petrolatum
	Cortizone-10 Thompson Medical	cream	1%	aluminum sulfate · calcium acetate	glycerin · light mineral oil · methylparaben · propylparaben · potato dextrin · sodium lauryl sulfate · water · white petrolatum · white wax · aloe · cetearyl alcohol
	Cortizone-10 Scalp Itch Thompson Medical	liquid	1%		benzyl alcohol · SD alcohol 40 · propylene glycol · water
	Cortizone-5 Thompson Medical	cream	0.5%	aluminum sulfate · calcium acetate	glycerin · light mineral oil · methylparaben · propylparaben · potato dextrin · sodium lauryl sulfate · water · white petrolatum · white wax · aloe · cetearyl alcohol
	Cortizone-5 Thompson Medical	ointment	0.5%		white petrolatum · aloe
	Dermarest DriCort Del Ph'cals	cream	1%		
	DermiCort Republic Drug	cream	0.5%		aloe
	Dermtex Pfeiffer Ph'cals	pump spray	1%		menthol, 1%
	Dermtex HC Pfeiffer Ph'cals	cream	1%		aloe vera gel
	Dr. Gordshell's Salve Thomas & Thompson	ointment			lard · tallow · beeswax · elder flowers · bayberry · sassafras oil · benzoic acid · rosin

See Chapter 26, "Dermatologic Products," for more information about these products.

DERMATITIS PRODUCTS - continued

	Product Manufacturer/Supplier	Dosage Form	Hydro-cortisone	Astringent	Other Ingredients
**	**Hytone** Dermik Labs	cream	1%	cetyl alcohol	isopropyl myristate · cholesterol & related sterols · polysorbate 60 · sorbitan monostearate · polyoxyl 40 stearate · glyceryl monostearate SE · propylene glycol · sorbic acid · purified water
**	**Hytone** Dermik Labs	lotion	1%	cetyl alcohol	carbomer 940 · propylene glycol · polysorbate 40 · propylene glycol stearate · cholesterol and related sterols · isopropyl myristate · sorbitan palmitate · triethanolamine · sorbic acid · simethicone · purified water
	Kericort 10 Bristol-Myers Products	cream	1%	stearyl alcohol · cetyl alcohol	citric acid, anhydrous · sodium citrate · methylparaben · sorbic acid · polyoxyl 40 stearate · glyceryl stearate · white wax · isopropyl myristate · sorbitan monostearate · polysorbate 60 · propylparaben · propylene glycol
	Lanacort Combe	cream	0.5%		
	Lanacort 10 Combe	cream · ointment	1%		
	Neutrogena T/Scalp Anti-Pruritic Neutrogena Dermatologics	liquid	1%		
PE	**No More Itchies** Johnson & Johnson Consumer	pump spray	1%	SD alcohol 40-B, 45%	
	Preparation H Hydrocortisone 1% Anti-Itch Whitehall-Robins Healthcare	cream	1%		BHA · cellulose gum · citric acid · disodium EDTA · glycerin · glyceryl oleate · glyceryl stearate · lanolin · methylparaben · petrolatum · propyl gallate · propylene glycol · propylparaben · simethicone · sodium benzoate · sodium lauryl sulfate · water · xanthan gum · cetyl alcohol · stearyl alcohol
	Procort Roberts Ph'cal	cream	1%		glycerin · glyceryl stearate · mineral oil · methylparaben · polysorbate 60 · propylparaben · sorbitan stearate · purified water · aloe vera gel
	Scalp Relief Medicine Goldline Labs	liquid	1%		
	Scalpicin Anti-Itch Combe	liquid	1%		SD alcohol 40 · menthol · propylene glycol · water
**	**Scalpmycin** Pfeiffer Ph'cals	liquid	1%		

** New listing

See Chapter 26, "Dermatologic Products," for more information about these products.

DRY SKIN PRODUCTS

	Product Manufacturer/Supplier	Dosage Form	Keratin Softener	Humectant	Other Ingredients
	ACID Mantle Creme Acid pH Sandoz Consumer	cream	citric acid	glycerin	aluminum acetate · aluminum sulfate · calcium acetate · cetearyl alcohol · light mineral oil · methylparaben · water · sodium lauryl sulfate · synthetic beeswax · white petrolatum · white potato dextrin · ammonium hydroxide
	ActiBath Soak Moisture Treatment Andrew Jergens	effervescent tablet	petrolatum		fumaric acid · sodium bicarbonate · sodium carbonate · dextrin · sorbitol · titanium dioxide · PEG-150 · cetyl octanoate · cholesteryl isostearate · fragrance · oleth-9 · isostearic/myristic glycerides · carragunan · sucrose stearate · tocopherol · color
	ActiBath Soak Oatmeal Treatment Andrew Jergens	effervescent tablet		colloidal oatmeal, 20%	fumaric acid · sodium carbonate · lactose · sodium bicarbonate · PEG-150 · magnesium oxide · sucrose stearate
** FR	**Alpha Glow Body Care** Fischer Ph'cals	lotion	glycolic acid, 10%		octyl methoxycinnamate, 7.5% · titanium dioxide, 2%
FR	**Alpha Glow Day** Fischer Ph'cals	cream	glycolic acid, 8%		octyl methoxycinnamate, 7.5% · titanium dioxide, 2%
	Alpha Keri Bristol-Myers Products	bar		glycerin	sodium tallowate · sodium cocoate · mineral oil · PEG-75 · titanium dioxide · lanolin oil · sodium chloride · BHT · EDTA · color · fragrance
	Alpha Keri Bristol-Myers Products	oil			mineral oil · lanolin oil · PEG-4-dilaurate · benzophenone-3 · fragrance · color
**	**Ambi Cocoa Butter** Kiwi	cream		glycerin · propylene glycol	dimethicone, 1% · water · cocoa butter · glyceryl stearate SE · mineral oil · stearic acid · steareth-21 · tocopheryl acetate · retinyl palmitate · cholecalciferol · carbomer · triethanolamine · BHT · corn oil · diazolidinyl urea · methylparaben · propylparaben · quaternium-15 · disodium EDTA · fragrance · FD&C yellow#5 · FD&C red#4
	Aqua A Baker Cummins Derm'cals	cream			water · caprylic/capric triglyceride · methyl gluceth-10 · glyceryl stearate squalene · mineral oil · PPG-20 methyl glucose ether distearate · dimethicone · stearic acid · PEG-50 stearate · retinyl palmitate · sodium hyaluronate · lecithin · sodium polyglutamate · magnesium aluminum silicate · carbomer 934 · dichlorobenzyl alcohol · cetyl alcohol · BHT · xanthan gum · menthol · sodium hydroxide · tetrasodium EDTA · diazolidinyl urea
	Aqua Care Menley & James Labs	lotion	urea, 10% · lactic acid	propylene glycol stearate	mineral oil · petrolatum · sorbitan stearate · cetyl alcohol · magnesium aluminum silicate · sodium lauryl sulfate · methylparaben · propylparaben · may contain sodium hydroxide

See Chapter 26, "Dermatologic Products," for more information about these products.

DRY SKIN PRODUCTS - continued

	Product Manufacturer/Supplier	Dosage Form	Keratin Softener	Humectant	Other Ingredients
	Aqua Care Menley & James Labs	cream	urea, 10%	glycerin	cetyl esters · DEA-oleth-3 phosphate · petrolatum · triethanolamine · carbomer · lanolin oil · mineral oil/lanolin alcohol · benzyl alcohol · fragrance · water
	Aquabase Paddock Labs	ointment			petrolatum · mineral oil · mineral wax · wool wax alcohol · cholesterol
	Aquaderm Baker Cummins Derm'cals	cream · lotion			water · caprylic/capric triglyceride · methyl gluceth-10 · glyceryl stearate · dimethicone · petrolatum · mineral oil · ether distearate · stearic acid · sodium hyaluronate · lecithin · sodium polyglutamate · magnesium aluminum silicate · carbomer 934 · dichlorobenzyl alcohol · cetyl alcohol · BHT · xanthan gum · menthol · tetrasodium EDTA · sodium hydroxide · diazolidinyl urea
	Aquaphilic Medco Lab	ointment		propylene glycol · sorbitol	stearyl alcohol · petrolatum · isopropyl palmitate · methylparaben · propylparaben · water · sodium lauryl sulfate
	Aquaphilic with Carbamide Medco Lab	ointment	urea, 10%; 20% · lactic acid	propylene glycol · sorbitol	stearyl alcohol · petrolatum · isopropyl palmitate · methylparaben · propylparaben · water · sodium lauryl sulfate
	Aveeno Bath Treatment Moisturizing Formula Rydelle Labs	powder		colloidal oatmeal, 43%	mineral oil
	Aveeno Bath Treatment Soothing Formula Rydelle Labs	powder		colloidal oatmeal, 100%	
FR	**Aveeno for Combination Skin** Rydelle Labs	cleansing bar	lactic acid	colloidal oatmeal, 38% · glycerin	sodium cocoyl isethionate · sodium lactate · magnesium aluminum silicate · potassium sorbate · titanium dioxide · PEG-14M · cetyl alcohol · benzaldehyde · C12-14 alkyl benzoate · iodopropynyl butylcarbamate · polyoxymethylene urea
FR	**Aveeno for Dry Skin** Rydelle Labs	cleansing bar	lactic acid	colloidal oatmeal, 38% · glycerin	sodium cocoyl isethionate · hydrogenated vegetable oil · vegetable shortening · PEG-75 · lauramide DEA · sodium lactate · sorbic acid · titanium dioxide · cetyl alcohol · benzaldehyde · polyoxymethylene urea · C12-14 alkyl benzoate
** FR	**Aveeno Gentle Skin Cleanser** Rydelle Labs	lotion	citric acid	oatmeal flour · sodium PCA	deionized water · disodium laureth sulfosuccinate · hydrogenated tallow glyceride · potassium cocoyl hydrolyzed collagen · disodium lauroamphodiacetate · ammonium lauryl sulfate · sodium citrate · phenylcarbinol · hexahydrohexamethyl cyclopentabenzopyran · musk ketone · PEG-150 distearate · diethyl phthalate
	Aveeno Moisturizing Rydelle Labs	cream · lotion		colloidal oatmeal, 1% · glycerin	petrolatum · distearyldimonium chloride · isopropyl palmitate · cetyl alcohol · dimethicone · sodium chloride · benzyl alcohol

See Chapter 26, "Dermatologic Products," for more information about these products.

DRY SKIN PRODUCTS - continued

	Product Manufacturer/Supplier	Dosage Form	Keratin Softener	Humectant	Other Ingredients
FR	**Aveeno Shower & Bath** Rydelle Labs	bath oil		colloidal oatmeal, 4%	mineral oil · laureth-4 · benzaldehyde · quaternium-18 hectorite · phenylcarbinol · silica
	Bagbalm Multisource	ointment	petrolatum		8-hydroxyquinoline sulfate, 0.3% · lanolin
	Candermyl Galderma Labs	cream		glycerin · propylene glycol	oleic/palmitoleic triglycerides · polyamidoacid · sodium lactate methylsilanol · polyglyceryl-3 · hexadecylether · cholesterol
	Carmol 10 Doak Dermatologics	lotion	urea, 10%		nonlipid base
**	**Carmol 20** Doak Dermatologics	lotion	urea, 20%		nonlipid base
	Cetaphil Galderma Labs	bar			sodium cocoyl isethionate · stearic acid · sodium tallowate
FR	**Cetaphil Gentle Cleanser** Galderma Labs	liquid		propylene glycol	cetyl alcohol · stearyl alcohol · sodium lauryl sulfate
** FR	**Cetaphil Moisturizing Cream** Galderma Labs	cream		polyglycerylmethacrylate · propylene glycol	petrolatum · dicapryl ether · PEG-5 glyceryl stearate · dimethicone · dimethiconol · sweet almond oil
** FR	**Cetaphil Moisturizing Lotion** Galderma Labs	lotion		glycerin	hydrogenated polyisorbutene · cetearyl alcohol · ceteareth-20 · macadamia nut oil · dimethicone · tocopheryl acetate
	ChapStick Plus Whitehall-Robins Healthcare	ointment			white petrolatum, 99% · aloe · butylated hydroxytoluene · flavor · lanolin · phenonip
	ChapStick Plus, Cherry Whitehall-Robins Healthcare	ointment			white petrolatum, 98.85% · aloe · butylated hydroxytoluene · D&C red#6 barium lake · flavors · lanolin · phenonip · saccharin
	ChapStick, Regular/Original Whitehall-Robins Healthcare	stick			petrolatum, 44% · padimate O, 1.5% · lanolin, 1% · isopropyl myristate, 1% · cetyl alcohol, 0.5% · arachidyl propionate · camphor · carnauba wax · D&C red#6 barium lake · FD&C yellow#5 aluminum lake · fragrance · isopropyl lanolate · methylparaben · mineral oil · 2-octyl dodecanol · oleyl alcohol · polyphenylmethylsiloxane 556 · propylparaben · titanium dioxide · paraffin wax · white wax
	ChapStick; Cherry, Mint, Orange, or Strawberry Whitehall-Robins Healthcare	stick			petrolatum, 44% · padimate O, 1.5% · lanolin, 1% · isopropyl myristate, 0.5% · cetyl alcohol · arachidyl propionate · camphor (Cherry · Strawberry) · carnauba wax · colors · flavors · isopropyl lanolate · methylparaben · mineral oil · 2-octyl dodecanol · polyphenylmethylsiloxane 556 · propylparaben · saccharin · paraffin wax · white wax

See Chapter 26, "Dermatologic Products," for more information about these products.

DRY SKIN PRODUCTS - continued

	Product Manufacturer/Supplier	Dosage Form	Keratin Softener	Humectant	Other Ingredients
	Clocream Roberts Ph'cal	cream		glycerin	cetyl palmitate · vitamin A palmitate · cottonseed oil · glyceryl monostearate · methylparaben · mineral oil · potassium stearate · propylparaben · sodium citrate · vitamins A & D · fragrance · purified water
	Complex 15 Therapeutic Moisturizing Schering-Plough HealthCare	cream · lotion		glycerin	lecithin
	Complex 15 Therapeutic Moisturizing Face Cream Schering-Plough HealthCare	cream		glycerin	lecithin
	Corn Huskers Warner Wellcome Consumer	lotion		glycerin	SD alcohol 40 · oleyl sarcosine · methylparaben · guar gum · calcium sulfate · calcium chloride · sodium calcium alginate · triethanolamine · fragrance · fumaric acid · boric acid · water
FR	**Curél Alpha Hydroxy** Bausch & Lomb	lotion	lactic acid · glycolic acid	glycerin	petrolatum · distearyl dimonium chloride · isopropylpalmitate · 1-hexadecanol · dimethicone · ammonium hydroxide · methylparaben · propylparaben
**	**Curél Nutrient Rich Severe Dry Skin** Bausch & Lomb	lotion		glycerin	petrolatum · quaternium-5 · isopropyl palmitate · 1-hexadecanol · dimethicone · nylon 12 · methylparaben · tocopheryl acetate · propylparaben · DL-panthenol · ascorbyl palmitate
FR	**Curél Therapeutic Moisturizing, Fragrance-Free or Scented** Bausch & Lomb	cream · lotion		glycerin	petrolatum · quaternium-5 · isopropyl palmitate · 1-hexadecanol · dimethicone · methylparaben · propylparaben · sodium chloride
	Cutemol Emollient Skin Cream Summers Labs	cream	allantoin		liquid petrolatum · acetylated lanolin · lanolin alcohols extract · isopropyl myristate wax · sorbitan sesquioleate
	Dermabase Paddock Labs	cream		propylene glycol	water · mineral oil · petrolatum · cetostearyl alcohol · sodium lauryl sulfate · isopropyl palmitate · methylparaben · propylparaben · imidazolidinyl urea
** FR	**Dermal Therapy Extra Strength Body** Bayer Diagnostics	lotion	urea · lactic acid	propylene glycol	deionized water · hydrogenated polyisobutene · isopropyl myristate · cetyl alcohol · GMS/PEG-100 stearate · triethanolamine · emulsifying wax · silk amino acid · imidazolidinyl urea · carbomer 941 · tetrasodium EDTA · sorbic acid · quaternium-15

See Chapter 26, "Dermatologic Products," for more information about these products.

DRY SKIN PRODUCTS - continued

	Product Manufacturer/Supplier	Dosage Form	Keratin Softener	Humectant	Other Ingredients
	Dermasil Dry Skin Treatment Chesebrough-Pond's	cream		glycerin	dimethicone, 1.1% · water · petrolatum · myreth-3myristate · sunflower seed oil · cetostearyl alcohol · dimethicone · triethanolamine · carbomer 934 · ceteareth-20 · methylparaben · DMDM hydantoin · propylparaben · cholesterol · stearic acid · lecithin · ethylene brassylate · palmarosa oil · rose extract · sandalwood oil · sweet almond oil · borage seed oil · vanilla
	Dermasil Dry Skin Treatment Chesebrough-Pond's	lotion		glycerin	dimethicone, 1.1% · water · petrolatum · mineral oil · stearic acid · sunflower seed oil · glycol stearate · dimethicone · triethanolamine · PEG-40 stearate · acetylated lanolin alcohol · magnesium aluminum silicate · methylparaben · propylparaben · cetyl alcohol · stearamide AMP · cholesterol · carbomer 934 · disodium EDTA · lecithin · ethylene brassylate · palmarosa oil · rose extract · sandalwood oil · sweet almond oil · borage seed oil · DMDM hydantoin · vanilla · ascorbyl palmitate
	Dermsol Parnell Ph'cals	lotion		glycerin · propylene glycol	dimethicone, 1% · mineral oil · yerba santa · cetyl alcohol · glyceryl stearate · isopropyl myristate · PEG-40 stearate · squalene · stearic acid · diazolidinyl urea · lecithin · PEG-12 oleate · benzoic acid · quaternized acetamide MEA · BHT · retinyl palmitate · tocopheryl acetate
FR	**DiabetiDerm** Health Care Products	cream	urea · lactic acid · allantoin		purified water · cetyl alcohol · hydrogenated apricot kernel oil · glyceryl stearate · PEG-100 stearate · polysorbate 60 · isostearyl alcohol · benzyl alcohol · wheat germ oil · soybean & calendula extract · dimethicone copolymer · St. John's Wart · silk protein · carbomer 940 · cosmedia polymer · may contain: sodium hydroxide
FR	**DiabetiDerm** Health Care Products	lotion	urea · lactic acid	glycerin · propylene glycol dipelargonate · propylene glycol	purified water · stearic acid · cetyl alcohol · PEG-8 dioleate · sodium lauryl sulfate · dimethicone copolymer · benzyl alcohol · PEG-8 distearate · silk protein · carbomer 940 · xanthan gum · may contain: sodium hydroxide
FR	**DML Facial Moisturizer** Person & Covey	cream		propylene glycol dioctanoate · glycerin	petrolatum · octyl methoxycinnamate, 8% · oxybenzone, 4% · water · DEA cetyl phosphate · glyceryl stearate · PEG-100 stearate · stearic acid · hyaluronic acid · benzyl alcohol · dimethicone · PVP/eicosene copolymer · sodium carbomer 941 · disodium EDTA · magnesium aluminum silicate

See Chapter 26, "Dermatologic Products," for more information about these products.

DRY SKIN PRODUCTS - continued

	Product Manufacturer/Supplier	Dosage Form	Keratin Softener	Humectant	Other Ingredients
FR	**DML Forte** Person & Covey	cream		propylene glycol dioctanoate · glycerin	petrolatum · water · glyceryl stearate · PEG-100 stearate · stearic acid · D-panthenol · DEA-cetyl phosphate · simethicone · PVP/eicosene copolymer · benzyl alcohol · cetyl alcohol · silica · disodium EDTA · magnesium aluminum silicate · sodium carbomer 1542
	Emollia Gordon Labs	lotion		propylene glycol	mineral oil · cetyl alcohol · white wax · sodium lauryl sulfate · oleic acid · methylparaben · propylparaben
	Eucerin Beiersdorf	lotion		sorbitol · propylene glycol	water · mineral oil · isopropyl myristate · PEG-40 sorbitan peroleate · lanolin acid glycerin ester · cetyl palmitate · magnesium sulfate · aluminum stearate · lanolin alcohol · BHT · methylchloroisothiazolinone-methylisothiazolinone
	Eucerin Beiersdorf	cleansing bar			disodium lauryl sulfosuccinate · sodium cocoyl isethionate · cetearyl alcohol · corn starch · glyceryl stearate · water · titanium dioxide · octyldodecanol · cyclopentadecanolide · lanolin alcohol · bisabolol
	Eucerin Creme Beiersdorf	cream			water · petrolatum · mineral oil · mineral wax · lanolin alcohol · methylchloroisothiazolinone-methylisothiazolinone
	Eucerin Plus Beiersdorf	lotion	urea	glycerin	water · mineral oil · PEG-7 hydrogenated castor oil · isohexadecane · sodium lactate · isopropyl palmitate · panthenol · magnesium sulfate · lanolin alcohol · bisabolol · methylchloroisothiazolinone-methylisothiazolinone
	Eucerin Plus Creme Beiersdorf	cream	urea		water · mineral oil · magnesium stearate · polyglyceryl-3 diisostearate · mineral wax · isopropyl palmitate · benzyl alcohol · panthenol · bisabolol · lanolin alcohol · magnesium sulfate · sodium lactate
**	**Facial Hydrating Fluid, Oil Free** C & M Pharmacal	lotion	allantoin	glycerin	purified water · soluble collagen · hydrolyzed elastin · hydroxyethyl ethylcellulose · sorbic acid · octoxynol-9
**	**Facial Hydrating Gel, Oil Free** C & M Pharmacal	gel	allantoin	glycerin	purified water · soluble collagen · hydrolyzed elastin · carbomer 940 · triethanolamine · disodium EDTA · sorbic acid · octoxynol-9 · hyaluronic acid
	Gormel Gordon Labs	cream	urea, 20%		
	Hydrisea Pedinol Pharmacal	lotion		dead sea salts, 8% · propylene glycol · propylene glycol stearate	polysorbate 40 · silicone oil · coloring agent
	Hydrisinol Pedinol Pharmacal	cream · lotion			sulfonated hydrogenated castor oil · hydrogenated vegetable oil

See Chapter 26, "Dermatologic Products," for more information about these products.

DRY SKIN PRODUCTS - continued

	Product Manufacturer/Supplier	Dosage Form	Keratin Softener	Humectant	Other Ingredients
	Hydrocream Base Paddock Labs	cream			water · petrolatum · cholesterol · mineral oil · mineral wax · woolwax alcohol · methylparaben · propylparaben · imidazolidinyl urea
**	**Jergens Advanced Therapy Dry Skin Care** Andrew Jergens	lotion		glycerin	water · cetearyl alcohol · isopropyl myristate · ceteareth-20 · tocopherol · cholesteryl isostearate · dimethicone · C12-15 alkyl benzoate · cyclomethicone · lanolin · stearic acid · cetyl alcohol · sodium carbomer · methylparaben · propylparaben · DMDM hydantoin · fragrance
** FR	**Jergens Advanced Therapy Dual Healing** Andrew Jergens	cream		glycerin	water · cyclomethicone · mineral oil · isopropyl palmitate · dimethicone · cetyl dimethicone copolyol · cetyl-PG hydroxyethyl palmitamide · sodium lactate · cholesteryl isostearate · petrolatum · cetyl dimethicone · isostearyl glyceryl ether · trihydroxystearin · dextrin palmitate · sodium chloride · diazolidinyl urea · pentasodium pentetate · tetrasodium etidronate
** FR	**Jergens Advanced Therapy Ultra Healing, Reg. or Frag. Free** Andrew Jergens	lotion		glycerin	water · cetearyl alcohol (Reg.) · stearyl alcohol (Frag. Free) · petrolatum · mineral oil · ceteareth-20 · cetyl-PG hydroxyethyl palmitamide · cholesteryl isostearate · allantoin · dimethicone · cyclomethicone · glyceryl dilaurate · stearic acid (Frag. Free) · aluminum starch octenylsuccinate · cetyl alcohol (Frag. Free) · sodium carbomer · methylparaben · propylparaben · DMDM hydantoin · fragrance (Reg.)
** DY FR PE	**Johnson's Ultra Sensitive Baby Cream** Johnson & Johnson Consumer	cream		glycerin	water · mineral oil · polyethylene · sorbitan isostearate · sodium lactate · methylparaben · propylparaben · ethylparaben · butylparaben · magnesium sulfate
** DY FR PE	**Johnson's Ultra Sensitive Baby Lotion** Johnson & Johnson Consumer	lotion		glycerin	water · mineral oil · PEG-55 lanolin · carbomer · ceteareth-6 · sodium citrate · methylparaben · stearyl alcohol · butylparaben · ethylparaben · propylparaben
	Keri Bristol-Myers Products	lotion		propylene glycol	mineral oil · lanolin oil · water · glyceryl monostearate SE · PEG-40 stearate · emulsifier · laureth-4 · methylparaben · propylparaben · carbomer 934 · triethanolamine · fragrance · sodium dioctyl sulfosuccinate · quaternium-15
FR	**Keri** Bristol-Myers Products	cream		glycerin · propylene glycol	water · petrolatum · dimethicone · steareth-2 · cetyl alcohol · benzyl alcohol · magnesium aluminum silicate · laureth-23 · carbomer · tocopheryl linoleate · methylparaben · propylparaben · sodium hydroxide · quaternium-15

See Chapter 26, "Dermatologic Products," for more information about these products.

DRY SKIN PRODUCTS - continued

	Product Manufacturer/Supplier	Dosage Form	Keratin Softener	Humectant	Other Ingredients
FR	**Keri Silky Smooth, Fragrance Free or Regular** Bristol-Myers Products	lotion		glycerin	petrolatum · dimethicone · steareth-2 · cetyl alcohol · benzyl alcohol · laureth-23 · carbomer 934 · magnesium aluminum silicate · fragrance (Regular) · quaternium 15 · sodium hydroxide · tocopheryl linoleate · BHT · disodium EDTA
FR	**Lac-Hydrin Five** Westwood-Squibb Ph'cals	lotion	lactic acid	propylene glycol dioctanoate · glycerin	petrolatum · squalene · steareth-2 · steareth-21 · cetyl alcohol · dimethicone · cetyl palmitate · magnesium aluminum silicate · kathon CG · ammonium hydroxide · water · diazolidinyl urea
	Lacti-Care Stiefel Labs	lotion	lactic acid	sodium PCA	water · mineral oil · isopropyl palmitate · stearyl alcohol · ceteareth-20 · sodium hydroxide · glyceryl stearate · PEG-100 stearate · myristyl lactate · cetyl alcohol · carbomer · DMDM hydantoin · fragrance · methylparaben · propylparaben
**	**Lanaphilic** Medco Lab	ointment		propylene glycol · sorbitol	stearyl alcohol · petrolatum · isopropyl palmitate · lanolin oil · methylparaben · propylparaben · sodium lauryl sulfate · water
	Lanaphilic with Urea Medco Lab	ointment	urea, 10%; 20% · lactic acid	propylene glycol · sorbitol	stearyl alcohol · petrolatum · isopropyl palmitate · lanolin oil · methylparaben · propylparaben · water · sodium lauryl sulfate
**	**Lantiseptic Therapeutic** Summit	cream			lanolin, 35% · beeswax (yellow wax) · emulsifiers · fragrance · HEEDTA · mineral oil · oxyquinoline · sodium borate · water
	Lazer Creme Pedinol Pharmacal	cream		propylene glycol	vitamin E, 3500 IU/oz · vitamin A, 100000 IU/oz · stearic acid · isopropyl palmitate · triethanolamine · PEG-2 stearate · PEG-2 stearate SE · borax · carbomer 934 · DMDM hydantoin · methylparaben · propylparaben · diazolidinyl urea
	Lip Treatment Pfeiffer Ph'cals	jelly			white petrolatum
FR PE	**Little Noses Saline Moisturizing** Vetco	gel	allantoin · citric acid	glycerin · propylene glycol · sodium chloride	water · PEG-100 · hydroxyethyl cellulose · aloe vera gel · methyl gluceth-10 · dimethicone copolyol · diazolidinyl urea · methylparaben · vitamin E acetate · olive oil · geranium oil · propylparaben
	Lowila Cake Westwood-Squibb Ph'cals	cleansing bar	urea · lactic acid	sorbitol	dextrin · sodium lauryl sulfoacetate · boric acid · mineral oil · PEG-14M · dioctyl sodium sulfosuccinate · cellulose gum · fragrance
**	**Lubricating Hand and Body** C & M Pharmacal	cream		propylene glycol · glycerin	purified water · cetostearyl alcohol · petrolatum · mineral oil · sodium lauryl sulfate · sorbic acid

See Chapter 26, "Dermatologic Products," for more information about these products.

DRY SKIN PRODUCTS - continued

	Product Manufacturer/Supplier	Dosage Form	Keratin Softener	Humectant	Other Ingredients
	Lubriderm Moisture Recovery Alpha Hydroxy Formula Warner Wellcome Consumer	cream · lotion	lactic acid		isostearic acid · sodium lactate · stearic acid · mineral oil (cream) · magnesium aluminum silicate · cetyl alcohol · potassium sorbate · fragrance · steareth-21 · PPG-12/SMDI copolymer · steareth-2 · xanthan gum · imidurea · water
	Lubriderm Moisture Recovery GelCreme Warner Wellcome Consumer	cream		glycerin · propylene glycol	cetyl alcohol · mineral oil · cyclomethicone fluid · emulsifying wax · BHT · carbomer 940 · tocopheryl acetate · sodium benzoate · dicaprylate/dicaprate · PEG-40 stearate · isopropyl isostearate · diazolidinyl urea · titanium dioxide · tri (PPG-3 myristyl ether) citrate · disodium edetate · retinyl palmitate · sodium pyruvate · iodopropynyl butylcarbamate · sodium hydroxide · xanthan gum · lecithin · water
	Lubriderm Seriously Sensitive Warner Wellcome Consumer	lotion		glycerin · propylene glycol	petrolatum · water · carbomer 940 · titanium dioxide · methylparaben · propylparaben · cetyl alcohol · emulsifying wax · dimethicone · glycerin stearate · butylene glycol · mineral oil · dicaprylate/dicaprate · xanthan gum · PEG-40 stearate · C11-C13 isoparaffin · ethylparaben · titanium dioxide · tri (PPG-3 myristyl ether) citrate · DMDM hydantoin · disodium EDTA · sodium hydroxide butylparaben
	Lubriderm Skin Conditioning Warner Wellcome Consumer	bath oil			mineral oil · PPG-15 stearyl ether · oleth-2 · nonoxynol-5 · fragrance · D&C green#6
	Lubriderm, Scented or Unscented Warner Wellcome Consumer	lotion		sorbitol	mineral oil · petrolatum · lanolin · lanolin alcohol · stearic acid · triethanolamine · cetyl alcohol · fragrance (Scented) · methylparaben · propylparaben · sodium chloride · water · tri (PPG-3 myristyl ether) citrate · methyldibromo glutaronitrile/phenoxyethanol · ethylparaben · butylparaben
	Mammol Abbott Labs	ointment			bismuth subnitrate, 40% · castor oil, 30% · anhydrous lanolin, 22% · ceresin wax, 7% · peruvian balsam, 1%
FR	**Moisturel** Westwood-Squibb Ph'cals	cream		glycerin	petrolatum · PG dioctanoate · cetyl alcohol · steareth-2 · dimethicone · PVP/hexadecene copolymer · laureth-23 · magnesium aluminum silicate · carbomer 934 · sodium hydroxide · kathon CG · diazolidinyl urea · water
FR	**Moisturel** Westwood-Squibb Ph'cals	lotion		glycerin	petrolatum · dimethicone · steareth-2 · cetyl alcohol · benzyl alcohol · laureth-23 · carbomer 934 · magnesium aluminum silicate · quaternium-15 · sodium hydroxide · water

See Chapter 26, "Dermatologic Products," for more information about these products.

DRY SKIN PRODUCTS - continued

	Product Manufacturer/Supplier	Dosage Form	Keratin Softener	Humectant	Other Ingredients
FR	**Moisturel Sensitive Skin** Westwood-Squibb Ph'cals	lotion			sodium laureth sulfate · laureth 6 carboxylic acid · disodium laureth sulfosuccinate · methyl gluceth 20 · cocamidopropyl betaine · kathon CG · diazolidinyl urea · water
**	**Moisturizing Lotion** C & M Pharmacal	lotion		propylene glycol · glycerin	purified water · cetearyl · petrolatum · PEG-40 stearate
	Mother's Friend S.S.S. Company	liquid			cottonseed oil · lecithin · camphor · menthol · BHT · oleic acid · fragrance
	Mother's Friend S.S.S. Company	cream	allantoin, 0.19%	propylene glycol	lanolin oil · isopropyl myristate · silicone fluid · glyceryl monostearate · stearic acid · cetyl alcohol · TEA-lauryl sulfate · trisaminomethane · fragrance
	Nephro-Derm R & D Labs	cream			water · eucerin · petrolatum · mineral oil · paraffin wax · Tween · camphor · menthol · methylparaben · propylparaben · vitamin B12 · glyceryl stearate
FR	**Neutrogena** Neutrogena Dermatologics	lotion			purified water · isopropyl myristate · butylene glycol · glyceryl stearate · PEG-100 stearate · cetyl alcohol · carbomer · triethanolamine · diazolidinyl urea · methylparaben · ethylparaben · propylparaben · tetrasodium EDTA
	Neutrogena Neutrogena Dermatologics	body oil			isopropyl myristate · sesame oil · PEG-40 sorbitan peroleate · methylparaben · propylparaben
	Neutrogena Norwegian Formula Neutrogena Dermatologics	cream		glycerin, 41%	
FR	**Neutrogena Norwegian Formula Emulsion** Neutrogena Dermatologics	emulsion		glycerin, 25%	
	Nivea Creme Ultra Moisturizing Beiersdorf	cream		glycerin	water · mineral oil · petrolatum · isohexadecane · microcrystalline wax · lanolin alcohol · paraffin · panthenol · magnesium sulfate · decyl oleate · octyldodecanol · aluminum stearate · fragrance · methylchloroisothiazolinone-methylisothiazolinone · citric acid · magnesium stearate
	Nivea Moisturizing Extra Enriched Beiersdorf	lotion		glycerin	purified water · mineral oil · isohexadecane · PEG-40 · sorbitan peroleate · polyglyceryl-3 diisostearate · petrolatum · isopropyl palmitate · cetyl palmitate · glyceryl lanolate · magnesium sulfate · fragrance · aluminum stearate · lanolin alcohol · phenoxyethanol · methyldibromo glutaronitrile

See Chapter 26, "Dermatologic Products," for more information about these products.

DRY SKIN PRODUCTS - continued

	Product Manufacturer/Supplier	Dosage Form	Keratin Softener	Humectant	Other Ingredients
	Nivea Shower & Bath Beiersdorf	cleansing bar		glycerin	sodium tallowate/sodium cocoate · fragrance · petrolatum · titanium dioxide · sodium chloride · octyldodecanol · macadamia nut oil · aloe extract · sodium thiosulfate · purified water · lanolin alcohol · pentasodium pentetate · tetrasodium etidronate · BHT · beeswax
	Nivea Skin Original Therapeutic Beiersdorf	body oil			mineral oil · water · lanolin · petrolatum · glyceryl lanolate · lanolin alcohol · fragrance · sodium borate · methylchloroisothiazolinone-methylisothiazolinone
**	**Noncomedogenic Facial Moisturizing Cream** C & M Pharmacal	cream		glycerin · sorbitol	purified water · polawax A-31 · isopropyl palmitate · castor oil · benzyl alcohol · polysorbate 20
	Noxzema Original Procter & Gamble	cream		propylene glycol	water · stearic acid · linseed oil · soybean oil · fragrance · ammonium hydroxide · gelatin · camphor · menthol · phenol · clove oil · eucalyptus oil · calcium hydroxide
	Noxzema Original Procter & Gamble	lotion		propylene glycol	water · stearic acid · soybean oil · fragrance · linseed oil · gelatin · calcium hydroxide · cetyl alcohol · camphor · menthol · phenol · clove oil · eucalyptus oil · carbomer · triethanolamine
	Noxzema Plus Cleansing Procter & Gamble	lotion		glycerin	water · stearic acid · caprylic/capric triglyceride · glycol distearate · cetyl alcohol · PEG-8 · fragrance · cetearyl alcohol · ceteareth-20 · cocamide DEA · castor oil · triethanolamine · methylparaben · imidazolidinyl urea · carbomer · propylparaben · PEG-10 soya sterol · disodium EDTA
	Noxzema Plus Cleansing Procter & Gamble	cream		glycerin · propylene glycol	water · stearic acid · linseed oil · soybean oil · gelatin · calcium hydroxide · ammonium hydroxide · fragrance · methylparaben · propylparaben · DMDM hydantoin · disodium EDTA · phenoxyethanol
	Noxzema Sensitive Cleansing Procter & Gamble	cream · lotion		glycerin	water · stearic acid · cetyl alcohol · caprylic/capric triglyceride · glycol distearate · PEG-8 · cetearyl alcohol · triethanolamine · carbomer · ceteareth-20 · DMDM hydantoin · iodopropynyl butylcarbamate · PEG-10 soya sterol · disodium EDTA
	Nutraderm Galderma Labs	bath oil			bath oil · mineral oil · lanolin oil · PEG-4 dilaurate · benzophenone-3 · butylparaben
	Nutraderm Galderma Labs	cream			mineral oil · sorbitan stearate · stearyl alcohol · sodium lauryl sulfate · cetyl alcohol · methylparaben · propylparaben · fragrance
	Nutraderm Galderma Labs	lotion			mineral oil · sorbitan stearate · stearyl and cetyl alcohol · carbomer 940

See Chapter 26, "Dermatologic Products," for more information about these products.

DRY SKIN PRODUCTS - continued

Product Manufacturer/Supplier	Dosage Form	Keratin Softener	Humectant	Other Ingredients
Nutraderm 30 Galderma Labs	lotion	lactic acid · malic acid	sodium PCA · glycerin	petrolatum · cetearyl alcohol · ceteareth-20 · dimethicone · C10-30 cholesterol/lanosterol esters · cyclomethicone · cetyl alcohol · sodium lactate · cetyl lactate · C12-C15 alcohols lactate · xanthan gum · sodium hydroxide · methylparaben · propylparaben · fragrance · diazolidinyl urea
Nutraplus Galderma Labs	lotion	urea, 10%		glyceryl stearate · acetylated lanolin alcohol · isopropyl palmitate · stearic acid · petrolatum · methylparaben · propylparaben · carbomer 940
Nutraplus Galderma Labs	cream	urea, 10%	propylene glycol	glyceryl stearate · mineral oil · methylparaben · propylparaben
Oil of Olay Bath Bar, Pink or White Procter & Gamble	cleansing bar			sodium cocoyl isethionate · sodium cetearyl sulfate · paraffin · stearic acid · water · sodium isethionate · coconut acid · sodium stearate · sodium cocoate · fragrance · sodium chloride · titanium dioxide · lauric acid · sodium laurate · trisodium EDTA · trisodium etidronate · colorant (Pink)
Oil of Olay Foaming Face Wash, Regular or Sensitive Procter & Gamble	liquid	citric acid	glycerin	water · sodium myristol sarcosinate · PEG-120 methyl glucose dioleate · sodium lauroamphoacetate · disodium lauroamphodiacetate · glycol distearate · PEG-150 pentaerythritol tetra stearate · sodium trideceth sulfate · polyquaternium-10 · sodium laureth sulfate · phenoxyethanol · cocamide MEA · DMDM hydantoin · disodium EDTA · laureth-9 · fragrance (Regular)
Oil of Olay Sensitive Skin Bath Bar Procter & Gamble	cleansing bar			sodium cocoyl isethionate · sodium cetearyl sulfate · paraffin · stearic acid · water · sodium isethionate · coconut acid · sodium stearate · sodium cocoate · sodium chloride · titanium dioxide · lauric acid · sodium laurate · trisodium EDTA · trisodium etidronate · masking fragrance
Oilatum Soap Stiefel Labs	cleansing bar	citric acid	propylene glycol	sodium tallowate · sodium cocoate · water · peanut oil · octyl hydroxystearate · lecithin · fragrance · sodium chloride · PEG-14M · titanium dioxide · o-tolyl biguanide · trisodium HEDTA · sodium borohydride · glyceryl oleate · corn oil · t-butyl hydroquinone · FD&C red#4 · D&C orange#4
Pacquin Medicated Hand and Body Pfizer Consumer	cream		glycerin, 12%	dimethicone, 1% · water · stearic acid · potassium stearate · sodium stearate · cetyl alcohol · fragrance · diisopropyl sebacate · carbomer 940 · methylparaben · propylparaben

See Chapter 26, "Dermatologic Products," for more information about these products.

DRY SKIN PRODUCTS - continued

	Product Manufacturer/Supplier	Dosage Form	Keratin Softener	Humectant	Other Ingredients
	Pacquin Plus Dry Skin Hand and Body Pfizer Consumer	cream		glycerin, 12%	lanolin anhydrous 0.5% · water · stearic acid · potassium stearate · sodium stearate · myristyl lactate · cetyl alcohol · cetyl esters · fragrance · diisopropyl sebacate · stearamide DZA · carbomer 940 · methylparaben · propylparaben
	Pacquin Plus with Aloe Pfizer Consumer	cream			aloe vera gel, 20% · dimethicone, 1% · lanolin anhydrous 0.5% · water · isopropyl palmitate · mineral oil · petrolatum, white synthetic beeswax · cetyl alcohol · triethanolamine · glyceryl stearate · carbomer 934 · stearic acid · fragrance · methylparaben · laureth-23 · quaternium-15 · D&C red#33 · imidazolidinyl urea
	Panthoderm Jones Medical	cream			dexpanthenol, 2% · water-miscible base
	Pedi-Vit-A Pedinol Pharmacal	cream			vitamin A, 100000 IU/30mg
FR	**Pen-Kera** B. F. Ascher	cream		glycerin	octyl palmitate · mineral oil · polysorbate 60 · sorbitan stearate · carbomer 940 · triethanolamine · wheat germ glycerides · polyamino sugar condensate · dehydroacetic acid · DMDMH iodo-propynyl-butylcarbamate · diazolidinyl urea · water
	Perry Shampoo Perry Products	shampoo			water · sodium laureth sulfate · cocamidopropyl betaine · hydrolyzed animal protein · sodium chloride · methylparaben · propylparaben · quaternium-15 · skin esters
**	**Plexo Hand** Alvin Last	cream		propylene glycol · glycerin	water · zinc stearate · stearic acid · lanolin benzyl alcohol · fragrance · potassium hydroxide · mineral oil · cetyl alcohol · bertylparaben
FR	**Plexolan Moisturizing** Alvin Last	cream			water · petrolatum · mineral oil · ceresin · lanolin · alcohol · methylparaben · propylparaben
	Polysorb Hydrate E. Fougera	cream			sorbitan sesquioleate · wax & petrolatum base · water
	Pro-Cute Ferndale Labs	cream		glycerin	water · stearic acid · cetyl alcohol · ceraphyl 230 · forlan-LM · deltyl prime · trolamine · silicone · povidone · dowicil 200 · perfume
	Q.O.D. Bath Additive Perry Products	liquid		propylene glycol	sodium laureth sulfate · water · PEG-7 glyceryl cocoate · lauramide DEA · dioctyl adipate · octyl stearate · octyl palmitate · methylparaben · imidazolidinyl urea · propylparaben · cetyl alcohol · petrolatum · lanolin · sodium PCA · polysorbate 85
	Sardo Schering-Plough HealthCare	bath oil			mineral oil · isopropyl palmitate
	Sardoettes Schering-Plough HealthCare	wipe			mineral oil · isopropyl palmitate

See Chapter 26, "Dermatologic Products," for more information about these products.

DRY SKIN PRODUCTS - continued

	Product Manufacturer/Supplier	Dosage Form	Keratin Softener	Humectant	Other Ingredients
	Sarna Stiefel Labs	lotion			camphor, 0.5% · menthol, 0.5% · emollient base
FR	**Shepards** Dermik Labs	cream · lotion		glycerin · citric acid	water · sesame oil · SD alcohol 40-B · stearic acid · propylene glycol · ethoxydiglycol · triethanolamine · glyceryl stearate · cetyl alcohol · simethicone · methylparaben · propylparaben · vegetable oil · monoglyceride citrate · BHT
FR	**Shepards Skin** Dermik Labs	cream	urea	glycerin · propylene glycol	water · glyceryl stearate · ethoxydiglycol · stearic acid · isopropyl myristate · cetyl alcohol · lecithin · methylparaben · propylparaben
FR	**Silk Solution** Thompson Medical	lotion		glycerin	dimethicone, 2.0% · cetyl alcohol · cyclomethicone · dimethiconol · dioctyl adipate · methyldibromoglutaronitrite · phenoxyethanol · stearic acid · triethanolamine · water
	Skin Cream or Lotion Perry Products	cream · lotion		propylene glycol	water · cetyl alcohol · petrolatum · lanolin · polysorbate 85 · glyceryl stearate · PEG-100 stearate · sodium lauryl sulfate · methylparaben · imidazolidinyl urea · sodium PCA
	Sofenol 5 C & M Pharmacal	lotion	allantoin	glycerin	purified water · petrolatum · cetostearyl alcohol · soluble collagen · PEG-40 stearate · dimethicone · kaolin · sunflower seed oil · sorbic acid · carbomer 940 · disodium EDTA · sodium hydroxide
** FR	**Soft Sense Alpha Hydroxy Moisturizing** Bausch & Lomb	lotion	lactic acid	glycerin	petrolatum · distearyl dimonium chloride · isopropyl palmitate · l-hexadecanol · ammonium hydroxide · tocopheryl acetate · dimethicone · titanium dioxide · methylparaben · propylparaben
FR	**Soft Sense Moisturizing, Fragrance Free or Original** Bausch & Lomb	lotion		glycerin	petrolatum · purified water · distearyldimonium chloride · isopropyl palmitate · vitamin E · aloe · keratin protein · dimethicone · titanium dioxide · methylparaben · propylparaben
	Softlips, Cool Cherry Mentholatum	stick			dimethicone, 2% · cetyl octanoate · fragrance · lanolin · menthol · ozokerite · squalene · vitamin E acetate
** PE	**Stevens Baby** Stevens Skin	cream		glycerin	deionized water · glyceryl stearate · stearic acid · jojoba oil · cetyl alcohol · cetyl alcohol · apricot kernel oil · castor oil · sweet almond oil · cetyl palmitate · cetearyl octanoate · squalene · methyl gluceth-20 · magnesium aluminum silicate · panthenol · diazolidinyl urea · propylparaben · avocado oil · allantoin · methylparaben · butylparaben · tetrasodium EDTA · tocopherol · fragrance · aloe vera gel

See Chapter 26, "Dermatologic Products," for more information about these products.

DRY SKIN PRODUCTS - continued

	Product Manufacturer/Supplier	Dosage Form	Keratin Softener	Humectant	Other Ingredients
**	**Stevens Skin Softener** Stevens Skin	cream		glycerin	deionized water · glyceryl stearate · stearic acid · jojoba oil · cetyl alcohol · apricot kernel oil · castor oil · sweet almond oil · cetyl palmitate · cetearyl octanoate · squalene · methyl gluceth-20 · magnesium aluminum silicate · panthenol · diazolidinyl urea · propylparaben · avocado oil · allantoin · methylparaben · butylparaben · tetrasodium EDTA · tocopherol · aloe vera gel
**	**Sustained Effect Hydrating Lotion** C & M Pharmacal	lotion	lactic acid · allantoin	propylene glycol · glycerin	purified water · cetearyl alcohol · petrolatum · PEG-40 storate · potassium hydroxide
	Therapeutic Bath Lotion Goldline Labs	lotion		propylene glycol	mineral oil · lanolin oil · glyceryl stearate · PEG-100 stearate · PEG-40 stearate · laureth-4 · PEG-4 dilaurate · methylparaben · carbomer 934 · propylparaben · quaternium-15 · trolamine · dioctyl sodium sulfosuccinate
	Therapeutic Bath Oil Goldline Labs	bath oil			mineral oil · lanolin oil · PEG-4-dilaurate · benzophenone-3
** FR	**Theraplex Hydrolotion** Medicis	lotion			water · dimethicone copolyol · cyclomethicone · special petrolatum fraction · SD alcohol 40 · benzyl alcohol · sodium chloride · sorbitan laurate
FR	**U-Lactin** Fischer Ph'cals	lotion	urea, 10% · lactic acid		
	Ultra Derm Baker Cummins Derm'cals	bath oil			mineral oil · lanolin oil · octoxynol-3
	Ultra Derm Moisturizer Baker Cummins Derm'cals	lotion		glycerin · propylene glycol	mineral oil · petrolatum · lanolin oil · glyceryl stearate · PEG-50-stearate · propylene glycol stearate SE · cetyl alcohol · sorbitan laurate · potassium sorbate · phosphoric acid · tetrasodium EDTA
	Ultra Mide 25 Moisturizer Baker Cummins Derm'cals	lotion	urea, 25%		
	Ureacin-10 Pedinol Pharmacal	lotion	urea, 10% · lactic acid		vegetable oil base
	Ureacin-20 Pedinol Pharmacal	cream	urea, 20% · lactic acid		vegetable oil base
	Vaseline Dermatology Formula Chesebrough-Pond's	lotion		glycerin	white petrolatum, 5% · mineral oil-4% · dimethicone-1% · water · stearic acid · glycol stearate · cetyl acetate · glyceryl stearate · triethanolamine · PEG-40 stearate · magnesium aluminum silicate · cetyl alcohol · acetylated lanolin alcohol · methylparaben · fragrance · propylparaben · stearamide AMP · carbomer 934 · disodium EDTA · DMDM hydantoin

See Chapter 26, "Dermatologic Products," for more information about these products.

DRY SKIN PRODUCTS - continued

Product Manufacturer/Supplier	Dosage Form	Keratin Softener	Humectant	Other Ingredients
Vaseline Intensive Care Extra Strength Chesebrough-Pond's	lotion	urea · lactic acid	glycerin · sodium PCA	petrolatum · dimethicone, 1.5% · water · stearic acid · C11-13 isoparaffin · glycol stearate · glyceryl stearate · triethanolamine · zinc oxide · cetyl alcohol · potassium cetyl phosphate · carbomer 934 · stearamide AMP · fragrance · sunflower seed oil · soya sterol · lecithin · sodium stearoyl lactylate · tolopherylacetate · retinyl palmitate · potassium lactate · collagen amino acids · magnesium aluminum silicate · corn oil · methylparaben · DMDM hydantoin · iodopropynyl butyl carbamate · disodium EDTA
Vaseline Medicated Anti-Bacterial Petrolatum Jelly Chesebrough-Pond's	ointment			petrolatum, 98.3% · chloroxylenol, 0.53% · lanolin · beta carotene · phenol
Vitacel Republic Drug	cream			retinyl palmitate · collagen · elastin · squalene
Wibi Galderma Labs	lotion		glycerin	SD alcohol 40 · PEG-4 · PEG-6-32 · stearate · glycol stearate · carbomer 940 · PEG-75 · methylparaben · triethanolamine · menthol · fragrance

** New listing

See Chapter 26, "Dermatologic Products," for more information about these products.

DANDRUFF, SEBORRHEA, AND PSORIASIS PRODUCTS [a]

	Product Manufacturer/Supplier	Dosage Form	Keratolytic	Cytostatic	Tar Product	Other Ingredients
	Balnetar Westwood-Squibb Ph'cals	bath oil			coal tar, 2.5%	mineral oil · lanolin oil · PEG-4-dilaurate · laureth 4 · fragrance · docusate sodium
	Brylcreem Anti-Dandruff J. B. Williams	cream		pyrithione zinc, 1%		mineral oil · propylene glycol · paraffin wax · excipients · water · trilaneth-4 phosphate · petrolatum · poloxamer 284 · triethanolamine · carbomer 940 · fragrance
**	**Creamy Dandruff Shampoo** C & M Pharmacal	shampoo	salicylic acid, 2% · sulfur, 2%			sodium lauryl sulfate · purified water · diglycol monostearate · lauramide DEA · cetearyl alcohol · petrolatum · fragrance
	Cutar Summers Labs	emulsion			coal tar, 1.5%	
**	**Dandruff Shampoo Maximum Strength** C & M Pharmacal	shampoo	sulfur, 5% · salicylic acid, 3%			sodium lauryl sulfate · purified water · diethylene glycol monostearate · lauramide DEA · cetostearyl alcohol · glycerin · fragrance · petrolatum · hydroxyethyl ethylcellulose · FD&C red#40
**	**Dandruff Wash, Medicated** C & M Pharmacal	cream	sulfur, 4% · salicylic acid, 2%			water · TEA-dodecylbenzene sulfonate · magnesium aluminum silicate · glycerin · stearic acid · cetearyl alcohol · polysorbate 20 · fragrance · FD&C red#40
	Denorex Dandruff for Dry Scalp, Shamp. & Cond. or Shampoo Whitehall-Robins Healthcare	shampoo · conditioner			coal tar extract, 2% (equivalent to 0.5% coal tar)	ammonium laureth sulfate · ammonium lauryl sulfate · avocado oil · citric acid · cocamide MEA · dimethicone copolyol · disodium EDTA · FD&C blue#1 · fragrance · glycol distearate · hydroxypropyl methylcellulose · imidurea · lauramide DEA · lauramidopropyl betaine · laureth-9 · menthol · methylparaben · panthenol (provitamin B5) · PEG-27 lanolin · quaternium-80 · ricinoleamidopropyl ethyldimonium ethosulfate (Shampoo & Conditioner) · sodium laureth sulfate · trolamine · vitamin E acetate · water
	Denorex Medicated Shampoo & Conditioner Whitehall-Robins Healthcare	shampoo · conditioner			coal tar solution, 9% (equivalent to 1.8% coal tar)	alcohol, 7.5% · chloroxylenol · citric acid · fragrance · hydroxypropyl methylcellulose · lauramide DEA · menthol · PEG-27 lanolin · polyquaternium-11 · TEA-lauryl sulfate · water
	Denorex Medicated Shampoo & Conditioner, Extra Strength Whitehall-Robins Healthcare	shampoo · conditioner			coal tar solution, 12.5% (equivalent to 2.5% coal tar)	alcohol, 10.4% · avocado oil · chloroxylenol · citric acid · dimethicone copolyol · FD&C red#40 · fragrance · glycol distearate · hydroxypropyl methylcellulose · lauramide DEA · menthol · panthenol (provitamin B5) · PEG-27 lanolin · quaternium-80 · ricinoleamidopropyl ethyldimonium ethosulfate · TEA-lauryl sulfate · vitamin E acetate · water

See Chapter 26, "Dermatologic Products," for more information about these products.

DANDRUFF, SEBORRHEA, AND PSORIASIS PRODUCTS [a] - continued

	Product Manufacturer/Supplier	Dosage Form	Keratolytic	Cytostatic	Tar Product	Other Ingredients
	Denorex Medicated, Extra Strength Whitehall-Robins Healthcare	shampoo			coal tar solution, 12.5% (equivalent to 2.5% coal tar)	alcohol, 10.4% · chloroxylenol · FD&C red#40 · fragrance · glycol distearate · hydroxypropyl methylcellulose · lauramide DEA · menthol · panthenol (provitamin B5) · TEA-lauryl sulfate · vitamin E acetate · water
	Denorex Medicated, Mountain Fresh Scent Whitehall-Robins Healthcare	shampoo			coal tar solution, 9% (equivalent to 1.8% coal tar)	alcohol, 7.5% · chloroxylenol · fragrance · hydroxypropyl methylcellulose · lauramide DEA · menthol · stearic acid · TEA-lauryl sulfate · water
**	**DHS Sal** Person & Covey	liquid	salicylic acid, 3%			sodium C14-16 · olefin sulfonate · TEA-lauryl sulfate · cocamidopropyl betaine · cocamide DEA · cocamide MEA · disodium EDTA · PEG-8 distearate · purified water
	DHS Tar Person & Covey	shampoo			coal tar, 0.5%	water · TEA-lauryl sulfate · sodium chloride · PEG-8 distearate · cocamide DEA · cocamide MEA · citric acid
	DHS Tar Gel Person & Covey	shampoo			coal tar, 0.5%	water · TEA lauryl sulfate · sodium chloride · PEG-8 distearate · cocamide DEA · cocamide MEA · hydroxypropyl methylcellulose · citric acid · fragrance
	DHS Zinc Person & Covey	shampoo		pyrithione zinc, 2%		water · TEA lauryl sulfate · PEG-8 distearate · sodium chloride · cocamide DEA · cocamide MEA · magnesium aluminum silicate · hydroxypropyl methylcellulose · fragrance · FD&C yellow#6
	Doak Oil Doak Dermatologics	bath oil			tar distillate, 2%	
	Doak Tar Doak Dermatologics	lotion			tar distillate, 5%	
	Doak Tar Doak Dermatologics	shampoo			tar distillate, 3%	
	Doctar Savage Labs	shampoo			tar, 2% (coal tar, 0.5%)	demineralized water · sodium laureth sulfate · TEA-lauryl sulfate · cocamidopropyl betaine · PEG-30 glyceryl stearate · polysorbate 80 · cocamidopropylamine oxide · cocamide DEA · fragrance
	Duplex-T C & M Pharmacal	shampoo			coal tar solution, 10%	purified water · sodium lauryl sulfate · lauramide DEA
	Estar Westwood-Squibb Ph'cals	gel			coal tar, 5%	alcohol, 15.6% · alanine · benzyl alcohol · carbomer 940 · glycereth-7 cocoanate · polysorbate 80 · simethicone · sorbitol · water
**	**Glover's Dandruff Control Medicine** J. K. Ph'cals	liquid	sulfur, 2.5%		pine tar oil	mineral oil · polysorbate 85 · quaternium-18-hectorite · fragrance

See Chapter 26, "Dermatologic Products," for more information about these products.

DANDRUFF, SEBORRHEA, AND PSORIASIS PRODUCTS [a] - continued

	Product Manufacturer/Supplier	Dosage Form	Keratolytic	Cytostatic	Tar Product	Other Ingredients
**	**Glover's Medicated** J. K. Ph'cals	shampoo			coal tar solution, 5% (equivalent to 0.75% coal tar)	water · TEA lauryl sulfate · potassium coco hydrolyzed animal protein · lauramide DEA · TEA coco hydrolyzed animal protein · fragrance · methylparaben · propylparaben
**	**Glover's Medicated Dandruff Soap** J. K. Ph'cals	cleansing bar	sulfur, 2.08%		pine tar	sodium tallowate · sodium cocoate · water · petroleum · trisodium HEDTA · BHT
**	**Glover's Medicated for Dandruff** J. K. Ph'cals	ointment	sulfur, 5% · salicylic acid, 3%			petrolatum · mineral oil · glyceryl tribehenate · arachidyl propionate · fragrance · polysorbate-20 · propylparaben · iron oxides · talc
	Grandpa's Pine Tar Shampooing (liquid) Grandpa Soap	shampoo			pine tar oil, 1%	water · sodium lauryl sulfate · sodium laureth sulfate · sodium chloride · cocamide DEA · di (hydrogenated) tallow phthalic acid amide · polymethoxy bicyclic oxazolidine · fragrance
	Grandpa's Pine Tar Soap Grandpa Soap	cleansing bar			pine tar oil, 2.7%	
	Head & Shoulders Dandruff 2-in-1 Procter & Gamble	shampoo		pyrithione zinc, 1%		ammonium laureth sulfate · ammonium lauryl sulfate · cocamide MEA · glycol distearate · ammonium xylenesulfonate · fragrance · FD&C blue#1 · dimethicone · tricetylmonium chloride · cetyl alcohol · stearyl alcohol · DMDM hydantoin · sodium chloride · monosodium phosphate · disodium phosphate
	Head & Shoulders Dandruff, Fine or Oily Hair Procter & Gamble	shampoo		pyrithione zinc, 1%		ammonium laureth sulfate · ammonium lauryl sulfate · cocamide MEA · glycol distearate · ammonium xylenesulfonate · fragrance · citric acid · FD&C blue#1 · DMDM hydantoin
	Head & Shoulders Dandruff, Normal to Dry Hair Procter & Gamble	shampoo		pyrithione zinc, 1%		ammonium laureth sulfate · ammonium lauryl sulfate · cocamide MEA · glycol distearate · ammonium xylenesulfonate · fragrance · FD&C blue#1 · dimethicone · tricetylmonium chloride · cetyl alcohol · stearyl alcohol · DMDM hydantoin · sodium chloride
	Head & Shoulders Dry Scalp, Regular or Conditioning Procter & Gamble	shampoo		pyrithione zinc, 1%		ammonium laureth sulfate · ammonium lauryl sulfate · cocamide MEA · glycol distearate · ammonium xylenesulfonate · fragrance · FD&C blue#1 · dimethicone · tricetylmonium chloride · cetyl alcohol · stearyl alcohol · DMDM hydantoin · sodium chloride

See Chapter 26, "Dermatologic Products," for more information about these products.

DANDRUFF, SEBORRHEA, AND PSORIASIS PRODUCTS [a] - continued

	Product Manufacturer/Supplier	Dosage Form	Keratolytic	Cytostatic	Tar Product	Other Ingredients
	Head & Shoulders Intensive Treatment, Regular or 2-in-1 Procter & Gamble	shampoo		selenium sulfide, 1%		ammonium laureth sulfate · ammonium lauryl sulfate · cocamide MEA · glycol distearate · ammonium xylensulfonate · fragrance · dimethicone · tricetylmonium chloride · cetyl alcohol · stearyl alcohol · DMDM hydantoin · sodium chloride · hydroxypropyl methylcellulose · FD&C red#4
	Ionil Galderma Labs	shampoo	salicylic acid, 2%			polyoxyethylene ethers · benzalkonium chloride · alcohol · tetrasodium edetate
	Ionil Plus Galderma Labs	shampoo	salicylic acid, 2%			sodium laureth sulfate · lauramide DEA · quaternium-22 · talloweth-60 · myristyl glycol · laureth-23 · TEA lauryl sulfate · glycol distearate · laureth-4 · TEA abietoyl hydrolyzed collagen · DMDM hydantoin · tetrasodium EDTA · sodium hydroxide · fragrance · FD&C blue#1
	Ionil T Galderma Labs	shampoo			coal tar solution, 5%	alcohol, 12% · isopropyl alcohol, 4% · benzalkonium chloride, 0.2% · polyoxyethylene ethers · EDTA
	Ionil T Plus Galderma Labs	shampoo			crude coal tar	sodium laureth sulfate · lauramide DEA · quaternium-22 · laureth-23 · talloweth-60 · myristyl glycol · TEA lauryl sulfate · glycol distearate · laureth-4 · TEA-abietoyl hydrolyzed collagen · DMDM hydantoin · EDTA · fragrance · FD&C blue#1 · FD&C yellow#7
	Meted GenDerm	shampoo	sulfur, 5% · salicylic acid, 3%			
	MG217 for Psoriasis Triton Consumer	ointment			coal tar solution, 10%	
	MG217 for Psoriasis Triton Consumer	lotion			coal tar solution, 5%	
**	**MG217 for Psoriasis Sal-Acid** Triton Consumer	ointment	salicylic acid, 3%			
	Neutrogena Healthy Scalp Anti-Dandruff Neutrogena Dermatologics	shampoo	salicylic acid, 1.8%			
	Neutrogena T/Derm Neutrogena Dermatologics	body oil			tar, 5% (coal tar, 1.2%)	
	Neutrogena T/Gel Extra Strength Therapeutic Neutrogena Dermatologics	shampoo			coal tar, 4%	
	Neutrogena T/Gel Shampoo or Conditioner Neutrogena Dermatologics	shampoo · conditioner			tar, 2% (coal tar, 0.5%)	

See Chapter 26, "Dermatologic Products," for more information about these products.

DANDRUFF, SEBORRHEA, AND PSORIASIS PRODUCTS [a] - continued

	Product Manufacturer/Supplier	Dosage Form	Keratolytic	Cytostatic	Tar Product	Other Ingredients
	Neutrogena T/Sal Maximum Strength Therapeutic Neutrogena Dermatologics	shampoo	salicylic acid, 3%			
	Oxipor VHC Whitehall-Robins Healthcare	lotion			coal tar solution, 25% (equivalent to coal tar, 5%)	alcohol, 79% · citric acid · PEG-8 · water
	P&S Baker Cummins Derm'cals	shampoo	salicylic acid, 2%			
	Pentrax GenDerm	shampoo			equivalent to coal tar, 4.3%	
	Pentrax Gold GenDerm	shampoo			equivalent to coal tar, 2%	
**	**Polytar** Stiefel Labs	cleansing bar			Polytar, 2.5% (coal tar, 0.5%)	
**	**Polytar** Stiefel Labs	shampoo			Polytar, 4.5% (coal tar, 0.5%)	
	Poslam Psoriasis Alvin Last	ointment	sulfur, 5% · salicylic acid, 2%			petrolatum · corn starch · lanolin · zinc oxide · ozokerite · phenol · menthol · fragrance · talc · iron oxides
	Psor-A-Set Hogil Ph'cal	shampoo	salicylic acid, 2%			sodium laureth sulfate · ammonium myreth sulfate · cocamide DEA · magnesium aluminum silicate · cocamidopropyl betaine · tocopheryl nicotinate · sodium PCA · TEA cocoylglutamate · acetamide MEA · hydroxypropyl methylcellulose · PEG-14M · disodium EDTA · sodium hydroxide · methylchloroisothiazolinone · methylisothizolinone · FD&C blue#1 · fragrance
	Psor-A-Set Hogil Ph'cal	lotion	salicylic acid, 2%			hydrogenated coconut oil · glycerin · beeswax · glyceryl stearate · laureth-23 · polysorbate 60 · polysorbate 80 · squalene · stearic acid · tocopheryl nicotinate · cetyl alcohol · PEG-40 stearate · fish liver oil · isopropyl myristate · pyridodine · niacin · lecithin · potassium hydroxide · methylparaben · propylparaben
	Psor-A-Set Hogil Ph'cal	cleansing bar	salicylic acid, 2%			tocopheryl acetate · titanium dioxide · alpha bisabolol · octylhydroxy stearate
**	**Psoriasin** Alva-Amco Pharmacal	gel			coal tar, 1.25%	isopropyl alcohol, 50% · polyethylene glycol · vitamin E · aloe vera
**	**Psoriasis Tar** C & M Pharmacal	lotion			coal tar solution, 5%	purified water · propylene glycol · ceto stearyl alcohol · petrolatum · glycerin · PEG-40 stearate
	Psorigel Galderma Labs	gel			coal tar solution, 8.8%	alcohol · laureth-4 · fragrance · propylene glycol · hydroxyethylcellulose

See Chapter 26, "Dermatologic Products," for more information about these products.

DANDRUFF, SEBORRHEA, AND PSORIASIS PRODUCTS [a] - continued

	Product Manufacturer/Supplier	Dosage Form	Keratolytic	Cytostatic	Tar Product	Other Ingredients
	Salicylic Acid & Sulfur Soap Stiefel Labs	cleansing bar	sulfur, 5% (precipitated) · salicylic acid, 3%			
**	**Scalpicin Maximum Strength** Combe	liquid	salicylic acid, 3%			menthol · propylene glycol · SD alcohol 40 · water
**	**Scalpicin Maximum Strength** Combe	foam	salicylic acid, 3%			emulsifying wax · isobutane · menthol · propylene glycol · SD alcohol 40 · water
	Sebucare Westwood-Squibb Ph'cals	lotion	salicylic acid, 1.8%			laureth-4, 4.5% · alcohol, 61% · PPG-40 · butyl ether · dihydroabietyl alcohol · fragrance
	Sebulex Conditioning with Protein Westwood-Squibb Ph'cals	shampoo	salicylic acid, 2% · sulfur, 2%			sodium octoxynol-3 sulfonate · sodium lauryl sulfate · lauramide DEA · acetamide MEA · amphoteric-2 · hydrolyzed animal protein · magnesium aluminum silicate · propylene glycol · methylcellulose · PEG-14M · fragrance · disodium EDTA · FD&C blue#1 · D&C yellow#10 · dioctyl sodium sulfosuccinate · water
	Sebulex Medicated Westwood-Squibb Ph'cals	shampoo	sulfur, 2% · salicylic acid, 2%			sodium octoxynol-2 ethane sulfonate · sodium dodecyl benzene sulfonate · PEG-6 lauramide · sodium dioctyl sulfosuccinate · PEG-14M · fragrance · EDTA · FD&C blue#1 · D&C yellow#10 · water
	Sebulon Westwood-Squibb Ph'cals	shampoo		pyrithione zinc, 2%		acetamide MEA · benzyl alcohol · cocamide DEA · D&C green#5 · disodium oleamido PEG-2 sulfosuccinate · FD&C green#3 · fragrance · guar gum · magnesium aluminum silicate · TEA lauryl sulfate · quaternium-15 · water
	Sebutone Westwood-Squibb Ph'cals	shampoo	sulfur, 1.5% · salicylic acid, 1.5%		coal tar, 0.5%	sodium dodecyl benzene sulfonate · sodium octoxynol-2-ethane sulfonate · PEG-6 lauramide · sodium dioctyl sulfosuccinate · titanium dioxide · sodium chloride · PEG-90M · fragrance · lanolin oil · EDTA · FD&C blue#1 · D&C yellow#10 · water
	Sebutone Cream Westwood-Squibb Ph'cals	shampoo	sulfur, 1.5% · salicylic acid, 1.5%		coal tar, 0.5%	sodium octoxynol-2 ethane sulfonate · PEG-6 lauramide · sodium dodecyl benzene sulfonate · dextrin · stearyl alcohol · sodium dioctyl sulfosuccinate · titanium dioxide · magnesium aluminum silicate · PEG-14M · fragrance · lanolin oil · FD&C blue#1 · D&C yellow#10 · EDTA · water
	Selsun Blue Ross Products/Abbott Labs	shampoo		selenium sulfide, 1%		
	Selsun Gold for Women Ross Products/Abbott Labs	shampoo		selenium sulfide, 1%		

See Chapter 26, "Dermatologic Products," for more information about these products.

DANDRUFF, SEBORRHEA, AND PSORIASIS PRODUCTS [a] - continued

	Product Manufacturer/Supplier	Dosage Form	Keratolytic	Cytostatic	Tar Product	Other Ingredients
**	**SLT Lotion** C & M Pharmacal	lotion			liquid coal tar distillate, 2.5%	isopropyl alcohol · purified water · lactic acid · glycolic acid · fragrance · benzalkonium chloride
**	**Sulfoam Medicated Antidandruff** Doak Dermatologics	shampoo	sulfur, 2%			
	Sulray Alvin Last	cleansing bar	sulfur, 5%			fragrance free natural soap base · aloe vera · trisodium HEDTA
	Sulray Dandruff Alvin Last	shampoo	sulfur, 2%			aloe vera gel · sodium lauryl sulfate · lauramide DEA · glycol stearate · methylparaben · propylparaben · citric acid
**	**Tar Scalp Solution** C & M Pharmacal	lotion			liquid coal tar distillate, 2.5%	isopropyl alcohol · purified water · lactic acid · glycolic acid · fragrance · benzalkonium chloride
**	**Tar Shampoo Maximum Strength** C & M Pharmacal	shampoo			coal tar solution, 25%	purified water · sodium lauryl sulfate · glycerin · citric acid · lauramide DEA · fragrance · hydroxyethyl ethylcellulose
	Taraphilic Medco Lab	ointment			coal tar distillate, 1%	white petrolatum · stearyl alcohol · sorbitol · propylene glycol · polysorbate 20 · sodium lauryl sulfate · methylparaben · propylparaben · isopropyl palmitate
	Tarsum Shampoo/Gel Summers Labs	shampoo			coal tar solution, 10%	
	Tegrin Block Drug	shampoo			coal tar solution, 7% (coal tar, 1.1%)	water · sodium laureth sulfate · ammonium lauryl sulfate · alcohol · glycol stearate · hexylene · citric acid · lauramide DEA · fragrance · hydroxypropyl methylcellulose · guar hydroxypropyl tramnonium chloride · methylparaben · propylparaben · FD&C blue#1
	Tegrin Block Drug	cleansing bar			coal tar extract, 2%	chromium hydroxide · green · D&C yellow#10 lake · fragrance · glycerin · soap · titanium dioxide · water
	Tegrin Block Drug	cream			coal tar solution, 5%	acetylated lanolin alcohol · alcohol · carbomer 934P · ceteth-2 · cetyl alcohol · 5-chloro-4 isothiazolin-2 methyl-3-one · D&C red#28 · fragrance · glyceryl tribehenate · laureth 16 · laureth 23 · methyl gluceth 20 · mineral oil · octyldodecanol · petrolatum · potassium hydroxide · stearyl alcohol · titanium dioxide · water
	X-Seb Baker Cummins Derm'cals	shampoo		pyrithione zinc, 1%		
	X-Seb Plus Baker Cummins Derm'cals	shampoo		pyrithione zinc, 1%		
	X-Seb T Pearl Baker Cummins Derm'cals	shampoo			coal tar solution, 10% (crude coal tar, 2%)	
	X-Seb T Plus Baker Cummins Derm'cals	shampoo			coal tar solution, 10% (crude coal tar, 2%)	

See Chapter 26, "Dermatologic Products," for more information about these products.

DANDRUFF, SEBORRHEA, AND PSORIASIS PRODUCTS [a] - continued

Product Manufacturer/Supplier	**Dosage Form**	**Keratolytic**	**Cytostatic**	**Tar Product**	**Other Ingredients**
Zetar Rhône-Poulenc Rorer Ph'cals	shampoo			whole colloidal coal tar, 1%	parachlorometaxylenol, 0.5% · cocoamphocarboxyglycinate EDTA · fragrance · hexylene glycol · lauramide DEA · linoleamide DEA · magnesium aluminum silicate · PEG-75 lanolin · polysorbate 20 · polysorbate 80 · purified water · sodium polynaphthalene sulfonate
Zincon Lederle Consumer	shampoo		pyrithione zinc, 1%		water · sodium methyl cocoyl taurate · cocamide MEA · sodium chloride · magnesium aluminum silicate · sodium cocoyl isethionate · fragrance · glutaraldehyde · D&C green#5 · may contain: citric acid · sodium hydroxide
ZNP Bar Stiefel Labs	cleansing bar		pyrithione zinc, 2%		

** New listing

[a] Topical hydrocortisone may also be used to relieve the itching associated with seborrhea. See the Dermatitis Products table for products containing hydrocortisone.

See Chapter 26, "Dermatologic Products," for more information about these products.

TOPICAL ANTIFUNGAL PRODUCTS

	Product Manufacturer/Supplier	Dosage Form	Antifungal	Other Ingredients
	Aerodine Graham-Field	aerosol spray	povidone-iodine	propellant nitrogen
	Aftate Schering-Plough HealthCare	aerosol spray powder	tolnaftate, 1%	SD alcohol 40-2, 14% · BHT · propellants · talc
	Aftate Jock Itch Schering-Plough HealthCare	aerosol spray powder	tolnaftate, 1%	alcohol, 14%
	Aftate Spray Liquid Schering-Plough HealthCare	aerosol spray	tolnaftate, 1%	SD alcohol 40-2, 36% · propellants · BHT
	Betadine Purdue Frederick	douche · gel · ointment	povidone-iodine, 10%	
	Betadine First Aid Purdue Frederick	aerosol spray · cream	povidone-iodine, 5%	
	Blis-To-Sol Chattem	liquid	tolnaftate, 1%	acetone · D&C red#22 · PEG-8 · thymol
	Blis-To-Sol Chattem	powder	zinc undecylenate, 12%	bentonite · talc · thymol · zinc oxide
	Breezee Mist Pedinol Pharmacal	aerosol spray	miconazole nitrate, 2%	aluminum chlorhydrate · menthol · micro kaolin
	Care-Creme Cream Care-Tech Labs	cream	chloroxylenol, 0.8%	cetyl alcohol · cod liver oil · lanolin oil · lanolin alcohol · propylene glycol · vitamins A, D3, and E
	Cruex Antifungal Ciba Self-Medication	cream	total undecylenate, 20% (as undecylenic acid and zinc undecylenate)	fragrance · glycol stearate SE · lanolin · methylparaben · PEG-8 laurate · PEG-6 stearate · propylparaben · sorbitol solution · stearic acid · trolamine · water · white petrolatum
	Cruex Antifungal Ciba Self-Medication	aerosol spray powder	total undecylenate, 19% (as undecylenic acid and zinc undecylenate)	fragrance · isobutane · isopropyl myristate · menthol · talc · trolamine
	Cruex Antifungal Squeeze Powder Ciba Self-Medication	powder	calcium undecylenate, 10%	talc · colloidal silicon dioxide · fragrance · isopropyl myristate
**	**Desenex AF** Ciba Self-Medication	cream	clotrimazole, 1%	cetostearyl alcohol · cetyl ester wax · 2-oxtyldodecanol · polysorbate 60 · sorbitan monostearate · purified water · benzyl alcohol
**	**Desenex AF** Ciba Self-Medication	aerosol spray powder	miconazole nitrate, 2%	aloe vera gel · aluminum starch octenylsuccinate · isopropyl myristate · propylene carbonate · SD alcohol 40B · sorbitan monooleate · stearalkonium hectorite · isobutane/propane
**	**Desenex AF Spray Liquid** Ciba Self-Medication	aerosol spray	miconazole nitrate, 2%	polyethylene glycol 300 · polysorbate 20 · SD alcohol 40-B · dimethyl ether
	Desenex Antifungal Ciba Self-Medication	cream · ointment	total undecylenate, 25% (as undecylenic acid and zinc undecylenate)	fragrance · glycol stearate SE · lanolin · methylparaben · PEG-8 laurate · PEG-6 stearate · propylparaben · purified water · sorbitol solution · stearic acid · trolamine · white petrolatum
	Desenex Antifungal Ciba Self-Medication	aerosol spray powder	total undecylenate, 25% (as undecylenic acid and zinc undecylenate)	fragrance · isobutane · isopropyl myristate · menthol · talc · trolamine
	Desenex Antifungal Ciba Self-Medication	powder	total undecylenate, 25% (as undecylenic acid and zinc undecylenate)	fragrance · talc

See Chapter 26, "Dermatologic Products," for more information about these products.

TOPICAL ANTIFUNGAL PRODUCTS - continued

	Product Manufacturer/Supplier	Dosage Form	Antifungal	Other Ingredients
	Desenex Antifungal Spray Liquid Ciba Self-Medication	aerosol spray	tolnaftate, 1%	BHT · fragrance · isobutane · PEG-400 · SD alcohol 40-B
	FungiCure Alva-Amco Pharmacal	liquid	undecylenic acid, 10%	isopropyl alcohol, 70% · aloe vera gel · vitamin E
	FungiCure Alva-Amco Pharmacal	gel	tolnaftate, 1%	isopropyl alcohol · vitamin E · aloe vera gel
**	**Fungoid Tincture** Pedinol Pharmacal	solution	miconazole nitrate, 2%	benzyl alcohol · isopropyl alcohol · water · acetic acid (glacial) · laureth-4
	Genaspor Goldline Labs	ointment	tolnaftate, 1%	
	Isodine Antiseptic Blair Labs	solution	povidone-iodine, 10%	
	Lagol Alvin Last	oil	8-hydroxyquinoline, 0.0377%	mineral oil · cottonseed oil · fragrance
	Lotrimin AF Schering-Plough HealthCare	solution	clotrimazole, 1%	PEG
	Lotrimin AF Schering-Plough HealthCare	aerosol spray powder	miconazole nitrate, 2%	SD alcohol 40, 10% · propellants · talc
	Lotrimin AF Schering-Plough HealthCare	cream	clotrimazole, 1%	benzyl alcohol
	Lotrimin AF Schering-Plough HealthCare	powder	miconazole nitrate, 2%	talc
	Lotrimin AF Jock Itch Schering-Plough HealthCare	lotion	clotrimazole, 1%	benzyl alcohol, 1% · cetearyl alcohol · cetyl esters wax · octyldodecanol · polysorbate · sodium biphosphate dibasic · sorbitan monostearate · water
	Lotrimin AF Jock Itch Schering-Plough HealthCare	aerosol spray powder	miconazole nitrate, 2%	SD alcohol 40, 10%
	Lotrimin AF Spray Liquid Schering-Plough HealthCare	aerosol spray	miconazole nitrate, 2%	SD alcohol 40, 10% · propellants
	Micatin Johnson & Johnson Consumer	aerosol spray powder	miconazole nitrate, 2%	alcohol, 10%
	Micatin Johnson & Johnson Consumer	cream · powder	miconazole nitrate, 2%	
	Micatin Liquid Johnson & Johnson Consumer	aerosol spray	miconazole nitrate, 2%	alcohol, 17%
	Minidyne Pedinol Pharmacal	solution	povidone-iodine, 10%	
	NP·27 Cream Thompson Medical	cream	tolnaftate, 1%	aloe · polyethylene glycol · carbopol · titanium dioxide · butylated hydroxytoluene · monoamylamine · propylene glycol · cocoa butter · fragrance
	NP·27 Solution Thompson Medical	solution	tolnaftate, 1%	polyethylene glycol · butylated hydroxytoluene · propylene glycol

See Chapter 26, "Dermatologic Products," for more information about these products.

TOPICAL ANTIFUNGAL PRODUCTS - continued

	Product Manufacturer/Supplier	Dosage Form	Antifungal	Other Ingredients
	NP-27 Spray Powder Thompson Medical	aerosol spray powder	tolnaftate, 1%	alcohol, 14% · aloe · cocoa butter · isobutane · isopropyl myristate · fragrance
	Polydine Century Ph'cals	solution	povidone-iodine, 10%	
	Tetterine S.S.S. Company	cream · ointment	miconazole nitrate, 2%	
	Tinactin Schering-Plough HealthCare	powder	tolnaftate, 1%	corn starch · talc
	Tinactin Schering-Plough HealthCare	cream	tolnaftate, 1%	BHT · titanium dioxide
	Tinactin Schering-Plough HealthCare	solution	tolnaftate, 1%	PEG · BHT
	Tinactin Jock Itch Schering-Plough HealthCare	aerosol spray powder	tolnaftate, 1%	SD alcohol 40-2, 14% · BHT · propellants · talc
	Tinactin Spray Liquid Schering-Plough HealthCare	aerosol spray	tolnaftate, 1%	SD alcohol 40-2, 36% · propellants · BHT
	Tinactin, Deodorant or Regular Schering-Plough HealthCare	aerosol spray powder	tolnaftate, 1%	SD alcohol 40-2, 14% · talc · propellants · BHT
	Ting Antifungal Ciba Self-Medication	cream	tolnaftate, 1%	BHT · fragrance · PEG-400 · PEG-3350 · titanium dioxide
	Ting Antifungal Ciba Self-Medication	powder	tolnaftate, 1%	corn starch · fragrance · talc
	Ting Antifungal Ciba Self-Medication	aerosol spray powder	tolnaftate, 1%	SD alcohol 40-B · BHT · fragrance · isobutane · PPG-12-buteth-16 · talc
	Ting Antifungal Spray Liquid Ciba Self-Medication	aerosol spray	tolnaftate, 1%	SD alcohol 40-B · BHT · fragrance · isobutane · PEG-400
**	**Undelenic** Gordon Labs	ointment	undecylenic acid · zinc undecylenate	
**	**Undelenic** Gordon Labs	tincture	undecylenic acid	isopropyl alcohol, 79% · propylene glycol · triethanolamine · chloroxylenol
	Vaseline Medicated Anti-Bacterial Petroleum Jelly Chesebrough-Pond's	ointment	chloroxylenol, 0.53%	petrolatum, 98.3% · phenol · lanolin · beta carotene
	Zeasorb-AF Stiefel Labs	powder	miconazole nitrate, 2%	

** New listing
[a] For products used to treat fungal infections of the feet, see the Athlete's Foot Products table.

See Chapter 26, "Dermatologic Products," for more information about these products.

HYPERPIGMENTATION PRODUCTS

	Product Manufacturer/Supplier	Dosage Form	Hydro- quinone	Other Ingredients
**	**Ambi Skin Discoloration Fade Cream, Dry Skin** Kiwi	cream	2%	padimate O · water · stearic acid · glycerin · isopropyl myristate · cetyl alcohol · DEA-cetyl phosphate · glyceryl stearate · PEG-100 stearate · BHA · sodium metabisulfite · tocopheryl acetate · methyl-, ethyl-, propyl-, and butylparaben · disodium EDTA · fragrance
**	**Ambi Skin Discoloration Fade Cream, Normal Skin** Kiwi	cream	2%	padimate O · water · stearic acid · isopropyl myristate · stearyl alcohol · glycerin · emulsifying wax · glyceryl stearate · myrtrimonium bromide · PEG-8 stearate · BHA · sodium metabisulfite · tocopheryl acetate · methyl-, ethyl-, propyl-, and butylparaben · disodium EDTA · fragrance
**	**Ambi Skin Discoloration Fade Cream, Oily Skin** Kiwi	cream	2%	padimate O · water · stearic acid · PPG-2 myristyl ether propionate · PEG-8 · isopropyl myristate · glyceryl myristate · stearyl alcohol · glyceryl stearate · emulsifying wax · myrtrimonium bromide · PEG-8 stearate · BHA · sodium metabisulfite · tocopheryl acetate · methyl-, ethyl-, propyl-, and butylparaben · disodium EDTA · fragrance
**	**Eldopaque** ICN Ph'cals	cream	2%	
**	**Eldoquin** ICN Ph'cals	cream	2%	
**	**Esotérica Facial Formula** Medicis	cream	2%	padimate O, 3.3% · oxybenzone, 2.5% · water · isopropyl myristate · stearyl alcohol · glyceryl monostearate · propylene glycol · ceresin · poloxamer 188 · steareth-20 · ceteareth-3 · dimethicone · fragrance · sodium bisulfite · methylparaben · propylparaben · sodium lauryl sulfate · BHA · citric acid · trisodium EDTA
**	**Esotérica Regular Formula** Medicis	cream	2%	water · glyceryl stearate · isopropyl palmitate · ceresin · mineral oil · propylene glycol · stearyl alcohol · PEG-6-32 stearate · poloxamer 188 · propylene glycol monostearate · steareth-20 · laureth-23 · sodium bisulfite · sodium lauryl sulfate · citric acid · dimethicone · fragrance · methylparaben · propylparaben · trisodium EDTA · BHA
**	**Nudit Fade Cream** Medtech Labs	cream	2%	
**	**Palmer's Skin Success** E. T. Browne	cream	2%	octyl salicylate
**	**Porcelana Original Formula** Dep	cream	2%	water · mineral oil · glyceryl stearate · PEG-50 stearate · isopropyl palmitate · cetyl alcohol · propylene glycol · stearic acid · hydroxyethyl cellulose · citric acid · sodium metabisulfite · disodium EDTA · BHA · propylparaben · methylparaben · diazolidinyl urea · fragrance
**	**Porcelana Sunscreen Formula** Dep	cream	2%	octyl methoxycinnamate, 2.5% · water · mineral oil · cetyl alcohol · propylene glycol · ceteth-2 · stearic acid · magnesium aluminum silicate · PEG-40 stearate · citric acid · hydroxyethyl cellulose · fragrance · sodium sulfite · imidazolidinyl urea · sodium metabisulfite · disodium EDTA · methylparaben · BHA
**	**Solaquin** ICN Ph'cals	cream	2%	

** New listing

See Chapter 26, "Dermatologic Products," for more information about these products.

HAIR REGROWTH PRODUCTS

	Product Manufacturer/Supplier	Dosage Form	Minoxidil	Other Ingredients
**	**Minoxidil Topical Solution** Barre-National	solution	2%	alcohol, 60% · propylene glycol · purified water
**	**Minoxidil Topical Solution** Lemmon	solution	2%	alcohol, 60% · propylene glycol · purified water
**	**Minoxidil Topical Solution** Bausch & Lomb Ph'cal	solution	2%	alcohol, 60% · propylene glycol · purified water
**	**Rogaine for Men** Pharmacia & Upjohn	solution	2%	alcohol, 60% · propylene glycol · purified water · packaged with two applicators: sprayer and child-resistant dropper
**	**Rogaine for Women** Pharmacia & Upjohn	solution	2%	alcohol, 60% · propylene glycol · purified water · packaged extender spray applicator (helps direct spray through hair onto scalp)

** New listing

See Chapter 26, "Dermatologic Products," for more information about these products.

ACNE PRODUCTS

	Product Manufacturer/Supplier	Dosage Form	Benzoyl Peroxide	Sulfur	Resorcinol/ Salicylic Acid	Other Ingredients
	Acne Cleansing Maximum Strength Goldline Labs	pad			salicylic acid, 2%	
**	**Acne Treatment Cleanser** C & M Pharmacal	liquid			salicylic acid, 2%	purified water · sodium lauryl sulfate · propylene glycol · lauramide DEA · fragrance · chloroxylenol · hydroxyethyl ethylcellulose
**	**Acne Treatment Wash** C & M Pharmacal	liquid		4%	resorcinol, 2%	purified water · magnesium aluminum silicate · TEA-dodecyl benzene sulfonate · glycerin · stearic acid · cetostearyl alcohol · polysorbate 20 · fragrance · FD&C red#40
**	**Acne Treatment, Tinted** C & M Pharmacal	lotion		8%	resorcinol, 2%	purified water · isopropyl alcohol · propylene glycol · titanium dioxide · acetone · magnesium aluminum silicate · iron oxide yellow · octoxynol 9 · chloroxylenol · iron oxide brown · iron oxide red · xanthan gum · fragrance
**	**Acne Treatment, Vanishing** C & M Pharmacal	lotion		10%		purified water · glycerin · magnesium aluminum silicate · sorbic acid · fragrance · FD&C red#40
	Acne- 5 Goldline Labs	lotion	5%			
	Acne-10 Goldline Labs	lotion	10%			
	Acno Baker Cummins Derm'cals	lotion		3%	salicylic acid, 2%	
	Acnomel Menley & James Labs	cream		8%	resorcinol, 2%	alcohol, 11% · bentonite · titanium dioxide · fragrance · iron oxide · potassium hydroxide · propylene glycol · water
	Acnotex C & M Pharmacal	lotion		8%	resorcinol, 2%	purified water · isopropyl alcohol · propylene glycol · titanium dioxide · acetone · magnesium aluminum silicate · iron oxide yellow · octoxynol 9 · chloroxylenol · iron oxide brown · iron oxide red · xanthan gum · fragrance
**	**AMBI 10 Acne Medication** Kiwi	cream	10%			aluminum hydroxide · bentonite · carbomer 940 · glyceryl stearate SE · isopropyl myristate · methylparaben · PEG-12 · potassium hydroxide · propylene glycol · propylparaben · purified water

See Chapter 27, "Acne Products," for more information about these products.

ACNE PRODUCTS - continued

	Product Manufacturer/Supplier	Dosage Form	Benzoyl Peroxide	Sulfur	Resorcinol/ Salicylic Acid	Other Ingredients
**	**AMBI 10 Acne Pads** Kiwi	pad			salicylic acid, 2%	SD alcohol, 44% · ammonium xylenesulfonate · citric acid · fragrance · simethicone emulsion · sodium carbonate · sodium dodecylbenzene sulfonate · water
**	**Aveeno Medicated Cleanser** Rydelle Labs	liquid			salicylic acid, 2%	water · sodium laureth sulfosuccinate · disodium lauroamphoacetate · ammonium lauryl sulfate · hydrogenated tallow glyceride · potassium cocoyl hydrolyzed collagen · benzyl alcohol · guar hydroxypropyl ammonium chloride · oatmeal flour · sodium PCA · sodium citrate · citric acid phantolid · galaxolide · PEG-150 distearatechloride
	Benoxyl 5 Stiefel Labs	lotion	5%			
	Benoxyl 10 Stiefel Labs	lotion	10%			
	Betadine Skin Cleanser Purdue Frederick	liquid				povidone-iodine, 7.5%
**	**Clean & Clear Invisible Blemish Treatment** Johnson & Johnson Consumer	gel			salicylic acid, 2%	butylene glycol · glycerin · hydroxyethyl cellulose · propylene glycol · SD alcohol 40B, 28% · sodium citrate · water
**	**Clean & Clear Invisible Blemish Treatment, Sensitive Skin** Johnson & Johnson Consumer	gel			salicylic acid, 0.5%	butylene glycol · citric acid · glycerin · hydroxyethyl cellulose · propylene glycol · SD alcohol 40B, 28% · sodium citrate · water
**	**Clean & Clear Oil Controlling Astringent** Johnson & Johnson Consumer	liquid			salicylic acid, 2%	water · alcohol, 42% · eucalyptus oil · benzoic acid · camphor · peppermint oil · clove oil · FD&C red#4 · denatonium benzoate
**	**Clean & Clear Oil Controlling Astringent Sensitive Skin** Johnson & Johnson Consumer	liquid			salicylic acid, 0.5%	water · alcohol, 36.5% · glycerin · PPG-5-ceteth 20 · eucalyptus oil · benzoic acid · camphor · peppermint oil · clove oil · benzophenone-4 · denatonium benzoate · FD&C blue#1
**	**Clean & Clear Persa-Gel Extra Strength** Johnson & Johnson Consumer	gel	5%			water · carbomer · laureth-4 · hydroxypropyl methylcellulose · sodium hydroxide

See Chapter 27, "Acne Products," for more information about these products.

ACNE PRODUCTS - continued

	Product Manufacturer/Supplier	Dosage Form	Benzoyl Peroxide	Sulfur	Resorcinol/ Salicylic Acid	Other Ingredients
**	**Clean & Clear Persa-Gel Maximum Strength** Johnson & Johnson Consumer	gel	10%			water · carbomer · laureth-4 · hydroxypropyl methylcellulose · sodium hydroxide
	Clear By Design SmithKline Beecham	gel	2.5%			carbomer 940 · dioctyl sodium sulfosuccinate · sodium hydroxide · EDTA
	Clearasil Clearstick Maximum Strength Procter & Gamble	liquid			salicylic acid, 2.0%	alcohol, 39% · water · aloe vera gel · triethanolamine · menthol · disodium EDTA · fragrance
	Clearasil Clearstick Regular Strength Procter & Gamble	liquid			salicylic acid, 1.25%	alcohol, 39% · water · aloe vera gel · triethanolamine · menthol · disodium EDTA · fragrance
	Clearasil Clearstick Sensitive Skin Procter & Gamble	liquid			salicylic acid, 2.0%	alcohol, 39% · water · glycerin · aloe vera gel · triethanolamine · menthol · disodium EDTA
	Clearasil Double Textured Maximum Strength Procter & Gamble	pad			salicylic acid, 2%	alcohol, 40% · water · isoceteth-20 · aloe vera gel · triethanolamine · fragrance · menthol · disodium EDTA
	Clearasil Double Textured Reg. Strength with Skin Soothers Procter & Gamble	pad			salicylic acid, 2%	alcohol, 40% · water · glycerin · aloe vera gel · triethanolamine · disodium EDTA
	Clearasil Maximum Strength, Tinted or Vanishing Procter & Gamble	cream	10%			water · propylene glycol · bentonite · aluminum hydroxide · glyceryl stearate SE · PEG-12 · isopropyl myristate · carbomer · dimethicone · methylparaben · propylparaben · titanium dioxide (Tinted) · iron oxides (Tinted)
	Clearasil Maximum Strength, Vanishing Procter & Gamble	lotion	10%			water · aluminum hydroxide · isopropyl stearate · PEG-100 stearate · glyceryl stearate · cetyl alcohol · glycereth-26 · isocetyl stearate · glycerin · dimethicone copolyol · sodium citrate · citric acid · methylparaben · propylparaben · fragrance
	Clearasil Medicated Deep Cleanser Procter & Gamble	liquid			salicylic acid, 0.5%	alcohol, 42% · water · aloe vera gel · menthol · allantoin · fragrance · sorbitol · sodium lactate · proline · sodium PCA · hydrolyzed collagen · PEG-40 hydrogenated castor oil · disodium EDTA

See Chapter 27, "Acne Products," for more information about these products.

ACNE PRODUCTS - continued

	Product Manufacturer/Supplier	Dosage Form	Benzoyl Peroxide	Sulfur	Resorcinol/ Salicylic Acid	Other Ingredients
	Drytex C & M Pharmacal	liquid			salicylic acid, 2%	purified water · isopropyl alcohol · acetone · polysorbate 20 · benzalkonium chloride · fragrance · FD&C red#40 · FD&C yellow#5
**	**ExACT Adult Medication** APS/Premier	cream	2.5%			water · glycerin · acrylates copolymer · sorbitol · cetyl alcohol · glyceryl dilaurate · stearyl alcohol · sodium lauryl sulfate · magnesium aluminum silicate · sodium citrate · silica · citric acid · methylparaben · xanthan gum · propylparaben
**	**ExACT Pore Treatment** APS/Premier	gel			salicylic acid, 2%	purified water · dimethicone · PEG-20 · polyacrylamide · C13-14 isoparaffin · laureth-7 · methyl gluceth-20 · aloe vera gel · acrylates copolymer · polysorbate 80 · propylene glycol · diazolidinyl urea · methylparaben · propylparaben · triethanolamine · panthenol · allantoin · disodium EDTA
	ExACT Vanishing APS/Premier	cream	5%			water · acrylates copolymer · glycerin · sorbitol · cetyl alcohol · glyceryl dilaurate · stearyl alcohol · sodium lauryl sulfate · magnesium aluminum silicate · sodium citrate · silica · citric acid · methylparaben · xanthan gum · propylparaben
**	**Exfoliating Astringent for Oily Skin** C & M Pharmacal	liquid			salicylic acid, 2%	purified water · isopropyl alcohol · acetone · polysorbate 20 · benzalkonium chloride · fragrance · FD&C red#40 · FD&C yellow#5
	Fostex 10% BPO Bristol-Myers Products	cleansing bar	10%			urea · dextrin · sodium lauryl sulfoacetate · boric acid · disodium EDTA · lactic acid
	Fostex 10% BPO Bristol-Myers Products	gel	10%			water · laureth-4 · diisopropanolamine · carbomer · disodium EDTA
	Fostex 10% BPO Wash Bristol-Myers Products	liquid	10%			sodium laureth sulfate · water · sodium dioctyl sulfosuccinate · magnesium aluminum silicate · hydroxypropyl methylcellulose · disodium EDTA · sodium chloride · citric acid
	Fostex Medicated Bristol-Myers Products	cleansing bar			salicylic acid, 2%	boric acid · urea · dextrin · sodium lauryl sulfoacetate · cake gel · sodium dioctyl sulfosuccinate · lactic acid · triton X-200 · disodium EDTA · ocher · water

See Chapter 27, "Acne Products," for more information about these products.

ACNE PRODUCTS - continued

Product Manufacturer/Supplier	Dosage Form	Benzoyl Peroxide	Sulfur	Resorcinol/ Salicylic Acid	Other Ingredients
Fostex Medicated Cleansing Bristol-Myers Products	cream			salicylic acid, 2%	triton X-200 · liquid sodium dodecylbenzene sulfonate · water · poloxamer 188 · sodium dioctyl sulfosuccinate · stearyl alcohol C-20 · methocel A4M · modified food starch · sodium chloride · fragrance · EDTA · color
Fostril Westwood-Squibb Ph'cals	lotion		2%		laureth-4 · zinc oxide · talc · PEG-40 stearate · magnesium aluminum silicate · PEG-8 stearate · bentonite · iron oxides · methylcellulose · methylparaben · citric acid · EDTA · fragrance · quaternium-15 · simethicone · water
Ionax Astringent Skin Cleanser Galderma Labs	liquid			salicylic acid	isopropyl alcohol, 48% · allantoin · acetone · polyoxyethylene ethers
Liquimat Summers Labs	lotion		4%		alcohol, 22% · tinted bases
Loroxide Summers Labs	lotion	5.5%			BHA · BHT · caprylic/capric triglyceride · caramel · cetyl alcohol · decyl oleate · disodium phosphate · eidetic acid · hydroxyethylcellulose · kaolin · methylparaben · mineral oil · lanolin alcohol · monoglyceride citrate · sodium phosphate · talc · tetrasodium EDTA · titanium dioxide · vegetable oil · polysorbate 20 · propylene glycol · propylene glycol stearate · propyl gallate · propylparaben · purified water · simethicone · stearyl heptanoate · sodium hydroxide
Neutrogena Acne Neutrogena Dermatologics	mask	5%			
Neutrogena Clear Pore Treatment Neutrogena Dermatologics	gel			salicylic acid, 2%	purified water · PEG-32 · PVM/MA decadiene crospolymer · sodium hydroxide · fragrance
Neutrogena Oil-Free Wash Neutrogena Dermatologics	liqui-gel			salicylic acid, 2%	
Noxzema 2 in 1 Maximum Strength Procter & Gamble	pad			salicylic acid, 2%	alcohol, 63% · water · PEG-4 · PPG-11 stearyl ether · camphor · clove oil · eucalyptus oil · menthol · fragrance
Noxzema 2 in 1 Regular Strength Procter & Gamble	pad			salicylic acid, 0.5%	alcohol, 63% · water · PPG-11 stearyl ether · camphor · clove oil · eucalyptus oil · menthol · fragrance

See Chapter 27, "Acne Products," for more information about these products.

ACNE PRODUCTS - continued

Product Manufacturer/Supplier	Dosage Form	Benzoyl Peroxide	Sulfur	Resorcinol/ Salicylic Acid	Other Ingredients
Noxzema Oily Astringent Procter & Gamble	liquid			salicylic acid, 2%	alcohol, 49% · water · triethanolamine · fragrance · menthol · disodium EDTA · FD&C yellow#5 · FD&C blue#1
On-the-Spot Neutrogena Dermatologics	lotion	2.5%			
Oxy Deep Cleansing, Maximum Strength SmithKline Beecham	pad			salicylic acid, 2%	alcohol, 50% · citric acid · fragrance · glycerin · menthol · sodium lauryl sulfate · water · propylene glycol · polyethylene glycol
Oxy Deep Cleansing, Regular Strength SmithKline Beecham	pad			salicylic acid, 0.5%	alcohol, 43% · citric acid · fragrance · glycerin · menthol · sodium lauryl sulfate · water · propylene glycol
Oxy Deep Cleansing, Sensitive Skin SmithKline Beecham	pad			salicylic acid, 0.5%	alcohol, 22% · disodium lauryl sulfosuccinate · fragrance · glycerin · menthol · PEG-4 · sodium lauryl sarcosinate · sodium PCA · trisodium EDTA · water
Oxy Medicated Cleanser SmithKline Beecham	liquid			salicylic acid, 0.5%	alcohol, 43% · citric acid · menthol · sodium lauryl sulfate · fragrance · glycerin · propylene glycol · water
Oxy Medicated Face Wash SmithKline Beecham	liquid	10%			citric acid · cocamidopropyl betaine · diazolidinyl urea · methylparaben · propylparaben · sodium citrate · sodium cocoyl isethionate · sodium laureth sulfate sarcosinate · water · xanthan gum
Oxy Medicated Soap SmithKline Beecham	cleansing bar				triclosan, 1.0% · bentonite · cocoamphodipropionate · fragrance · glycerin · iron oxides · magnesium silicate · sodium chloride · sodium borohydride · sodium cocoate · sodium tallowate · talc · tetrasodium EDTA · titanium dioxide · trisodium HEDTA · water
Oxy Moisturizing Face Wash SmithKline Beecham	lotion				triclosan, 0.6% · cocamidopropyl betaine · diazolidinyl urea · sodium cocoyl isethionate · sodium laureth sulfate · water · FD&C blue#1 · glycerin

See Chapter 27, "Acne Products," for more information about these products.

ACNE PRODUCTS - continued

Product Manufacturer/Supplier	Dosage Form	Benzoyl Peroxide	Sulfur	Resorcinol/ Salicylic Acid	Other Ingredients
Oxy Night Watch Maximum Strength SmithKline Beecham	lotion			salicylic acid, 2%	cetyl alcohol · disodium EDTA · methylparaben · propylene glycol · propylparaben · silica · sodium lauryl sulfate · stearyl alcohol · water
Oxy Sensitive Skin, Vanishing SmithKline Beecham	gel	2.5%			acrylates copolymer · carbomer 940 · citric acid · diazolidinyl urea · dimethicone · dioctyl sodium sulfosuccinate · edetate disodium · glycerin · propylene glycol · silica · sodium citrate · sodium hydroxide · water · xanthan gum
Oxy-10 Maximum Strength, Tinted SmithKline Beecham	lotion	10%			carbomer 940 · dioctyl sulfosuccinate · edetate disodium · iron oxides · sodium hydroxide · titanium dioxide · water
Oxy-10 Maximum Strength, Vanishing SmithKline Beecham	lotion	10%			acrylates copolymer · carbomer 940 · citric acid · diazolidinyl urea · dimethicone · dioctyl sodium sulfosuccinate · edetate disodium · glycerin · propylene glycol · silica · sodium citrate · sodium hydroxide · water · xanthan gum
Pan Oxyl 5 Stiefel Labs	cleansing bar	5%			mild surfactant base
Pan Oxyl 10 Stiefel Labs	cleansing bar	10%			mild surfactant base
Pernox Westwood-Squibb Ph'cals	lotion		2%	salicylic acid, 1.5%	polyethylene granules · sodium octoxynol-2 · ethane sulfonate · sodium dodecylbenzene sulfonate · fragrance · docusate sodium · modified starch · magnesium aluminum · silicate · methylcellulose · EDTA · water
Pernox, Lemon or Regular Westwood-Squibb Ph'cals	abrasive		2%	salicylic acid, 1.5%	polyethylene granules · sodium octoxynol-2 · ethane sulfonate · sodium dodecylbenzene sulfonate · poloxamer 184 · docusate sodium · methylcellulose · food starch · fragrance · EDTA · D&C yellow#10 · FD&C blue#1 (Regular) · water
Propa pH Acne Medication Del Ph'cals	cream			salicylic acid, 2%	

See Chapter 27, "Acne Products," for more information about these products.

ACNE PRODUCTS - continued

	Product Manufacturer/Supplier	Dosage Form	Benzoyl Peroxide	Sulfur	Resorcinol/ Salicylic Acid	Other Ingredients
**	**Propa pH Astringent Cleanser** Del Ph'cals	lotion			salicylic acid, 0.5%	aloe vera gel · benzophenone-4 · disodium EDTA · fragrance · menthol · citric acid · green tea extract · lactic acid · malic acid · peppermint oil · SD alcohol 40-A · sodium citrate · sodium laureth-12 sulfate · triclosan · water
**	**Propa pH Astringent Cleanser Maximum Strength** Del Ph'cals	lotion			salicylic acid, 2%	aloe vera gel · benzophenone-4 · disodium EDTA · fragrance · menthol · citric acid · green tea extract · lactic acid · malic acid · peppermint oil · polysorbate 20 · SD alcohol 40-A · sodium citrate · triclosan · water
	Propa pH Foaming Face Wash Del Ph'cals	liquid			salicylic acid, 2%	aloe vera gel · disodium EDTA · fragrance · glycol distearate · citric acid · green tea extract · lactic acid · malic acid · polyol alkoxy esters · polyoxyethylene-15-cocoamine phosphate/oleate complex · menthol · quaternium-15 · sodium laureth sulfate · sodium lauryl sarcosinate · water
**	**Propa pH Peel-off** Del Ph'cals	mask			salicylic acid, 2%	aloe vera gel · FD&C red#4 · FD&C yellow#5 · fragrance · methylparaben · citric acid · green tea extract · lactic acid · malic acid · polyethylene glycol · polysorbate 80 · polyvinyl alcohol · PPG-5-ceteth-20 · propylparaben · purified water · SD alcohol 40 · sodium carbonate · tocopheryl acetate
**	**Propa pH Perfectly Clear Cleansing, Oily Skin** Del Ph'cals	lotion			salicylic acid, 0.6%	purified water · SD alcohol 40 · sodium laureth-12 sulfate · aloe vera gel · triclosan · sodium carbonate · benzophenone-4 · disodium EDTA · menthol · fragrance
**	**Propa pH Perfectly Clear Cleansing, Sensitive Skin** Del Ph'cals	lotion			salicylic acid, 0.5%	purified water · SD alcohol 40 · sodium laureth-12 sulfate · aloe vera gel · triclosan · sodium carbonate · benzophenone-4 · disodium EDTA · menthol · fragrance
	Rezamid Acne Lotion Summers Labs	liquid		5%	resorcinol, 2%	
	SalAc Cleanser GenDerm	liquid			salicylic acid, 2%	

See Chapter 27, "Acne Products," for more information about these products.

ACNE PRODUCTS - continued

	Product Manufacturer/Supplier	Dosage Form	Benzoyl Peroxide	Sulfur	Resorcinol/ Salicylic Acid	Other Ingredients
	SAStid Soap Stiefel Labs	cleansing bar		10%		
	Seales Lotion-Modified C & M Pharmacal	lotion		6.4%		purified water · acetone · zinc oxide · sodium borate · bentonite
	Sebasorb Summers Labs	liquid			salicylic acid, 2%	attapulgite, 10% · polysorbate 80
	Stri-Dex Clear Blistex	gel			salicylic acid, 2%	SD alcohol, 9.3% · glycerin
	Stri-Dex Maximum Strength, Single or Dual Textured Blistex	pad			salicylic acid, 2%	SD alcohol, 44%
	Stri-Dex Regular Strength, Dual Textured Blistex	pad			salicylic acid, 0.5%	SD alcohol, 28%
	Stri-Dex Sensitive Skin, Dual Textured Blistex	pad			salicylic acid, 0.5%	SD alcohol, 28% · aloe vera gel
	Stri-Dex Super Scrub Blistex	pad			salicylic acid, 2%	SD alcohol, 54%
	Sulforcin Galderma Labs	lotion		5%	resorcinol, 2%	alcohol, 11.65%
	Sulmasque C & M Pharmacal	mask		6.4%		purified water · bentonite · kaolin · isopropyl alcohol · zinc oxide · calcium oxide · sodium lauryl sulfate · lauramide DEA · fragrance · methylparaben
**	**Sulpho-Lac** Doak Dermatologics	cream		5%		
**	**Sulpho-Lac Soap** Doak Dermatologics	cleansing bar		5%		
**	**Sulray Acne Treatment** Alvin Last	cream		3%		water · kaolin · glyceryl stearate · laureth-23 · PEG-8 stearate · aloe vera gel · glycerin · PEG-8 distearate · silica · methylparaben · propylparaben · caramel
	Sulray Facial Cleanser Alvin Last	liquid		3%		aloe vera gel · sodium lauryl sulfate · lauramide DEA · glycol stearate · methylparaben · propylparaben · citric acid
	Sulray Soap Alvin Last	cleansing bar		5%		fragrance free natural soap base · aloe vera · trisodium HEDTA
	Therac C & M Pharmacal	lotion		10% (colloidal)	salicylic acid, 2.35%	purified water · glycerin · magnesium aluminum silicate · sorbic acid · fragrance · FD&C red#40

See Chapter 27, "Acne Products," for more information about these products.

ACNE PRODUCTS - continued

Product Manufacturer/Supplier	Dosage Form	Benzoyl Peroxide	Sulfur	Resorcinol/ Salicylic Acid	Other Ingredients
Thylox Acne Treatment Soap C. S. Dent	cleansing bar		3%		sodium tallowate · sodium cocoate · water · glycerin · fragrance · titanium dioxide · tetrasodium etidronate · pentasodium pentetate · cosmetic orange oxide
Vanoxide Dermik Labs	lotion	5%			BHA/BHT · caprylic/capric triglyceride · cetyl alcohol · colloidal silicon dioxide · decyl oleate · dibasic sodium phosphate · eidetic acid · hydroxyethyl cellulose · methylparaben · mineral oil · lanolin oil · monobasic sodium phosphate · polysorbate 20 · polysorbate 80 · cetyl acetate · acetylated lanolin alcohol · propylene glycol · propylene glycol monostearate · propylparaben · purified water · simethicone · sodium hydroxide · stearyl heptanoate · tetrasodium EDTA

** New listing

See Chapter 27, "Acne Products," for more information about these products.

FIRST-AID ANTIBIOTIC AND ANTISEPTIC PRODUCTS

	Product Manufacturer/Supplier	Dosage Form	Antibiotic	Antiseptic	Other Ingredients
	Aerocaine Graham-Field	aerosol spray		benzethonium chloride, 0.5%	benzocaine, 13.6% · isobutane
	B.F.I. Menley & James Labs	powder		bismuth formic iodide, 16%	bismuth subgallate · boric acid · magnesium carbonate · potassium alum · talc · zinc phenylsulfonate · eucalyptol · menthol · thymol
	Baciguent Roberts Ph'cal	ointment	bacitracin, 500 IU/g		white petroleum · mineral oil
	Bactine Bayer Consumer	spray		benzalkonium chloride, 0.13%	lidocaine HCl, 2.5% · disodium edetate · fragrance · octoxynol-9 · propylene glycol · water
	Benzalkonium Chloride Multisource	liquid		benzalkonium chloride, 17% · bismuth formic iodide, 16%	
**	**Betadine First Aid Antibiotics + Moisturizer** Purdue Frederick	ointment	polymyxin B sulfate, 10000 IU/g · bacitracin zinc, 500 IU/g		
	Buro-Sol Antiseptic Doak Dermatologics	powder		sodium diacetate, 0.23% · benzethonium chloride, 4.4%	aluminum acetate, 46.8%
	Campho-phenique Pain Relieving Antiseptic Bayer Consumer	gel · liquid		camphor, 10.8% · phenol, 4.7%	eucalyptus oil
	Campho-phenique Triple Antibiotic Bayer Consumer	ointment	polymyxin B sulfate, 10000 IU/g · bacitracin zinc, 500 IU/g · neomycin sulfate, 5mg/g (equivalent to neomycin base, 3.5mg)		lidocaine HCl, 40mg
**	**Castellani Paint, Modified** Pedinol Pharmacal	liquid		phenol, 1.5% · SD alcohol 40B	water · resorcinol · acetone · basic fuschin (color)
	Clomycin Roberts Ph'cal	cream	polymyxin B sulfate, 5000 IU/g · bacitracin, 500 IU/g · neomycin sulfate, 3.5mg/g		lidocaine, 40mg/g · yellow petrolatum · anhydrous lanolin · mineral oil
	Dakins 1/2 Strength Century Ph'cals	solution		sodium hypochlorite, 0.25%	
	Dakins Full Strength Century Ph'cals	solution		sodium hypochlorite, 0.5%	
**	**Dr. Tichenor's Antiseptic** Dr. G. H. Tichenor	liquid		SDA alcohol 38B, 70%	oil of peppermint · extract of arnica · water
	Efodine E. Fougera	ointment		available iodine, 1%	anhydrous carbowax base
**	**First Aid Cream** Johnson & Johnson Consumer	cream		cetylpyridinium chloride	water · cetyl alcohol · glyceryl stearate · isopropyl palmitate · stearyl alcohol · benzyl alcohol · synthetic beeswax · lapyrium chloride · hydroxypropyl methylcellulose · trisodium phosphate

See Chapter 28, "First-Aid Products and Minor Wound Care," for more information about these products.

FIRST-AID ANTIBIOTIC AND ANTISEPTIC PRODUCTS - continued

	Product Manufacturer/Supplier	Dosage Form	Antibiotic	Antiseptic	Other Ingredients
**	**First Aid Medicated Powder** Johnson & Johnson Consumer	powder			zinc oxide · menthol · corn starch · dipropylene glycol · eucalyptol · thymol · methyl salicylate
	Hibiclens Zeneca Ph'cals	liquid		chlorhexidine gluconate, 4%	
	Hibiclens Sponge Brush Zeneca Ph'cals	sponge		chlorhexidine gluconate, 4%	
	Hibistat Towelette Zeneca Ph'cals	liquid		chlorhexidine gluconate, 0.5%	
	Hydrogen Peroxide Multisource	solution		hydrogen peroxide, 3%	
	Iodine Topical Multisource	solution		sodium iodide, 2.5% · iodine, 2%	
	Lanabiotic Combe	ointment	polymyxin B sulfate, 10000 IU/g · bacitracin, 500 IU/g · neomycin sulfate, 5mg/g		
	Medi-Quik Triple Antibiotic Mentholatum	ointment	polymyxin B sulfate, 5000 IU/g · bacitracin, 500 IU/g · neomycin sulfate, 3.5mg/g		mineral oil · petrolatum
	Mercurochrome Multisource	solution		merbromin, 2%	
	Mersol Century Ph'cals	liquid · ointment		alcohol, 52.5% · thimerosal, 0.1%	
	Myciguent Roberts Ph'cal	cream	neomycin sulfate, 3.5mg/g		anhydrous lanolin · mineral oil · white petroleum
	Mycitracin Pharmacia & Upjohn	ointment	polymyxin B sulfate, 10000 IU/g · bacitracin zinc, 500 IU/g · neomycin sulfate, 5mg (equivalent to neomycin, 3.5mg)		butylparaben · cholesterol · methylparaben · microcrystalline wax · mineral oil · white petrolatum
	Mycitracin Plus Pharmacia & Upjohn	ointment	polymyxin B sulfate, 10000 IU/g · bacitracin zinc, 500 IU/g · neomycin sulfate (equivalent to neomycin, 3.5mg)		lidocaine, 40mg · butylparaben · cholesterol · methylparaben · microcrystalline wax · mineral oil · white petrolatum
	Neosporin Warner Wellcome Consumer	ointment	polymyxin B sulfate, 5000 IU/g · bacitracin zinc, 400 IU/g · neomycin base, 3.5mg/g		white petrolatum
	Neosporin Plus Maximum Strength Warner Wellcome Consumer	cream	polymyxin B sulfate, 10000 IU/g · neomycin base, 3.5mg/g		lidocaine, 40mg/g · methylparaben, 0.25% · emulsifying wax · mineral oil · poloxamer 188 · purified water · white petrolatum
	Neosporin Plus Maximum Strength Warner Wellcome Consumer	ointment	polymyxin B sulfate, 10000 IU/g · bacitracin zinc, 500 IU/g · neomycin base, 3.5mg/g		lidocaine, 40mg/g · white petrolatum

See Chapter 28, "First-Aid Products and Minor Wound Care," for more information about these products.

FIRST-AID ANTIBIOTIC AND ANTISEPTIC PRODUCTS - continued

Product Manufacturer/Supplier	Dosage Form	Antibiotic	Antiseptic	Other Ingredients
New Skin Liquid Bandage Medtech Labs	liquid · spray		8-hydroxyquinoline, 1%	proxylin (collodion), 98% · clove oil, 1%
Oxyzal Wet Dressing Gordon Labs	solution		benzalkonium chloride, 0.05%	oxyquinoline sulfate
Polysporin Warner Wellcome Consumer	ointment · powder	polymyxin B sulfate, 10000 IU/g · bacitracin zinc, 500 IU/g		white petrolatum (ointment) · lactose (powder)
Povidone-Iodine Multisource	ointment · solution		povidone-iodine, 10%	
ST 37 Menley & James Labs	liquid		hexylresorcinol, 0.1%	glycerin · propylene glycol · citric acid · disodium edetate · sodium bisulfite · sodium citrate
Tribiotic Plus Thompson Medical	ointment	polymyxin B sulfate, 5500 IU/g · bacitracin, 600 IU/g · neomycin sulfate, 3.85mg/g		lidocaine, 40mg/g · petrolatum · anhydrous lanolin · light mineral oil
Unguentine Mentholatum	ointment		phenol, 1%	eucalyptus oil · oleostearine · petrolatum · thyme oil · zinc oxide
Unguentine Plus Mentholatum	cream		phenol, 0.5%	lidocaine HCl, 2% · fragrance · glyceryl · stearate · isoceteth-20 · isopropyl palmitate · methylparaben · mineral oil · poloxamer 407 · propylparaben · quaternium-15 · sorbitan stearate · tetrasodium EDTA · water

** New listing

See Chapter 28, "First-Aid Products and Minor Wound Care," for more information about these products.

DIAPER RASH AND PRICKLY HEAT PRODUCTS

	Product Manufacturer/Supplier	Dosage Form	Protectant	Powder Base	Antimicrobial	Other Ingredients
PE	**A and D Medicated Ointment** Schering-Plough HealthCare	ointment	white petrolatum · zinc oxide · cholecalciferol · cod liver oil · mineral oil			benzyl alcohol · cyclomethicone · glyceryl monostearate · magnesium aluminum silicate · ozokerite · propylparaben · benzoic acid
** PE	**A and D Medicated Powder** Schering-Plough HealthCare	powder	zinc oxide	corn starch · kaolin	benzethonium chloride	aloe
	A and D Ointment Schering-Plough HealthCare	ointment	vitamins A & D · cholecalciferol · fish liver oil · mineral oil · petrolatum			fragrance · paraffin
	ActiBath Soak Oatmeal Treatment Andrew Jergens	effervescent tablet	colloidal oatmeal, 20%	sodium bicarbonate		fumaric acid · sodium carbonate · lactose · PEG-150 · magnesium oxide · sucrose stearate
	Ammens Medicated Original Fragrance Bristol-Myers Products	powder	zinc oxide, 9.1%	talc · corn starch	8-hydroxyquinoline · 8-hydroxyquinoline sulfate	PPG methyl glucose ether · isostearic acid · fragrance
	Ammens Medicated Shower Fresh Scent Bristol-Myers Products	powder	zinc oxide, 9.1%	talc · corn starch		fragrance · PPG-20 methyl glucose ether · isostearic acid · fragrance
	Aveeno Bath Treatment Moisturizing Formula Rydelle Labs	powder	colloidal oatmeal, 43% · mineral oil			
	Aveeno Bath Treatment Soothing Formula Rydelle Labs	powder	colloidal oatmeal, 100%			
PE	**Balmex** Block Drug	ointment	zinc oxide			beeswax · silicone · synthetic white wax · purified water · balsam · benzoic acid · bismuth subnitrate · mineral oil · others
	Calamine Goldline Labs	lotion	calamine, 8% · zinc oxide, 8%			
PE	**Caldesene Medicated** Ciba Self-Medication	ointment	white petrolatum, 53.9% · zinc oxide, 15%	talc		fragrance · methylparaben · propylparaben · cod liver oil · lanolin oil
PE	**Caldesene Medicated** Ciba Self-Medication	powder	talc		calcium undecylenate, 10%	fragrance
	Care-Creme Cream Care-Tech Labs	cream	petrolatum · cod liver oil · lanolin oil · vitamins A & D		chloroxylenol, 0.8%	cetyl alcohol · lanolin alcohol · propylene glycol · vitamin E
	Clocream Roberts Ph'cal	cream	vitamins A & D			
PE	**Desitin** Pfizer Consumer	ointment	zinc oxide, 40% · cod liver oil · petrolatum · lanolin	talc		water · methylparaben · BHA · fragrance
PE	**Desitin Cornstarch Baby Powder** Pfizer Consumer	powder	zinc oxide, 10%	corn starch, 88.2%		fragrance · tribasic calcium phosphate

See Chapter 29, "Diaper Rash, Prickly Heat, and Adult Incontinence Products," for more information about these products.

DIAPER RASH AND PRICKLY HEAT PRODUCTS - continued

	Product Manufacturer/Supplier	Dosage Form	Protectant	Powder Base	Antimicrobial	Other Ingredients
PE	**Desitin Daily Care** Pfizer Consumer	ointment	zinc oxide, 10% · dimethicone · petrolatum · mineral oil			water · white wax · cyclomethicone · sorbitan sesquioleate · sodium borate · fragrance · methylparaben · propylparaben
PE	**Diapa-Kare** Perry Products	powder		corn starch · sodium bicarbonate	methylbenzethonium chloride	fragrance
PE	**Diaparene Cornstarch Baby Powder** Reckitt & Colman	powder		corn starch, 88%		aloe vera extract · chamomile · evening primrose extract · tricalcium phosphate · fragrance
PE	**Diaparene Diaper Rash** Reckitt & Colman	ointment	zinc oxide, 15.8%		methylparaben · propylparaben · imidazolidinyl urea	trihydroxystearin · bisabolol · petrolatum
PE	**Diaper Guard** Del Ph'cals	ointment	white petrolatum, 66% · dimethicone, 1% · cocoa butter · colloidal oatmeal · cholecalciferol · zinc oxide		benzalkonium chloride	colloidal silicon dioxide · fragrance · magnesium silicate · methylparaben · paraffin · propylparaben · retinyl palmitate · d-alpha tocopheryl acetate
PE	**Diaper Rash Ointment** G & W Labs	ointment	zinc oxide, 40% · cod liver oil			
**	**DML Lotion** Person & Covey	lotion	petrolatum · glycerin			PPG-2 · myristyl ether propionate · glyceryl stearate · simethicone · benzyl alcohol · silica · EDTA · sodium carbomer 1342
PE	**Dyprotex** Blistex	ointment · pad	micronized zinc oxide, 40% · petrolatum, 31.1% dimethicone, 2.5% · cod liver oil	zinc stearate		aloe extract
**	**First Aid Medicated Powder** Johnson & Johnson Consumer	powder	zinc oxide	corn starch		menthol · dipropylene glycol · eucalyptol · thymol · methyl salicylate
PE	**Flanders Buttocks** Flanders	ointment	zinc oxide · white petrolatum · peruvian balsam			castor oil
PE	**Gold Bond Baby Powder** Chattem	powder	zinc oxide	talc		fragrance
	Gold Bond Medicated, Regular or Extra Strength Chattem	powder	zinc oxide · zinc stearate	talc		menthol · eucalyptol · methyl salicylate · salicylic acid · thymol · boric acid
	Hydropel C & M Pharmacal	ointment	silicone, 30% · petrolatum			aluminum starch octenyl succinate
PE	**Johnson's Baby Cream** Johnson & Johnson Consumer	cream	dimethicone, 2% · lanolin · mineral oil			fragrance · glyceryl stearate · paraffin · propylparaben · sodium borate · water
PE	**Johnson's Baby Diaper Rash Ointment** Johnson & Johnson Consumer	ointment	petrolatum · zinc oxide		benzethonium chloride	trihydroxystearin · bisabolol · fragrance

See Chapter 29, "Diaper Rash, Prickly Heat, and Adult Incontinence Products," for more information about these products.

DIAPER RASH AND PRICKLY HEAT PRODUCTS - continued

	Product Manufacturer/Supplier	Dosage Form	Protectant	Powder Base	Antimicrobial	Other Ingredients
PE	**Johnson's Baby Powder** Johnson & Johnson Consumer	powder		talc		fragrance
PE	**Johnson's Baby Powder Cornstarch** Johnson & Johnson Consumer	powder		corn starch, 95%		tricalcium phosphate · fragrance
** PE	**Johnson's Baby, Medicated** Johnson & Johnson Consumer	powder	zinc oxide	corn starch		fragrance
**	**Lantiseptic Skin Protectant** Summit	ointment	lanolin, 50%			beeswax (yellow wax) · fragrance · HEEDTA · oxyquinoline · petrolatum · water · sodium borate · sorbitan sesquioleate
PE	**Little Bottoms** Vetco	ointment	zinc oxide, 15%· balsam peru · mineral oil · petrolatum · dimethicone			aloe · PEG-40 · sorbitan peroleate · beeswax · titanium dioxide · bismuth subnitrate · benzoic acid · deionized water
**	**Lobana Derm-ADE** Lobana Labs	cream	vitamins A, D, & E · silicone			
**	**Lobana Peri-Gard** Lobana Labs	ointment	petrolatum · vitamins A & D		chloroxylenol	
	Mexsana Medicated Schering-Plough HealthCare	powder	zinc oxide, 10.8%	corn starch · kaolin	benzethonium chloride	camphor · eucalyptus oil
	Nutra Soothe Medicated Brimms Labs	powder	colloidal oatmeal · zinc oxide	corn starch · oat starch		tricalcium phosphate · fragrance
	Panthoderm Jones Medical	lotion	dexpanthenol, 2%			water-miscible base
	Plexolan Lanolin Alvin Last	cream	lanolin, 15.5% · zinc oxide · petrolatum · mineral oil			water · ozokerite · PEG-400 distearate · fragrance · methylparaben
**	**Protective Barrier** C & M Pharmacal	ointment	silicone, 30% · petrolatum			aluminum starch octenyl succinate
** PE	**Resinol Diaper Rash** Mentholatum	ointment	zinc oxide, 12% · calamine			lanolin · petrolatum · starch
**	**Schamberg's Anti-itch** C & M Pharmacal	lotion	zinc oxide			purified water · refined peanut oil · propylene glycol · magnesium aluminum silicate · phenol · cellulose gum · calcium oxide · octoxynol-9 · menthol
	Spectro-Jel Recsei Labs	gel			cetylpyridinium chloride, 0.1%	isopropyl alcohol, 5% · methylcellulose, 1.5% · glycol-polysiloxane, 1%
	Triple Paste Summers Labs	ointment	white petrolatum, 52% · zinc oxide ·			aluminum acetate solution
	Vaseline Pure Petroleum Jelly Chesebrough-Pond's	ointment	white petrolatum, 100%			
	Velvet Fresh Powder Care-Tech Labs	powder		corn starch		tricalcium phosphate · fragrance

See Chapter 29, "Diaper Rash, Prickly Heat, and Adult Incontinence Products," for more information about these products.

DIAPER RASH AND PRICKLY HEAT PRODUCTS - continued

	Product Manufacturer/Supplier	Dosage Form	Protectant	Powder Base	Antimicrobial	Other Ingredients
PE	**ZBT Baby Powder** Glenwood	powder	mineral oil	talc · magnesium stearate		propylene glycol · BHT · fragrance
	Zeasorb Stiefel Labs	powder		talc · microporous cellulose	chloroxylenol	carbohydrate acrylic copolymer · imidazolidinyl urea · aldioxa · fragrance

** New listing

See Chapter 29, "Diaper Rash, Prickly Heat, and Adult Incontinence Products," for more information about these products.

ADULT INCONTINENCE GARMENTS

	Product Manufacturer/Supplier	Product Form	Absorbency	Comments
**	**Attends Briefs** Procter & Gamble	pad	heavy	small, medium, large sizes · refastenable tapes
**	**Attends Guards** Procter & Gamble	pad	light/moderate	curved
**	**Attends Pads** Procter & Gamble	pad	light	
**	**Attends Undergarments** Procter & Gamble	pad	moderate: regular · super	reusable elastic belts
**	**Depend Fitted Briefs** Kimberly-Clark	pad	heavy/complete: regular · overnight (absorbs 30% more)	regular absorbency in small, medium, large sizes · overnight absorbency in medium size · each has six refastenable tapes · elastic leg and waist
**	**Depend Guards for Men** Kimberly-Clark	pad	light/moderate: one absorbency	one size · anatomical design with elasticized pouch · cup-like fit
**	**Depend Poise** Kimberly-Clark	pad	light: thin · regular · extra · extra plus	maxi pad size · elasticized sides
**	**Depend Poise Guards** Kimberly-Clark	pad	light/moderate: super · super plus	thermo-formed shell creates a reservoir
**	**Depend Poise Shields** Kimberly-Clark	pad	light: regular · extra	one size · cup-shaped design
**	**Depend Undergarments** Kimberly-Clark	pad	moderate: EasyFit - regular, extra · Elastic Leg - regular, extra · Non-Elastic Leg - extra	soft, cloth-like outer cover · three styles, each in one size: EasyFit with reusable strap tabs, Elastic Leg with reusable button strap tabs, and Non-Elastic Leg with reusable button strap tabs
**	**Stayfree Serenity Curved Pads** McNeil Consumer	pad	extra (light to moderate) · extra plus (moderate)	
**	**Stayfree Serenity Guards** McNeil Consumer	pad	regular (moderate) · super (moderate to heavy) · super plus (heavy)	
**	**Stayfree Serenity Pads** McNeil Consumer	pad	thin pads (light) · pads (light to moderate)	

** New listing

See Chapter 29, "Diaper Rash, Prickly Heat, and Adult Incontinence Products," for more information about these products.

SUNSCREEN AND SUNTAN PRODUCTS

	Product Manufacturer/Supplier	Dosage Form	SPF Value	Sunscreen	Other Ingredients
	A-Fil GenDerm	cream	8 · 15	menthyl anthranilate, 5% · titanium dioxide, 5%	
	Aquaderm Sunscreen Moisturizer Baker Cummins Derm'cals	cream	15	octyl methoxycinnamate, 7.5% · oxybenzone, 6%	
**	**Aquaray** Harold Pharmacal	lotion	20	octyl methoxycinnamate, 7.5% · oxybenzone, 5% · octyl salicylate, 5%	water · steareth-100 · isodecyl isononanoate · olive oil · stearyl alcohol · cetyl alcohol · sorbitol · TEA-carbomer · benzyl alcohol
** PE	**Baby Sunblock** Goldline Labs	lotion	30	octyl methoxycinnamate · octyl salicylate · homosalate · oxybenzone	
PE	**Bain de Soleil All Day for Kids Waterproof Sunblock** Pfizer Consumer	lotion	30	octyl methoxycinnamate · octocrylene · oxybenzone · titanium dioxide	water · PVP/eicosene copolymer · isohexadecane · butylene glycol · dimethicone · cyclomethicone · panthenol · triethanolamine · cetyl palmitate · tribehenin · stearoxytrimethylsilane · stearyl alcohol · tocopheryl acetate · DEA-cetyl phosphate · carbomer · acrylates/C10-30 alkyl acrylate crosspolymer · disodium EDTA · DMDM hydantoin · iodopropynyl butylcarbamate
	Bain de Soleil All Day Six Hour Waterproof Sunfilter Pfizer Consumer	lotion	4 · 8	octocrylene · octyl methoxycinnamate · titanium dioxide	water · PVP/eicosene copolymer · isohexadecane · butylene glycol · dimethicone · cyclomethicone · panthenol · triethanolamine · cetyl palmitate · tribehenin · stearoxytrimethylsilane · stearyl alcohol · tocopheryl acetate · DEA-cetyl phosphate · carbomer · acrylates/C10-30 alkyl acrylate crosspolymer · disodium EDTA · DMDM hydantoin · iodopropynyl butylcarbamate
	Bain de Soleil All Day Waterproof Sunblock Pfizer Consumer	lotion	15	octyl methoxycinnamate · octocrylene · oxybenzone · titanium dioxide	water · PVP/eicosene copolymer · isohexadecane · butylene glycol · dimethicone · cyclomethicone · panthenol · triethanolamine · cetyl palmitate · tribehenin · stearoxytrimethylsilane · stearyl alcohol · tocopheryl acetate · DEA-cetyl phosphate · carbomer · acrylates/C10-30 alkyl acrylate crosspolymer · disodium EDTA · DMDM hydantoin · iodopropynyl butylcarbamate
**	**Bain de Soleil Mega Tan** Pfizer Consumer	lotion	4	octyl methoxycinnamate · octocrylene	water · dihydroxyacetone · cyclomethicone · butylene glycol · PVP/eicosene copolymer · isohexadecane · fragrance · polyquarternium-37 · mineral oil · PPG-1-tridegeth-6 · cetyl palmitate · tribehenin · extracts of aloe, lanolin, cocoa butter, palm, chamomile, eucalyptus, and guava · cetyl alcohol · cetyl hydroxyethyl cellulose · distearyldimonium chloride · DMDM hydantoin · iodopropynyl butylcarbamate · disodium EDTA
**	**Bain de Soleil Orange Gelee** Pfizer Consumer	gel	4	octyl methoxycinnamate · octyl salicylate	mineral oil · petrolatum · paraffin · ozokerite · isopropyl myristate · fragrance · propylparaben · butylparaben · D&C red#17 · D&C yellow#10 aluminum lake

See Chapter 30, "Sunscreen and Suntan Products," for more information about these products.

SUNSCREEN AND SUNTAN PRODUCTS - continued

	Product Manufacturer/Supplier	Dosage Form	SPF Value	Sunscreen	Other Ingredients
**	**Bain de Soleil Sand Buster** Pfizer Consumer	oil	2	octyl methoxycinnamate · octyl salicylate	mineral oil · cyclomethicone · polybutene · coconut oil · lanolin oil · fragrance · extracts of aloe, lanolin, cocoa butter, eucalyptus, palm, chamomile, and guava · propylparaben · D&C red#17 · D&C violet#2
	Bain de Soleil SPF+Color Pfizer Consumer	lotion	8 ·15 ·30	octyl methoxycinnamate · octocrylene · oxybenzone	dihydroxyacetone
**	**Bain de Soleil Tropical Deluxe Tanning** Pfizer Consumer	lotion	4	octyl methoxycinnamate · octyl salicylate	water · mineral oil · stearic acid · cyclomethicone · butylene glycol · cetyl alcohol · fragrance · myristyl myristate · shea butter · triethanolamine · extracts of aloe, lanolin, cocoa butter, palm oil, chamomile, eucalyptus, and guava · glycol stearate · DMDM hydantoin · iodopropynyl butylcarbamate · carbomer · acrylates/C10-30 alkyl acrylate crosspolymer · disodium EDTA
PE	**Banana Boat Active Kids Sunblock** Sun Ph'cals	lotion	30 · 50	octyl methoxycinnamate · octocrylene (SPF50) · oxybenzone · octyl salicylate · titanium dioxide (SPF50)	
PE	**Banana Boat Baby Sunblock** Sun Ph'cals	lotion	50	octyl methoxycinnamate · oxybenzone · octocrylene · octyl salicylate · titanium dioxide	
	Banana Boat Deep Tanning Sun Ph'cals	oil	4	phenylbenzimidazole sulfonic acid	
**	**Banana Boat Faces Plus Sunblock, Normal/Combination Skin** Sun Ph'cals	lotion	23	octyl methoxycinnamate · oxybenzone · octyl salicylate	
**	**Banana Boat Faces Plus Sunscreen, Normal to Oily Skin** Sun Ph'cals	lotion	14	octyl methoxycinnamate · oxybenzone · octyl salicylate	
	Banana Boat Faces Sensitive Skin Sunblock Sun Ph'cals	lotion	15 · 23	octyl methoxycinnamate · oxybenzone · octyl salicylate	
	Banana Boat Faces Sunblock Spot Stick Sun Ph'cals	stick	30	octocrylene · homosalate · octyl methoxycinnamate · oxybenzone · octyl salicylate	
	Banana Boat Maximum Sunblock Sun Ph'cals	lotion	50	octyl methoxycinnamate · octocrylene · oxybenzone · octyl salicylate · titanium dioxide	
	Banana Boat Natural Chemical Free Sunblock Sun Ph'cals	lotion	25	titanium dioxide · zinc oxide	

See Chapter 30, "Sunscreen and Suntan Products," for more information about these products.

SUNSCREEN AND SUNTAN PRODUCTS - continued

	Product Manufacturer/Supplier	Dosage Form	SPF Value	Sunscreen	Other Ingredients
	Banana Boat Sport Sunblock Sun Ph'cals	lotion	15 · 50	octyl methoxycinnamate · octocrylene (SPF50) · oxybenzone · octyl salicylate · titanium dioxide (SPF50)	
	Banana Boat Sunscreen or Sunblock Sun Ph'cals	lotion	8 (Sunscreen) · 15 (Sunblock)	padimate O · oxybenzone · octyl methoxycinnamate (Sunblock)	
	Banana Boat Tanning Sun Ph'cals	oil	4 · 8	padimate O · octyl methoxycinnamate	
**	**Blistex DCT Daily Conditioning Treatment for Lips** Blistex	cream	20	octyl methoxycinnamate, 7.3% · benzophenone-3, 4.5%	petrolatum, 56.26% · aloe extract · cetyl alcohol · cocoa butter · flavor · lanolin · mixed waxes · phenol · vitamins A and E
	Blistex Lip Balm; Berry, Mint or Regular Blistex	stick	10	padimate O, 6.6% · oxybenzone, 2.5%	dimethicone, 2% · cocoa butter · color · flavor · isopropyl esters · lanolin · methylparaben · mineral oil · mixed waxes · petrolatum · propylparaben
**	**Blistex Lip Tone Lip Balm** Blistex	stick	15	octyl methoxycinnamate, 7.3% · menthyl anthranilate, 4%	dimethicone, 2% · abc extract · arginine · glycine · mixed waxes · petrolatum · vitamins A and E · color
	Blistex Ultra Protection Lip Balm Blistex	stick	30	octyl methoxycinnamate, 7.4% · oxybenzone, 5.2% · octyl salicylate, 5% · menthyl anthranilate, 4.8% · homosalate, 4.5%	dimethicone, 3% · flavors · isopropyl myristate · mixed waxes · myristyl myristate
	Bull Frog Chattem	gel	36	octyl methoxycinnamate, 7.5% · octocrylene, 10% · benzophenone-3, 3%	isostearyl alcohol
	Bull Frog Chattem	stick	18	octyl methoxycinnamate, 7.5% · benzophenone-3, 2.5%	isostearyl alcohol
PE	**Bull Frog for Kids** Chattem	gel	36	octyl methoxycinnamate, 7.5% · octocrylene, 10% · benzophenone-3, 3%	isostearyl alcohol
**	**Bull Frog Quik** Chattem	gel	18	octyl methoxycinnamate, 7.5% · octyl salicylate, 5% · benzophenone-3, 5%	SD alcohol 40
	Bull Frog Sport Chattem	lotion	18	octyl methoxycinnamate, 7.5% · octocrylene, 7% · octyl salicylate, 5% · benzophenone-3, 4% · titanium dioxide, 2%	
	Bull Frog Sunblock Chattem	gel	18	octyl methoxycinnamate, 7.5% · octocrylene, 7% · benzophenone-3, 2%	aloe extract · beeswax · cyclomethicone · fragrance · isostearyl alcohol · panthenol · silica · tocopheryl acetate

See Chapter 30, "Sunscreen and Suntan Products," for more information about these products.

SUNSCREEN AND SUNTAN PRODUCTS - continued

	Product Manufacturer/Supplier	Dosage Form	SPF Value	Sunscreen	Other Ingredients
**	**ChapStick Lip Moisturizer** Whitehall-Robins Healthcare	ointment · stick	15	octyl methoxycinnamate, 7.5% · oxybenzone, 3.5%	petrolatum, 40.7% (stick) or 33% (ointment) · aloe vera oil · carnauba wax (stick) · cetyl alcohol (stick) · fragrance · isocetyl stearate · isopropyl lanolate (stick) · isopropyl myristate (stick) · lanolin · methylparaben · microcrystalline wax (ointment) · paraffin wax (stick) · propylparaben · vitamin E acetate · vitamin E linoleate · white wax (stick)
	ChapStick Sunblock 15 Whitehall-Robins Healthcare	stick	15	padimate O, 7% · oxybenzone, 3%	petrolatum, 44% · cetyl alcohol, 0.5% · lanolin, 0.5% · isopropyl myristate, 0.5% · camphor · carnauba wax · D&C red#6 barium lake · FD&C yellow#5 aluminum lake · fragrance · isopropyl lanolate · methylparaben · mineral oil · propylparaben · titanium dioxide · paraffin wax · white wax
	ChapStick Sunblock 15 Petroleum Jelly Plus Whitehall-Robins Healthcare	ointment	15	padimate O, 7% · oxybenzone, 3%	white petrolatum, 89% · aloe · butylated · hydroxytoluene · flavor · lanolin · phenonip
**	**ChapStick Ultra** Whitehall-Robins Healthcare	stick	30	octocrylene, 10% · octyl methoxycinnamate, 7.5% · octyl salicylate, 5% · oxybenzone, 5%	white petrolatum, 30% · aloe vera oil · arachidyl propionate · carnauba wax · cetyl alcohol · fragrance · isopropyl lanolate · isopropyl myristate · lanolin · methylparaben · octyldodecanol · oleyl alcohol · paraffin wax · phenyl trimethicone · propylparaben · titanium dioxide · vitamin E acetate · vitamin E linoleate · white wax
	Coppertone Dry Schering-Plough HealthCare	oil	2	homosalate	
** PE	**Coppertone Kids Sunblock** Schering-Plough HealthCare	lotion	40	octyl methoxycinnamate · octyl salicylate · oxybenzone · homosalate	
PE	**Coppertone Kids Sunblock** Schering-Plough HealthCare	lotion	15 · 30	octyl methoxycinnamate · oxybenzone · octyl salicylate · homosalate (SPF 15)	
	Coppertone LipKote Sunblock Lip Balm Schering-Plough HealthCare	stick	15	octyl methoxycinnamate · oxybenzone	
	Coppertone Moisturizing Sunblock Schering-Plough HealthCare	lotion	30	octyl methoxycinnamate · oxybenzone · octyl salicylate · homosalate	
	Coppertone Moisturizing Sunblock Schering-Plough HealthCare	lotion	45	octyl methoxycinnamate · octyl salicylate · octocrylene · oxybenzone	
	Coppertone Moisturizing Sunblock or Suntan Schering-Plough HealthCare	lotion	4 (Suntan) · 15 (Sunblock)	octyl methoxycinnamate · oxybenzone	
	Coppertone Moisturizing Sunscreen Schering-Plough HealthCare	lotion	6 · 8	octyl methoxycinnamate · oxybenzone	
**	**Coppertone Oil-Free Sunblock** Schering-Plough HealthCare	lotion	4 · 8 · 15	octyl methoxycinnamate · oxybenzone	

See Chapter 30, "Sunscreen and Suntan Products," for more information about these products.

SUNSCREEN AND SUNTAN PRODUCTS - continued

	Product Manufacturer/Supplier	Dosage Form	SPF Value	Sunscreen	Other Ingredients
	Coppertone Protect & Tan Schering-Plough HealthCare	lotion	15 · 25	octyl methoxycinnamate · octyl salicylate · oxybenzone · homosalate	
**	**Coppertone Protect and Tan** Schering-Plough HealthCare	lotion	8	octyl methoxycinnamate · octyl salicylate · oxybenzone	
**	**Coppertone Skin Selects Dry Skin Sunblock** Schering-Plough HealthCare	lotion	15	octyl methoxycinnamate · oxybenzone	
**	**Coppertone Skin Selects Oily Skin Sunblock** Schering-Plough HealthCare	lotion	15	octyl methoxycinnamate · oxybenzone	
**	**Coppertone Skin Selects Sensitive Skin Sunblock** Schering-Plough HealthCare	lotion	15	titanium dioxide · octyl methoxycinnamate	
	Coppertone Sport Schering-Plough HealthCare	lotion	4 · 8 · 15 · 30	octyl methoxycinnamate · oxybenzone · octyl salicylate (SPF30)	
	Dermsol-30 Parnell Ph'cals	lotion	30	octyl methoxycinnamate, 7.5% · oxybenzone, 6.0% · octyl salicylate, 5.0%	octyldodecyl neopentanoate · glycerin · TEA stearate · DEA-cetyl phosphate · ceteth-25 · cetyl alcohol · laneth-25 · oleth-25 · steareth-25 · diazolidinyl urea · methylparaben · propylparaben · yerba santa · hyaluronic acid · hydrolyzed collagen · sodium PCA · carbomer
**	**DuraScreen** Schwarz Pharma	lotion	15	octyl methoxycinnamate · octyl salicylate · oxybenzone	algae extract · carbomer 940 · cetyl alcohol · chamomile · DEA cetyl phosphate · dimethicone · imidurea · isoarachidyl neopentanoate · methylparaben · PPG-12/SMDI copolymer · propylparaben · propylene glycol · purified water · sodium dehydroacetate · stearic acid · titanium dioxide · trolamine
**	**DuraScreen** Schwarz Pharma	lotion	30	octyl methoxycinnamate · octyl salicylate · oxybenzone · phenylbenzimidazole sulfonic acid · titanium dioxide	acrylates/C10-30 alkyl acrylate crosspolymer · aluminum stearate · ceteareth-20 · cetearyl alcohol · diazolidinyl urea · dimethicone · fluornalkyldimethicone (copolyol) · isoarachidyl neopentanoate · methylparaben · phenoxyethanol · PPG-12/SMDI copolymer · propylene glycol · propylparaben · purified water · shea butter · trimethylsiloxysilicate · trolamine · xanthan gum
**	**Facial Moisturizing Sunscreen** C & M Pharmacal	cream	20	octyl methoxycinnamate, 7.5% · benzophenone-4, 5%	purified water · dioctyl maleate · emulsifying wax · propylene glycol · glycerin · sodium lauryl sulfate · soluble collagen · DEA-cetyl phosphate · PVP/eicosene copolymer · benzyl alcohol · hydrolyzed elastin · magnesium aluminum silicate · titanium dioxide micronized · xanthan gum
**	**Full Body Sunscreen** C & M Pharmacal	lotion	15	octyl methoxycinnamate, 7.5% · benzophenone-4	purified water · dioctyl maleate · glycerin · PVP/eicosene · stearic acid · DEA-cetyl phosphate · cetyl alcohol · titanium dioxide · fragrance · methylparaben · carbomer 940 · triethanolamine · propylparaben

See Chapter 30, "Sunscreen and Suntan Products," for more information about these products.

SUNSCREEN AND SUNTAN PRODUCTS - continued

	Product Manufacturer/Supplier	Dosage Form	SPF Value	Sunscreen	Other Ingredients
PE	**Hawaiian Tropic Baby Faces Sunblock** Hawaiian Tropic	lotion	25	2-octyl p-methoxycinnamate · oxybenzone · menthyl anthranilate · octyl salicylate	
	Hawaiian Tropic Dark Tanning with Sunscreen Hawaiian Tropic	lotion	4	2-octyl p-methoxycinnamate · menthyl anthranilate	
**	**Hawaiian Tropic Facial Sunblock** Hawaiian Tropic	lotion	15	octyl methoxycinnamate · benzophenone-3 · octyl salicylate	
	Hawaiian Tropic Sunblock Hawaiian Tropic	lotion	15	2-octyl p-methoxycinnamate · oxybenzone · menthyl anthranilate	
	Hawaiian Tropic Sunblock Hawaiian Tropic	lotion	30	homosalate · octyl methoxycinnamate · benzophenone-3 · menthyl anthranilate · octyl salicylate	
**	**Hawaiian Tropic Tan Amplifier** Hawaiian Tropic	gel	2	phenylbenzimidazole sulfonic acid	
AL	**Herpecin-L Cold Sore Lip Balm** Campbell Labs	stick	15	padimate O · titanium dioxide	allantoin
PE	**Johnson's Baby Sunblock** Johnson & Johnson Consumer	lotion	30	octyl methoxycinnamate · octyl salicylate · oxybenzone · titanium dioxide	
	Lip Treatment Jelly Pfeiffer Ph'cals	jelly	15	padimate O · oxybenzone	petrolatum
	Mentholatum Lipbalm Mentholatum	stick	14	padimate O, 8%	petrolatum · camphor · fragrance · lanolin · menthol · mineral oil · ozokerite · dimethicone, 1%
**	**Mentholatum Lipbalm, Cherry Ice** Mentholatum	stick	12	padimate O, 8%	dimethicone, 1% · fragrance · lanolin · menthol · mineral oil · ozokerite · petrolatum
	Neutrogena Chemical-Free Sunblocker Neutrogena Dermatologics	lotion	17	titanium dioxide	
	Neutrogena Lip Moisturizer Neutrogena Dermatologics	stick	15	octyl methoxycinnamate, 7.5% · benzophenone-3, 4%	castor oil · corn oil · ozokerite · petrolatum · beeswax · octyl palmitate · paraffin · stearyl alcohol · carnauba · BHT
	Neutrogena Moisture for the Face, Tinted and Untinted Neutrogena Dermatologics	lotion	15	octyl methoxycinnamate, 7.5 % · oxybenzone, 5%	

See Chapter 30, "Sunscreen and Suntan Products," for more information about these products.

SUNSCREEN AND SUNTAN PRODUCTS - continued

	Product Manufacturer/Supplier	Dosage Form	SPF Value	Sunscreen	Other Ingredients
	Neutrogena Sunblock Neutrogena Dermatologics	cream	15	octyl methoxycinnamate · octyl salicylate · menthyl anthranilate	
	Neutrogena Sunblock Neutrogena Dermatologics	cream	30	octocrylene · octyl methoxycinnamate · menthyl anthranilate	
	Neutrogena Sunblock Neutrogena Dermatologics	stick	25	octyl methoxycinnamate · benzophenone-3 · octyl salicylate	
	Neutrogena Sunblock Neutrogena Dermatologics	cream	8	octyl methoxycinnamate · menthyl anthranilate	
	Nivea Hand Therapy Beiersdorf	lotion	15	octyl methoxycinnamate · phenylbenzimidazole sulfonic acid · oxybenzone	
	Nivea Sun Beiersdorf	lotion	15	octyl methoxycinnamate · octyl salicylate · benzophenone-3 · phenoxylbenzimidazole sulfonic acid	
FR	**Oil of Olay Daily UV Protectant Fragrance Free** Procter & Gamble	cream · lotion	15	octyl methoxycinnamate · phenylbenzimidazole sulfonic acid · titanium dioxide	water · isohexadecane · butylene glycol · triethanolamine · glycerin · stearic acid · cetyl alcohol · cetyl palmitate · DEA-cetyl phosphate · aluminum starch octenylsuccinate · imidazolidinyl urea · methylparaben · propylparaben · carbomer · acrylates/C10-30 alkyl acrylate crosspolymer · PEG-10 soya sterol · disodium EDTA · castor oil
	Oil of Olay Daily UV Protectant Original Procter & Gamble	cream · lotion	15	octyl methoxycinnamate · phenylbenzimidazole sulfonic acid · titanium dioxide	water · isohexadecane · butylene glycol · triethanolamine · glycerin · stearic acid · cetyl alcohol · cetyl palmitate · DEA-cetyl phosphate · aluminum starch octenylsuccinate · imidazolidinyl urea · methylparaben · propylparaben · carbomer · acrylates/C10-30 alkyl acrylate crosspolymer · PEG-10 soya sterol · disodium EDTA · castor oil · fragrance · FD&C red#4 · FD&C yellow#5
	PreSun 15 or 30 Active Westwood-Squibb Ph'cals	gel	15 · 30	benzophenone-3 · octyl methoxycinnamate · octyl salicylate	SD alcohol · PPG-15 stearyl ether · acrylates/t-octylpropenamide · hydroxypropylcellulose
	PreSun 15 Sensitive Skin Westwood-Squibb Ph'cals	lotion	15 · 29	octyl methoxycinnamate · benzophenone-3 · oxybenzone (29) · octyl salicylate	carbomer 940 · cetyl alcohol · DEA-cetyl phosphate · diazolidinyl urea · dimethicone · isopropyl myristate · isodecyl neopentanoate · kathon CG · PG dioctanoate · PVP/eicosene copolymer · stearic acid · triethanolamine · water
**	**PreSun 21** Westwood-Squibb Ph'cals	lotion	21	titanium dioxide	phenyl trimethicone · C12-15 alcohol benzoate · polyglyceryl-4-isostearate · cetyl dimethicone copolyol · hexyl laurate · isopropyl myristate · octyl dodecyl neopentanoate · propylene glycol · magnesium stearate · magnesium sulfate · sodium chloride · dioctyl sodium sulfosuccinate · diazolidinyl urea · dichlorobenzyl alcohol · BHT · aluminum hydroxide · lauric acid · water

See Chapter 30, "Sunscreen and Suntan Products," for more information about these products.

SUNSCREEN AND SUNTAN PRODUCTS - continued

	Product Manufacturer/Supplier	Dosage Form	SPF Value	Sunscreen	Other Ingredients
	PreSun 23 Westwood-Squibb Ph'cals	spray	23	octyl dimethyl PABA · octyl methoxycinnamate · benzophenone-3 · octyl salicylate	cyclomethicone · SD alcohol · C12-15 alcohol benzoate · PG dioctanoate · PVP/hexadecene copolymer
	PreSun 25 Moisturizing Westwood-Squibb Ph'cals	lotion	25	octyl methoxycinnamate · benzophenone-3 · octyl salicylate	dimethicone · diazolidinyl urea · carbomer 940 · triethanolamine · kathon CG · petrolatum · isopropyl myristate · PG dioctanoate · isodecyl neopentanoate · DEA-cetyl phosphate · PVP/eicosene copolymer · stearic acid · cetyl alcohol
	PreSun 46 Moisturizing Westwood-Squibb Ph'cals	lotion	46	octyl dimethyl PABA · benzophenone	carbomer 940 · cetyl alcohol · DEA-cetyl phosphate · diazolidinyl urea · dimethicone · isopropyl myristate · isodecyl neopentanoate · kathon CG · PG dioctanoate · PVP/eicosene copolymer · stearic acid · triethanolamine · fragrance · water
PE	**PreSun for Kids** Westwood-Squibb Ph'cals	lotion	29	octyl methoxycinnamate · octyl salicylate · benzophenone-3	carbomer 940 · cetyl alcohol · DEA-cetyl phosphate · diazolidinyl urea · dimethicone · isopropyl myristate · isodecyl neopentanoate · kathon CG · PG dioctanoate · PVP/eicosene copolymer · stearic acid · triethanolamine · water
PE	**PreSun for Kids** Westwood-Squibb Ph'cals	spray	23	octyl dimethyl PABA · octyl methoxycinnamate · benzophenone-3 · octyl salicylate	cyclomethicone · SD alcohol · C12-15 alcohol benzoate · PG dioctanoate · PVP/hexadecene copolymer
**	**RV Paque** ICN Ph'cals	cream	27	octyl methoxycinnamate, 7% · zinc oxide	sorbitol solution · purified water · cetyl alcohol · mineral oil · petrolatum · Arlacel 186 · sodium lauryl sulfate · yellow ochre · ceresin · white wax · iron oxide red
	Shade Sunblock Schering-Plough HealthCare	stick	30	octyl methoxycinnamate · octyl salicylate · oxybenzone · homosalate	
	Shade Sunblock Schering-Plough HealthCare	lotion	45	octyl methoxycinnamate · octyl salicylate · oxybenzone · octocrylene	
	Shade Sunblock Oil-Free Schering-Plough HealthCare	gel	30	octyl methoxycinnamate · homosalate · oxybenzone	SD alcohol 40, 73%
	Shade UVAGuard Schering-Plough HealthCare	lotion	15	octyl methoxycinnamate, 7.5% · avobenzone, 3% · oxybenzone, 3%	
	Softlips, Crystal Ice Mentholatum	stick	6	padimate O, 3%	petrolatum, 12% · BHT · camphor · ceresin · lanolin · dimethicone, 2% · menthol · squalene · vitamin E acetate
**	**Softlips, Sparkle Mint** Mentholatum	stick	7	padimate O, 3%	cetyl octanoate · dimethicone, 2% · fragrance · lanolin · menthol · ozokerite · petrolatum · squalene · vitamin E acetate
**	**Softlips, UV** Mentholatum	stick	17	octyl methoxycinnamate, 7.5% · padimate O, 7% · oxybenzone, 3%	butylated hydroxytoluene · dimethicone, 2% · lanolin · menthol · ozokerite · petrolatum · squalene · vitamin E acetate
**	**Solbar PF 50** Person & Covey	cream	50	oxybenzone · octyl methoxycinnamate · octocrylene	
	Solbar PF PABA Free Person & Covey	liquid	15	octyl methoxycinnamate, 7.5% · oxybenzone, 6%	SD alcohol 40, 76%

See Chapter 30, "Sunscreen and Suntan Products," for more information about these products.

SUNSCREEN AND SUNTAN PRODUCTS - continued

	Product Manufacturer/Supplier	Dosage Form	SPF Value	Sunscreen	Other Ingredients
	Solbar PF PABA Free Person & Covey	gel	30	octocrylene 10% · octyl methoxycinnamate, 7.5% · oxybenzone, 6%	SD alcohol 40
**	**Sport Sunblock** Goldline Labs	lotion	15	octyl methoxycinnamate · oxybenzone	
	Stay Moist Moisturizing Lip Conditioner Stanback	stick	15	padimate O, 7% · oxybenzone, 3%	petrolatums · isopropyl myristate · aloe vera oil · wax · flavor
**	**Stevens Sun Block** Stevens Skin	cream	15	octyl methoxycinnamate · benzophenone-3	deionized water · glyceryl stearate · PEG-100 stearate · C21-15 alkyl benzoate · glycerin · jojoba oil · apricot kernel oil · stearic acid · dimethyl stearamine · sweet almond oil · cetearyl octanoate · methyl gluceth-20 · castor oil · acrylates/octylacrylamide copolymer · squalene · dimethicone · panthenol · cetyl alcohol · cetyl palmitate · propylparaben · diazolidinyl urea · triethanolamine · methylparaben · butylparaben · fragrance · tocopherol · allantoin · tetrasodium EDTA · avocado oil · magnesium aluminum silicate · aloe vera gel
	Sundown Sunblock Johnson & Johnson Consumer	lotion	15	octyl methoxycinnamate · octyl salicylate · oxybenzone · titanium dioxide	
PE	**TI-Baby Natural** Fischer Ph'cals	lotion	16	titanium dioxide, 5%	
	TI-Screen Fischer Ph'cals	gel	20	octyl methoxycinnamate, 7.5% · oxybenzone, 5% · octyl salicylate, 5%	ethanol, 68%
	TI-Screen Fischer Ph'cals	lotion	15	octyl methoxycinnamate, 7.5% · oxybenzone, 3%	
	TI-Screen Fischer Ph'cals	lotion	30	octyl methoxycinnamate, 7.5% · octyl cyano diphenyl acrylate, 7.5% · oxybenzone, 6% · octyl salicylate, 5%	
	TI-Screen Lip Protectant Fischer Ph'cals	stick	15	octyl methoxycinnamate, 7.5% · oxybenzone, 5%	
	TI-Screen Natural Fischer Ph'cals	lotion	16	titanium dioxide, 5%	
	Tropical Blend Dark Tanning Schering-Plough HealthCare	lotion	4	octyl methoxycinnamate · oxybenzone	
	Tropical Blend Dark Tanning Schering-Plough HealthCare	oil	4	padimate O · oxybenzone	
	Tropical Blend Dark Tanning Schering-Plough HealthCare	lotion · oil	2	homosalate	
	Tropical Blend Dry Schering-Plough HealthCare	oil	2 · 4	homosalate · oxybenzone (SPF4)	

See Chapter 30, "Sunscreen and Suntan Products," for more information about these products.

SUNSCREEN AND SUNTAN PRODUCTS - continued

	Product Manufacturer/Supplier	Dosage Form	SPF Value	Sunscreen	Other Ingredients
	Tropical Blend Tan Magnifier Schering-Plough HealthCare	oil	2	triethanolamine salicylate	
	Vaseline Lip Therapy Balm, Advanced or Cherry Chesebrough-Pond's	stick	8	octyl methoxycinnamate · oxybenzone	white petrolatum · paraffin · hydrogenated castor oil · triisostearin esters · dimethicone · borage seed oil · sunflower seed oil · nylon-12 · tocopheryl acetate · bisabolol · retinyl palmitate · panthenol · aloe extract · kukui nut oil · lecithin · stearic acid · soya sterol · carnauba · corn oil · zinc sulfate · saccharin sodium · flavor
	Vaseline Lip Therapy, Advanced or Cherry Chesebrough-Pond's	ointment	8	octyl methoxycinnamate · oxybenzone	white petrolatum · borage seed oil · sunflower seed oil · tocopheryl acetate · bisabolol · retinyl palmitate · panthenol · aloe extract · kukui nut oil · lecithin · stearic acid · soya sterol · corn oil · zinc sulfate · flavor
PE	**Water Babies Little Licks Sunblock Lip Balm** Schering-Plough HealthCare	stick	30	octyl methoxycinnamate · oxybenzone · octyl salicylate	
PE	**Water Babies UVA/UVB Sunblock** Schering-Plough HealthCare	lotion	15	octyl methoxycinnamate · oxybenzone	
PE	**Water Babies UVA/UVB Sunblock** Schering-Plough HealthCare	lotion	30	octyl methoxycinnamate · octyl salicylate · homosalate	
PE	**Water Babies UVA/UVB Sunblock** Schering-Plough HealthCare	lotion	45	octyl methoxycinnamate · octyl salicylate · oxybenzone · octocrylene	

** New listing

See Chapter 30, "Sunscreen and Suntan Products," for more information about these products.

BURN AND SUNBURN PRODUCTS

	Product Manufacturer/Supplier	Dosage Form	Anesthetic	Antimicrobial	Other Ingredients
	A and D Ointment Schering-Plough HealthCare	effervescent tablet			vitamins A & D · cholecalciferol · fish liver oil · mineral oil · petrolatum · fragrance · paraffin
	ActiBath Soak Oatmeal Treatment Andrew Jergens	effervescent tablet			colloidal oatmeal, 20% · fumaric acid · sodium carbonate · lactose · sodium bicarbonate · PEG-150 · magnesium oxide · sucrose stearate
	Aerocaine Graham-Field	aerosol spray	benzocaine, 13.6%	benzethonium chloride, 0.5%	isobutane
	Aerotherm Graham-Field	aerosol spray	benzocaine, 13.6%	benzethonium chloride, 0.5%	isobutane
	Americaine First Aid Ciba Self-Medication	ointment	benzocaine, 20%	benzethonium chloride, 0.1%	PEG 300 · PEG 3350
	Americaine Topical Anesthetic Ciba Self-Medication	aerosol	benzocaine, 20%		isobutane · PEG 300 · propane
	Anti-Itch Blistex	lotion	pramoxine HCl, 1%	benzethonium chloride	dimethicone, 1% · glyceryl stearate · PEG-100 stearate · petrolatum · polysorbate 60 · polyquaternium-24 · water · sesame oil · stearic acid · stearyl alcohol
	Aveeno Bath Treatment Moisturizing Formula Rydelle Labs	powder			colloidal oatmeal, 43% · mineral oil
	Aveeno Bath Treatment Soothing Formula Rydelle Labs	powder			colloidal oatmeal, 100%
	Bactine First Aid Bayer Consumer	liquid · spray	lidocaine HCl, 2.5%	benzalkonium chloride, 0.13%	disodium edetate · fragrance · octoxynol 9 · propylene glycol · water
**	**Banana Boat Sooth-A-Caine** Sun Ph'cals	gel	lidocaine		menthol · SD alcohol 40, 5% · purified water · aloe vera gel · tocopherol · glycerin · polysorbate-20
	Bicozene External Analgesic Creme Sandoz Consumer	cream	benzocaine, 6%	resorcinol, 1.67%	stearic acid · glycerin · glyceryl monostearate · castor oil · triglycerol diisostearate · parachlorometaxylenol · sodium borate · ethanolamine stearates · polysorbate 80 · chlorothymol · fragrance · water
	Boil Ease Del Ph'cals	ointment	benzocaine, 5%	phenol	anhydrous lanolin · camphor · eucalyptus oil · ichthammol · juniper tar · menthol · paraffin · petrolatum · precipitated sulfur · rosin · sexadecyl alcohol · thymol · yellow wax · zinc oxide
	Burn-O-Jel S.S.S. Company	gel	lidocaine, 0.5%		menthol · aloe vera gel
	Burnamycin Pfeiffer Ph'cals	pump spray	lidocaine, 0.5%		aloe vera gel
	Burntame Otis Clapp & Son	spray	benzocaine, 20%	8-hydroxyquinoline	

See Chapter 31, "Burn and Sunburn Products," for more information about these products.

BURN AND SUNBURN PRODUCTS - continued

	Product Manufacturer/Supplier	Dosage Form	Anesthetic	Antimicrobial	Other Ingredients
	Butesin Picrate Abbott Labs	ointment	butamben picrate, 1%		anhydrous lanolin · ceresin wax · mineral oil · mixed triglycerides · methylparaben · propylparaben · potassium chloride · sodium borate · white wax
	Cala-gel Clearly Calamine Tec Labs	liquid		benzethonium chloride, 15%	diphenhydramine HCl, 1.8% · zinc acetate, 0.21% · menthol, 0.11%
**	**Delazinc** Mericon	ointment			zinc oxide, 25%
	Dermacoat Century Ph'cals	aerosol	benzocaine	chloroxylenol	menthol · propylene glycol
	Dermoplast Whitehall-Robins Healthcare	spray	benzocaine, 20%		menthol, 0.5% · acetylated lanolin alcohol · aloe vera gel · butane · cetyl acetate · hydrofluorocarbon · methylparaben · PEG-8 laurate · polysorbate 85
	Dibucaine Multisource	ointment	dibucaine, 1%		
**	**DML Lotion** Person & Covey	lotion	benzyl alcohol		petrolatum · PPG-2 · myristyl ether propionate · glyceryl stearate · glycerin · simethicone · silica · EDTA · sodium carbomer 1342
	Family Medic Tender	liquid · pump spray · wipe	lidocaine HCl, 2.5%	benzalkonium chloride, 0.13%	aloe vera gel, 80% · fragrance, 0.05%
**	**Family Medic Afterburn** Tender	gel	lidocaine HCl, 0.5%		aloe vera gel, 80%
**	**First Aid Cream** Johnson & Johnson Consumer	cream		cetylpyridinium chloride	water · cetyl alcohol · glyceryl stearate · isopropyl palmitate · stearyl alcohol · benzyl alcohol · synthetic beeswax · lapyrium chloride · hydroxypropyl methylcellulose · trisodium phosphate
**	**First Aid Medicated Powder** Johnson & Johnson Consumer	powder			zinc oxide · menthol · corn starch · dipropylene glycol · eucalyptol · thymol · methyl salicylate
	Foille Medicated First Aid Blistex	ointment	benzocaine, 5% · benzyl alcohol	chloroxylenol, 0.1% · oxyquinoline	calcium disodium EDTA · corn oil · fragrance · mixed waxes · water
	Foille Medicated First Aid Blistex	aerosol	benzocaine, 5% · benzyl alcohol	chloroxylenol, 0.6% · oxyquinoline	corn oil · fragrance · lecithin · water
	Foille Plus Blistex	aerosol	benzocaine, 5%	benzethonium chloride, 0.15%	water-washable base
	Foille Plus Medicated First Aid Blistex	cream	benzocaine, 5%	chloroxylenol, 0.4%	water-washable base BHA · carbomer 934 · cetyl alcohol · fragrance · isopropyl myristate · isopropyl palmitate · isopropyl stearate · methylparaben · mineral oil · polysorbate 60 · propylparaben · water · stearic acid · sorbitan tristearate · triethanolamine

See Chapter 31, "Burn and Sunburn Products," for more information about these products.

BURN AND SUNBURN PRODUCTS - continued

	Product Manufacturer/Supplier	Dosage Form	Anesthetic	Antimicrobial	Other Ingredients
	Gold Bond Medicated Anti-Itch Chattem	cream	lidocaine		menthol · cetearyl alcohol · DMDM hydantoin · eucalyptol · glyceryl stearate · methyl salicylate · methylparaben · petrolatum · propylene glycol · simethicone · sorbic acid · sorbitol · thymol · tocopherol · water · zinc oxide
	Itch-X B. F. Ascher	gel · pump spray	benzyl alcohol, 10% · pramoxine HCl, 1%		aloe vera gel
	Lagol Alvin Last	ointment	benzocaine, 5%		petrolatum · corn starch · allantoin
	Lanacane Combe	aerosol	benzocaine, 20%	benzethonium chloride, 0.1%	
	Medi-Quik First Aid Mentholatum	aerosol spray	lidocaine, 2%	benzalkonium chloride, 0.13%	camphor · benzyl alcohol · BHA · isobutane · isopropyl palmitate · methyl gluceth-20 sesquistearate · methyl glucose sesquistearate · phosphoric acid · polyglyceryl-6 distearate · water
	Medicated First Aid Burn Blistex	cream	benzocaine, 5%	chloroxylenol, 0.4%	BHA · carbomer 934 · cetyl alcohol · fragrance · isopropyl myristate · isopropyl palmitate · isopropyl stearate · methylparaben · mineral oil · polysorbate 60 · propylparaben · water · stearic acid · sorbitan tristearate · triethanolamine
	Neosporin Plus Maximum Strength Warner Wellcome Consumer	ointment	lidocaine, 40mg/g		polymyxin B sulfate, 10000 IU/g · bacitracin zinc, 500 IU/g · neomycin base, 3.5mg/g · white petrolatum
	Neosporin Plus Maximum Strength Warner Wellcome Consumer	cream	lidocaine, 40mg/g		polymyxin B sulfate, 10000 IU/g · neomycin base, 3.5mg/g · methylparaben, 0.25% · emulsifying wax · mineral oil · poloxamer 188 · purified water · white petrolatum
PE	**No More Burn** Johnson & Johnson Consumer	pump spray	lidocaine HCl, 2.3%	benzethonium chloride, 0.13%	
PE	**No More Ouchies** Johnson & Johnson Consumer	pump spray	lidocaine HCl, 2.3%	benzethonium chloride, 0.13%	
	Outgro Pain Relieving Whitehall-Robins Healthcare	liquid	benzocaine, 20%		alcohol, 61.3% · D&C yellow#10 · FD&C blue#1 · FD&C red#40 · PEG-8
	Pramegel GenDerm	gel	pramoxine HCl, 1% · benzyl alcohol		menthol, 0.5% · carbomer 940 · methyl gluceth-20 · SD alcohol 40 · sodium hydroxide · water
	Prax Ferndale Labs	lotion	pramoxine HCl, 1%		hydrophilic base
**	**Solarcaine Aloe Extra Burn Relief** Schering-Plough HealthCare	cream	lidocaine, 0.5%		aloe extract
**	**Solarcaine Aloe Extra Burn Relief Gel or Mist** Schering-Plough HealthCare	gel · pump spray	lidocaine HCl, 0.5%		aloe vera gel · isopropyl alcohol, 0.05%

See Chapter 31, "Burn and Sunburn Products," for more information about these products.

BURN AND SUNBURN PRODUCTS - continued

Product Manufacturer/Supplier	Dosage Form	Anesthetic	Antimicrobial	Other Ingredients
Solarcaine Medicated First Aid Schering-Plough HealthCare	aerosol spray	benzocaine, 20%		SD alcohol, 35% · triclosan, 0.13% · propellants
Tronothane Hydrochloride Abbott Labs	cream	pramoxine HCl, 1%		cetyl alcohol · glycerin sodium · lauryl sulfate · methylparaben · propylparaben · cetyl esters wax
Unguentine Mentholatum	ointment		phenol, 1%	eucalyptus oil · oleostearine · petrolatum · thyme oil · zinc oxide
Unguentine Plus Mentholatum	cream	lidocaine HCl, 2%	phenol, 0.5%	fragrance · glyceryl stearate · isoceteth-20 · isopropyl palmitate · methylparaben · mineral oil · poloxamer 407 · propylparaben · quaternium-15 · sorbitan stearate · tetrasodium EDTA · water
Vaseline Medicated Anti-Bacterial Petroleum Jelly Chesebrough-Pond's	ointment		chloroxylenol, 0.53% · phenol	petrolatum, 98.3% · lanolin · beta carotene

** New listing

See Chapter 31, "Burn and Sunburn Products," for more information about these products.

POISON IVY, OAK, AND SUMAC PRODUCTS

	Product Manufacturer/Supplier	Dosage Form	Hydro-cortisone	Antipruritic/ Anesthetic	Antihistamine	Astringent	Other Ingredients
	ActiBath Soak Oatmeal Treatment Andrew Jergens	effervescent tablet		colloidal oatmeal, 20%			fumaric acid · sodium carbonate · lactose · sodium bicarbonate · PEG-150 · magnesium oxide · sucrose stearate
	Anti-Itch Blistex	lotion		pramoxine HCl, 1%			dimethicone, 1% · benzethonium chloride · glyceryl stearate · PEG-100 stearate · petrolatum · polysorbate 60 · polyquaternium-24 · water · sesame oil · stearic acid · stearyl alcohol
	Aveeno Anti-Itch Rydelle Labs	cream · lotion		pramoxine HCl, 1% · camphor, 0.3% · oatmeal flour		calamine, 3%	glycerin · distearyldimonium chloride · petrolatum · isopropyl palmitate · 1-hexadecanol · dimethicone · sodium chloride
	Aveeno Bath Treatment Moisturizing Formula Rydelle Labs	powder		colloidal oatmeal, 43%			mineral oil
	Aveeno Bath Treatment Soothing Formula Rydelle Labs	powder		colloidal oatmeal, 100%			
	Aveeno Moisturizing Rydelle Labs	cream · lotion		colloidal oatmeal, 1% · benzyl alcohol			glycerin · distearyldimonium chloride · petrolatum · isopropyl palmitate · dimethicone · sodium chloride · cetyl alcohol
	Bactine Hydrocortisone 1% Bayer Consumer	cream	1%			cetearyl alcohol	aluminum sulfate · beeswax · calcium acetate · dextrin · glycerin · hydrocortisone alcohol · light mineral oil · methylparaben · water · sodium lauryl sulfate · white petrolatum
**	**Benadryl Itch Stopping Extra Strength** Warner Wellcome Consumer	gel		camphor	diphenhydramine HCl, 2%	zinc acetate, 1% · SD alcohol 38B	citric acid · diazolidinyl urea · glycerin · hydroxypropyl methylcellulose · methylparaben · propylene glycol · propylparaben · sodium citrate · purified water
**	**Benadryl Itch Stopping Extra Strength** Warner Wellcome Consumer	stick			diphenhydramine HCl, 2%	alcohol, 73.5% · zinc acetate, 0.1%	glycerin · povidone · tromethamine

See Chapter 32, "Poison Ivy, Oak, and Sumac Products," for more information about these products.

POISON IVY, OAK, AND SUMAC PRODUCTS - continued

	Product Manufacturer/Supplier	Dosage Form	Hydro-cortisone	Antipruritic/ Anesthetic	Antihistamine	Astringent	Other Ingredients
	Benadryl Itch Stopping Extra Strength Warner Wellcome Consumer	spray			diphenhydramine HCl, 2%	alcohol, 73.5% · zinc acetate, 0.1%	glycerin · povidone · tromethamine
	Benadryl Itch Stopping Extra Strength Warner Wellcome Consumer	cream			diphenhydramine HCl, 2%	zinc acetate, 0.1% · cetyl alcohol	diazolidinyl urea · methylparaben · polyethylene glycol monostearate 1000 · propylene glycol · propylparaben · purified water
**	**Benadryl Itch Stopping Regular Strength** Warner Wellcome Consumer	cream			diphenhydramine HCl, 1%	zinc acetate, 0.1% · cetyl alcohol	diazolidinyl urea · methylparaben · polyethylene glycol monostearate 1000 · propylene glycol · propylparaben
**	**Benadryl Itch Stopping Regular Strength** Warner Wellcome Consumer	spray			diphenhydramine HCl, 1%	alcohol, 73.6% · zinc acetate, 0.1%	glycerin · povidone · tromethamine · purified water
**	**Benadryl Itch Stopping Regular Strength** Warner Wellcome Consumer	gel		camphor	diphenhydramine HCl, 1%	zinc acetate, 1% · SD alcohol 38B	citric acid · diazolidinyl urea · glycerin · hydroxypropyl methylcellulose · methylparaben · propylene glycol · propylparaben · sodium citrate
	Bluboro Allergan	powder					aluminum sulfate, 53.9% · calcium acetate, 43% · boric acid · FD&C blue#1
**	**Blue Star** McCue	ointment		camphor			salicylic acid · benzoic acid · methyl salicylate · lanolin oil · petrolatum
	Buro-Sol Antiseptic Doak Dermatologics	powder				aluminum acetate, 0.23%	sodium diacetate, 48.8% · benzethonium chloride, 4.4%
	Cala-gel Clearly Calamine Tec Labs	gel		menthol, 0.11%	diphenhydramine HCl, 1.8%	zinc acetate, 0.21%	benzethonium chloride, 0.15% · purified water · polysorbate 20 · hydroxypropyl methylcellulose · disodium EDTA · fragrance
	Cala-gen Clear Goldline Labs	solution			diphenhydramine HCl, 1%	zinc oxide, 2%	
	Caladryl Warner Wellcome Consumer	lotion		pramoxine HCl, 1%		calamine, 8% · SD alcohol 38B	propylene glycol · polysorbate 80 · xanthan gum · hydroxypropyl methylcellulose · fragrance · diazolidinyl urea · methylparaben · propylparaben

See Chapter 32, "Poison Ivy, Oak, and Sumac Products," for more information about these products.

POISON IVY, OAK, AND SUMAC PRODUCTS - continued

	Product Manufacturer/Supplier	Dosage Form	Hydro-cortisone	Antipruritic/ Anesthetic	Antihistamine	Astringent	Other Ingredients
	Caladryl Warner Wellcome Consumer	cream		pramoxine HCl, 1%		calamine, 8% · cetyl alcohol	propylene glycol · polysorbate 60 · sorbitan stearate · soya sterol · cyclomethicone · fragrance · diazolidinyl urea · methylparaben · camphor · propylparaben · purified water
	Caladryl Clear Warner Wellcome Consumer	lotion		pramoxine HCl, 1%		zinc acetate, 0.1% · SD alcohol 38B	camphor · polysorbate 40 · glycerin · fragrance · sodium citrate · citric acid · diazolidinyl urea · hydroxypropyl methylcellulose · methylparaben · propylene glycol · propylparaben · purified water
**	**Calamycin** Pfeiffer Ph'cals	pump spray		pramoxine HCl, 1%		zinc acetate, 0.1%	
	CaldeCORT Ciba Self-Medication	cream	1%				cetostearyl alcohol · sodium lauryl sulfate · white petrolatum · propylene glycol · purified water
**	**Cortaid FastStick** Pharmacia & Upjohn	stick	1%			alcohol, 55%	butylated hydroxytoluene · methylparaben · purified water
	Cortaid Maximum Strength Pharmacia & Upjohn	spray	1%			alcohol, 55%	glycerin · methylparaben · water
	Cortaid Maximum Strength Pharmacia & Upjohn	cream	1%			cetyl alcohol	glycerin · methylparaben · water · aloe · ceteareth-20 · cetyl palmitate · isopropyl myristate · isopropyl pentanoate
	Cortaid Sensitive Skin Formula Pharmacia & Upjohn	cream	0.5%				aloe · butylparaben · cetyl palmitate · glyceryl stearate · methylparaben · polyethylene glycol · stearamidoethyl diethylamine · water
	Cortaid Sensitive Skin Formula Pharmacia & Upjohn	ointment	0.5%				aloe · butylparaben · cholesterol · methylparaben · mineral oil · white petrolatum · microcrystalline wax
	Cortizone-10 Thompson Medical	ointment	1%				white petrolatum

See Chapter 32, "Poison Ivy, Oak, and Sumac Products," for more information about these products.

POISON IVY, OAK, AND SUMAC PRODUCTS - continued

	Product Manufacturer/Supplier	Dosage Form	Hydro-cortisone	Antipruritic/ Anesthetic	Antihistamine	Astringent	Other Ingredients
	Cortizone-10 Thompson Medical	cream	1%				aluminum sulfate · calcium acetate · glycerin · light mineral oil · methylparaben · propylparaben · potato dextrin · sodium lauryl sulfate · water · white petrolatum · white wax · aloe · cetyl alcohol
	Cortizone-5 Thompson Medical	cream	0.5%				glycerin · mineral oil · white petrolatum · propylparaben · methylparaben · aluminum sulfate · calcium acetate · potato dextrin · sodium lauryl sulfate · water · white wax · aloe · cetyl alcohol
	Cortizone-5 Thompson Medical	ointment	0.5%				white petrolatum · aloe
PE	**Cortizone-5 for Kids** Pfizer Consumer	cream	0.5%				aloe vera gel · aluminum sulfate · calcium acetate · cetearyl alcohol · glycerin · light mineral oil · methylparaben · potato dextrin · propylparaben · sodium C12-15 alcohols sulfate · sodium lauryl sulfate · water · white petrolatum
	Dermamycin Pfeiffer Ph'cals	cream			diphenhydramine HCl, 1%		
	Dermamycin Pfeiffer Ph'cals	pump spray		menthol, 1%	diphenhydramine HCl, 2%		
	Dermapax Recsei Labs	spray		benzyl alcohol, 1%	diphenhydramine HCl, 0.5%	isopropyl alcohol, 35%	chlorobutanol, 1%
	Dermarest Del Ph'cals	gel			diphenhydramine HCl, 2%		
	Dermarest DriCort Del Ph'cals	cream	1%				
	Dermarest Plus Del Ph'cals	gel		menthol, 1%	diphenhydramine HCl, 2%		
	DermiCort Republic Drug	cream	1%				greaseless base
	Dermoplast Whitehall-Robins Healthcare	spray		benzocaine, 20% · menthol, 0.5%		alcohol	acetylated lanolin · aloe vera gel · butane · cetyl acetate · hydrofluorocarbon · methylparaben · PEG-8 laurate · polysorbate 85
	Dermtex Pfeiffer Ph'cals	pump spray	1%	menthol, 1%			

See Chapter 32, "Poison Ivy, Oak, and Sumac Products," for more information about these products.

POISON IVY, OAK, AND SUMAC PRODUCTS - continued

	Product Manufacturer/Supplier	Dosage Form	Hydro-cortisone	Antipruritic/ Anesthetic	Antihistamine	Astringent	Other Ingredients
	Dermtex HC Pfeiffer Ph'cals	cream	1%				aloe vera gel
	Di-Delamine Del Ph'cals	gel · spray		menthol, 0.1%	diphenhydramine HCl, 1% · tripelennamine HCl, 0.5%		benzalkonium chloride, 0.12%
**	**Dickinson's Witch Hazel Formula** E. E. Dickinson	liquid				witch hazel distillate · witch hazel extract · alcohol, 14%	water
	Domeboro Bayer Consumer	powder					aluminum sulfate, 1191mg · calcium acetate, 938mg · dextrin
	FoilleCort Blistex	cream	0.5%			cetyl alcohol	BHA · carbomer 934 · fragrance · isopropyl palmitate · isopropyl myristate · isopropyl stearate · methylparaben · mineral oil · polysorbate 60 · propylparaben · purified water · stearic acid · sorbitan tristearate · triethanolamine
	Gold Bond Medicated Anti-Itch Chattem	cream		lidocaine · menthol	methyl salicylate	cetearyl alcohol · zinc oxide	DMDM hydantoin · eucalyptol · glyceryl stearate · methylparaben · petrolatum · propylene glycol · simethicone · sorbic acid · sorbitol · thymol · tocopherol · water
	Gold Bond Medicated, Regular or Extra Strength Chattem	powder		menthol	methyl salicylate	zinc oxide	boric acid · eucalyptol · salicylic acid · talc · thymol · zinc stearate
	HC-DermaPax Recsei Labs	spray	0.5%	benzyl alcohol, 1%	diphenhydramine HCl, 0.5%		isopropanol, 35%
**	**Hydrosal** Hydrosal	ointment			diphenhydramine HCl, 1%	zinc oxide	aloe · D&C red#33 · lanolin · mineral oil · petrolatum · water · sorbitan sesquioleate · ceresin wax
	Itch-X B. F. Ascher	gel · pump spray		benzyl alcohol, 10% · pramoxine HCl, 1%			aloe vera gel
	Ivarest 8-Hour Medicated Blistex	cream			diphenhydramine HCl, 2%	calamine, 14%	fragrance · hydroxyethylcellulose · lanolin oil · petrolatum · polysorbate 60 · propylene glycol · purified water · sorbitan stearate

See Chapter 32, "Poison Ivy, Oak, and Sumac Products," for more information about these products.

POISON IVY, OAK, AND SUMAC PRODUCTS - continued

	Product Manufacturer/Supplier	Dosage Form	Hydro-cortisone	Antipruritic/ Anesthetic	Antihistamine	Astringent	Other Ingredients
	Kericort 10 Bristol-Myers Products	cream	1%			stearyl alcohol · cetyl alcohol	citric acid, anhydrous · sodium citrate · methylparaben · sorbic acid · polyoxyl 40 stearate · glyceryl stearate · white wax · isopropyl myristate · sorbitan monostearate · polysorbate 60 · propylparaben · propylene glycol
	Lanacane Combe	spray		benzocaine, 20%			benzethonium chloride
	Lanacane Creme Combe	cream		benzocaine, 6%			benzethonium chloride
	Lanacort 10 Combe	cream · ointment	1%				
	Lanacort 5 Combe	ointment	0.5%				lanolin alcohols · aloe · petrolatum
	Lanacort 5 Combe	cream	0.5%				aloe · methylparaben · propylparaben
PE	**No More Itchies** Johnson & Johnson Consumer	pump spray	1%			SD alcohol 40-B, 45%	
	Nutra Soothe Oatmeal Bath Brimms Labs	powder		colloidal oatmeal 100%			
**	**Ostiderm** Pedinol Pharmacal	paste		phenol · camphor		zinc oxide	water · glycerin · sorbitol · magnesium carbonate · bentonite 670 · cabosil · acetic acid · kelcoloid HVF · Tween 20 · aluminum sulfate · calcium carbonate · fragrance · Thomasett Nu color blend
**	**Ostiderm Roll-on** Pedinol Pharmacal	lotion		phenol · camphor			water · SD alcohol 40 · aluminum chlorohydrate · glycerin · sorbitol · propylene glycol · aluminum sulfate · calcium carbonate · bentonite · hydroxypropyl cellulose · polysorbate-20 · fragrance · EDTA · diazolidinyl urea · sodium benzoate · potassium sorbate
	Pedi-Boro Soak Paks Pedinol Pharmacal	powder					aluminum sulfate · calcium acetate
	Pramegel GenDerm	gel		pramoxine HCl, 1% · menthol, 0.5% · benzyl alcohol		SD alcohol 40	carbomer 940 · methyl gluceth-20 · sodium hydroxide · water

See Chapter 32, "Poison Ivy, Oak, and Sumac Products," for more information about these products.

POISON IVY, OAK, AND SUMAC PRODUCTS - continued

	Product Manufacturer/Supplier	Dosage Form	Hydro-cortisone	Antipruritic/ Anesthetic	Antihistamine	Astringent	Other Ingredients
	Preparation H Hydrocortisone 1% Anti-Itch Whitehall-Robins Healthcare	cream	1%				BHA · cellulose gum · citric acid · disodium EDTA · glycerin · glyceryl oleate · glyceryl stearate · lanolin · methylparaben · petrolatum · propyl gallate · propylene glycol · propylparaben · cetyl alcohol · stearyl alcohol · simethicone · sodium benzoate · sodium lauryl sulfate · water · xanthan gum
**	**Resinol Medicated** Mentholatum	ointment		resorcinol, 2%		zinc oxide, 12% · calamine, 6%	lanolin · petrolatum · starch
	Rhuli Rydelle Labs	spray		benzocaine, 5% · camphor, 0.7% · benzyl alcohol		alcohol, 70% · calamine, 13.8%	hydrated silica · isobutane · isopropyl · sorbitan trioleate · oleyl alcohol
	Rhuli Rydelle Labs	gel		benzyl alcohol, 2% · menthol, 0.3% · camphor, 0.3%		SD alcohol 23A, 31%	propylene glycol · carbomer 940 · triethanolamine · benzophenone-4 · EDTA
	Sarna Stiefel Labs	lotion		camphor, 0.5% · menthol, 0.5%			
	Tronothane Hydrochloride Abbott Labs	cream		pramoxine HCl, 1%		cetyl alcohol	glycerin · sodium lauryl sulfate · methylparaben · propylparaben · cetyl esters wax
	Witch Hazel T. N. Dickinson					distilled witch hazel extract, 86% · alcohol, 14%	

** New listing

See Chapter 32, "Poison Ivy, Oak, and Sumac Products," for more information about these products.

PEDICULICIDE PRODUCTS

	Product Manufacturer/Supplier	Dosage Form	Active Ingredients	Other Ingredients
**	**A-200 Lice Control for Dogs and Household** Hogil Ph'cal	aerosol spray	permethrin, 0.5%	
**	**A-200 Lice Killing** Hogil Ph'cal	gel	piperonyl butoxide, 4% · pyrethrum extract, 0.33%	
	A-200 Lice Killing Hogil Ph'cal	shampoo	piperonyl butoxide, 4% · pyrethrum extract, 0.33%	benzyl alcohol · C13-C14 isoparaffin · isopropyl alcohol · fragrance · octylphenoxypolyethoxyenthanol · water · packaged with patented nit comb
**	**A-200 Lice Treatment Kit** Hogil Ph'cal	shampoo · aerosol spray	piperonyl butoxide, 4% (shampoo) · pyrethrum extract, 0.33% (shampoo) · permethrin, 0.5% (spray)	packaged with patented nit comb
	Barc Del Ph'cals	liquid	piperonyl butoxide, 2.2% · pyrethrins, 0.18%	
	End-Lice Thompson Medical	liquid	piperonyl butoxide, 4% · pyrethrins, 0.33%	benzyl alcohol · C13-C14 isoparaffin · polyoxyethylene (1,1,3,3,-tetramethylbutylphenyl ether) · water
	InnoGel Plus Hogil Ph'cal	gel	piperonyl butoxide, 4% · pyrethrum extract, 0.33%	carbomer 934 · D&C red#33 · FD&C blue#1 · water · benzyl alcohol · C13-C14 isoparaffin · isopropyl alcohol
	Lice Treatment Goldline Labs	liquid	piperonyl butoxide technical, 3% · pyrethrins, 0.3%	petroleum distillate
	Lice Treatment Kit Goldline Labs	liquid · aerosol spray	resmethrin-cyclopropanecarboxylate, 0.5%	packaged with nit comb
**	**Licetrol** Republic Drug	shampoo	piperonyl butoxide technical, 4% · pyrethrum extract, 0.33%	inert, 95.67%
	Licetrol 600 Republic Drug	liquid	piperonyl butoxide, 3% · pyrethrins, 0.3%	
	Licide Reese Chemical	shampoo	piperonyl butoxide, 3% · pyrethrins, 0.3%	benzyl alcohol, 2.4%
	Licide Reese Chemical	spray	piperonyl butoxide, 1% · pyrethrins, 0.2%	
	Licide Blue Reese Chemical	gel	pyrethrins, 0.2%	
	Nix Warner Wellcome Consumer	cream rinse	permethrin, 1%	isopropyl alcohol, 20% · balsam canada · cetyl alcohol · citric acid · FD&C yellow#6 · fragrance · hydrolyzed animal protein · hydroxyethylcellulose · polyoxyethylene 10 cetyl ether · propylene glycol · stearalkonium chloride · methylparaben · propylparaben · packaged with nit comb
	Pronto Lice Killing Del Ph'cals	shampoo	piperonyl butoxide, 4% · pyrethrins, 0.33%	
**	**Pronto Lice Killing** Del Ph'cals	aerosol spray	pyrethrins, 0.4%	inert, 99.6%
	R&C Shampoo Block Drug	shampoo	piperonyl butoxide, 3% · pyrethrins, 0.33%	C-13-14 isoparaffin · fragrance · isocetyl alcohol · isopropyl alcohol · lauramine oxide · laureth-4 · laureth-23 · petroleum distillate · polyquaternium · TEA-lauryl sulfate · water

See Chapter 33, "Insect Sting and Bite Products," for more information about these products.

PEDICULICIDE PRODUCTS - continued

	Product Manufacturer/Supplier	Dosage Form	Active Ingredients	Other Ingredients
	R&C Spray Block Drug	spray	pyrethrins, 0.4%	inert, 99.6%
**	**RID Lice Control for Dogs and Household** Pfizer Consumer	aerosol spray	permethrin, 0.5%	inert, 99.5%
**	**RID Lice Elimination Kit** Pfizer Consumer	aerosol spray · shampoo	permethrin, 0.5% (spray) · piperonyl butoxide, 4% · pyrethrum, 0.33% (shampoo)	spray: inert, 99.5% · shampoo: C13-C14 isoparaffin · fragrance · isopropyl alcohol · PEG-25 hydrogenated castor oil · water · xanthan gum
	RID Lice Killing Pfizer Consumer	shampoo	piperonyl butoxide, 4% · pyrethrum, 0.33%	C13-C14 isoparaffin · fragrance · isopropyl alcohol · PEG-25 hydrogenated castor oil · water · xanthan gum
**	**Tegrin-LT Lice Treatment** Block Drug	shampoo · conditioner	piperonyl butoxide, 3% · pyrethrum extract, 0.33%	inert, 96.67% · packaged with nit comb
	Tisit Pfeiffer Ph'cals	liquid	piperonyl butoxide, 2% · pyrethrins, 0.3%	
	Tisit Pfeiffer Ph'cals	shampoo	piperonyl butoxide, 3% · pyrethrins, 0.3%	benzyl alcohol, 2.4% · petroleum distillate, 1.2%
	Tisit Blue Pfeiffer Ph'cals	gel	piperonyl butoxide, 3% · pyrethrins, 0.3%	petroleum distillate, 1.2%

** New listing

See Chapter 33, "Insect Sting and Bite Products," for more information about these products.

INSECT STING AND BITE PRODUCTS

	Product Manufacturer/Supplier	Dosage Form	Antipruritic/Anesthetic/Counterirritant	Hydrocortisone	Other Ingredients
	ActiBath Soak Oatmeal Treatment Andrew Jergens	effervescent tablet	colloidal oatmeal, 20%		fumaric acid · sodium carbonate · lactose · sodium bicarbonate · PEG-150 · magnesium oxide · sucrose stearate
	Aerocaine Graham-Field	aerosol spray	benzocaine, 13.6%		benzethonium chloride, 0.5% · isobutane
	After-Bite Tender	liquid · wipe	ammonia, 3.6%		
	Americaine First Aid Ciba Self-Medication	ointment	benzocaine, 20%		benzethonium chloride · PEG-300 · PEG-3350
	Americaine Topical Anesthetic Ciba Self-Medication	aerosol spray	benzocaine, 20%		isobutane · PEG-300 · propane
	Anti-Itch Blistex	lotion	pramoxine HCl, 1%		dimethicone, 1% · benzethonium chloride · glyceryl stearate · PEG-100 stearate · petrolatum · polysorbate 60 · polyquaternium-24 · water · sesame oil · stearic acid · stearyl alcohol
	Aveeno Anti-Itch Rydelle Labs	cream · lotion	pramoxine HCl, 1% · camphor, 0.3% · oatmeal flour		calamine, 3% · glycerin · distearyldimonium chloride · petrolatum · isopropyl palmitate · 1-hexadecanol · dimethicone · sodium chloride
	Bactine Antiseptic/Anesthetic First Aid Bayer Consumer	spray	lidocaine HCl, 2.5%		benzalkonium chloride, 0.13% · disodium edetate · fragrance · octoxynol 9 · propylene glycol · water
	Bactine Hydrocortisone 1% Bayer Consumer	cream		1%	aluminum sulfate · beeswax · calcium acetate · cetearyl alcohol · dextrin · glycerin · hydrocortisone alcohol · light mineral oil · methylparaben · water · sodium lauryl sulfate · white petrolatum
	Bicozene External Analgesic Creme Sandoz Consumer	cream	benzocaine, 6% · resorcinol, 1.67%		stearic acid · glycerin · glyceryl monostearate · castor oil · triglycerol diisostearate · parachlorometaxylenol · sodium borate · ethanolamine stearates · polysorbate 80 · chlorothymol · fragrance · water
	Bluboro Allergan	powder			aluminum sulfate, 53.9% · calcium acetate, 43% · boric acid · FD&C blue#1
**	**Blue Star** McCue	ointment	camphor		salicylic acid · benzoic acid · methyl salicylate · lanolin oil · petrolatum
	Burnamycin Pfeiffer Ph'cals	pump spray	lidocaine, 5%		aloe vera gel
	Buro-Sol Antiseptic Doak Dermatologics	powder	aluminum acetate, 46.8%		sodium diacetate, 0.23% · benzethonium chloride, 4.4%
	Cala-gel Clearly Calamine Tec Labs	gel	menthol, 0.11%		diphenhydramine HCl, 1.8% · zinc acetate, 0.21% · benzethonium chloride, 0.15%

See Chapter 33, "Insect Sting and Bite Products," for more information about these products.

INSECT STING AND BITE PRODUCTS - continued

	Product Manufacturer/Supplier	Dosage Form	Antipruritic/Anesthetic/Counterirritant	Hydrocortisone	Other Ingredients
	Caladryl [b] Warner Wellcome Consumer	cream	pramoxine HCl, 1%		calamine, 8% · cetyl alcohol · propylene glycol · polysorbate 60 · sorbitan stearate · soya sterol · cyclomethicone · diazolidinyl urea · methylparaben · fragrance · camphor
	Caladryl [b] Warner Wellcome Consumer	lotion	pramoxine HCl, 1%		calamine, 8% · propylene glycol · polysorbate 80 · SD alcohol 38B · xanthan gum · hydroxypropyl methylcellulose · fragrance · diazolidinyl urea · methylparaben · propylparaben · camphor
	Caladryl Clear [b] Warner Wellcome Consumer	lotion	pramoxine HCl, 1%		SD alcohol 38B, 2.5% · zinc acetate, 0.1% · camphor · polysorbate 40 · glycerin · fragrance · sodium citrate · citric acid · diazolidinyl urea · hydroxypropyl methylcellulose · methylparaben · propylene glycol · propylparaben · purified water
	Chigger-Tox Scherer Labs	liquid	benzocaine, 2.1%		isopropyl alcohol, 53% · benzyl benzoate, 21.4% · soft soap, 21.4%
	Chiggerex Scherer Labs	ointment	benzocaine, 2%		pegosperse 100, 12% · camphor, 0.008% · olive oil, 0.008% · menthol, 0.005% · peppermint oil, 0.005% · methylparaben, 0.002% · clove oil, 0.002% · aloe vera
**	**Cortaid FastStick** Pharmacia & Upjohn	stick		1%	alcohol, 55% · butylated hydroxytoluene · glycerin · methylparaben · purified water
	Cortaid Maximum Strength Pharmacia & Upjohn	cream		1%	cetyl alcohol · glycerin · methylparaben · purified water · aloe · ceteareth-20 · cetyl palmitate · isopropyl myristate · isopropyl pentanoate
	Cortaid Maximum Strength Pharmacia & Upjohn	ointment		1% (as acetate)	butylparaben · cholesterol · methylparaben · microcrystalline wax · mineral oil · white petrolatum
	Cortaid Maximum Strength Pharmacia & Upjohn	spray		1%	alcohol, 55% · glycerin · methylparaben · water
	Cortaid Sensitive Skin Formula Pharmacia & Upjohn	ointment		0.5% (as acetate)	aloe · butylparaben · cholesterol · methylparaben · mineral oil · white petrolatum · microcrystalline wax
	Cortaid Sensitive Skin Formula Pharmacia & Upjohn	cream		0.5% (as acetate)	aloe · butylparaben · cetyl palmitate · glyceryl stearate · methylparaben · polyethylene glycol · stearamidoethyl diethylamine · water
	Dermamycin Pfeiffer Ph'cals	pump spray	menthol, 1%		diphenhydramine HCl, 2%
	Dermamycin Pfeiffer Ph'cals	cream			diphenhydramine HCl, 1%
	Dermarest Del Ph'cals	gel			diphenhydramine HCl, 2%
	Dermarest DriCort Del Ph'cals	cream		1%	
	Dermarest Plus Del Ph'cals	gel	menthol, 1%		diphenhydramine HCl, 2%

See Chapter 33, "Insect Sting and Bite Products," for more information about these products.

INSECT STING AND BITE PRODUCTS - continued

Product Manufacturer/Supplier	Dosage Form	Antipruritic/Anesthetic/Counterirritant	Hydrocortisone	Other Ingredients
Dermoplast Whitehall-Robins Healthcare	spray	benzocaine, 20% · menthol, 0.5%		acetylated lanolin alcohol · aloe vera gel · butane · cetyl acetate · hydrofluorocarbon · methylparaben · PEG-8 laurate · polysorbate 85
Dermtex Pfeiffer Ph'cals	pump spray	menthol, 1%	1%	
Dermtex HC Pfeiffer Ph'cals	cream		1%	aloe vera gel
Di-Delamine Double Antihistamine Del Ph'cals	gel · spray	menthol, 0.1%		diphenhydramine HCl, 1% · tripelennamine HCl, 0.5% · benzalkonium chloride, 0.12%
Domeboro Bayer Consumer	powder			aluminum sulfate, 1191mg · calcium acetate, 938mg · dextrin
Gold Bond Medicated Anti-Itch Chattem	cream	lidocaine · menthol		cetearyl alcohol · DMDM hydantoin · eucalyptol · glyceryl stearate · methyl salicylate · methylparaben · petrolatum · propylene glycol · simethicone · sorbic acid · sorbitol · thymol · tocopherol · water · zinc oxide
Gold Bond Medicated, Regular or Extra Strength Chattem	powder	methyl salicylate · menthol		boric acid · eucalyptol · salicylic acid · talc · thymol · zinc stearate · zinc oxide
HC-DermaPax Recsei Labs	spray	benzyl alcohol, 1% · diphenhydramine HCl, 0.5%	0.5%	isopropanol, 35%
Itch-X B. F. Ascher	gel · pump spray	benzyl alcohol, 10% · pramoxine HCl, 1%		aloe vera gel
Kericort 10 Bristol-Myers Products	cream		1%	citric acid · sodium citrate · methylparaben · sorbic acid · polyoxyl 40 stearate · glyceryl stearate · white wax · stearyl alcohol · isopropyl myristate · cetyl alcohol · sorbitan monostearate · polysorbate 60 · propylparaben · propylene glycol
Lanacort 10 Combe	cream · ointment		1%	
Nupercainal Ciba Self-Medication	cream	dibucaine, 0.5%		acetone sodium bisulfite · glycerin · potassium hydroxide · stearic acid · fragrance · trolamine · purified water
Nupercainal Ciba Self-Medication	ointment	dibucaine, 1%		acetone sodium bisulfite · lanolin · light mineral oil · white petrolatum · purified water
Outgro Pain Relieving Whitehall-Robins Healthcare	liquid	benzocaine, 20%		alcohol, 61.3% · D&C yellow#10 · FD&C blue#1 · FD&C red#40 · PEG-8
Pedi-Boro Soak Paks Pedinol Pharmacal	powder			aluminum sulfate · calcium acetate
Pramegel GenDerm	gel	pramoxine HCl, 1% · menthol, 0.5% · benzyl alcohol		carbomer 940 · methyl gluceth-20 · SD alcohol 40 · sodium hydroxide · water

See Chapter 33, "Insect Sting and Bite Products," for more information about these products.

INSECT STING AND BITE PRODUCTS - continued

Product Manufacturer/Supplier	**Dosage Form**	**Antipruritic/Anesthetic/Counterirritant**	**Hydrocortisone**	**Other Ingredients**
Preparation H Hydrocortisone 1% Anti-Itch Whitehall-Robins Healthcare	cream		1%	BHA · cellulose gum · cetyl alcohol · citric acid · disodium EDTA · glycerin · glyceryl oleate · glyceryl stearate · lanolin · methylparaben · petrolatum · propyl gallate · propylene glycol · propylparaben · simethicone · sodium benzoate · sodium lauryl sulfate · stearyl alcohol · water · xanthan gum
Rhuli Rydelle Labs	gel	benzyl alcohol, 2% · menthol, 0.3% · camphor, 0.3%		SD alcohol 23A, 31% · propylene glycol · carbomer 940 · triethanolamine · benzophenone-4 · EDTA
Rhuli Rydelle Labs	spray	benzocaine, 5% · camphor, 0.7% · benzyl alcohol		isopropyl alcohol, 70% (concentrate) · calamine, 13.8% · hydrated silica · isobutane · oleyl alcohol · sorbitan trioleate
Rhuli Bite-Aid Rydelle Labs	stick	benzocaine, 10% · benzyl alcohol, 10%		propylene glycol · sodium stearate · polyoxyethylene 20 isohexadecyl ether
Sarna Stiefel Labs	lotion	camphor, 0.5% · menthol, 0.5%		emollient base
Solarcaine Medicated First Aid Schering-Plough HealthCare	aerosol spray	benzocaine, 20%		SD alcohol 40, 35% · triclosan, 0.13% · isobutane
Sting-Eze Wisconsin Pharmacal	drops	camphor · phenol · benzocaine		diphenhydramine HCl · eucalyptol

** New listing
[a] For additional hydrocortisone products, see Poison Ivy, Oak, and Sumac Products table.
[b] This product is labeled for use on insect bites but not insect stings.

See Chapter 33, "Insect Sting and Bite Products," for more information about these products.

INSECT REPELLENT PRODUCTS

	Product Manufacturer/Supplier	Dosage Form	Active Ingredients	Other Ingredients
	Ben's Backyard Tender	lotion · pump spray	n,n-diethyl-meta-toluamide, 23%	
	Ben's Max Tender	lotion · pump spray	n,n-diethyl-meta-toluamide, 95%	
	Ben's Wilderness Tender	aerosol spray	n,n-diethyl-meta-toluamide, 27.5%	other isomers, 10.5% · inert ingredients, 62%
**	**Cutter Pleasant Protection** Spectrum	pump spray	n,n-diethyl-meta-toluamide, 9.5%	other isomers, 0.5% · inert ingredients, 90%
**	**Cutter with Sunscreen** Spectrum	lotion	n,n-diethyl-meta-toluamide, 9.5%	other isomers, 0.5% · inert ingredients, 90% · octyl methoxycinnamate, 7.5% · oxybenzone, 5%
	Muskol Schering-Plough HealthCare	aerosol spray	n,n-diethyl-meta-toluamide, 23.75%	other isomers, 1.25% · inert ingredients, 75%
	Muskol Maximum Strength Schering-Plough HealthCare	lotion · pump spray	n,n-diethyl-meta-toluamide, 95%	other isomers, 5%
	Muskol Ultra Extra Strength Schering-Plough HealthCare	aerosol spray	n,n-diethyl-meta-toluamide, 38%	other isomers, 2% · inert ingredients, 60%
	Natrapel Tender	lotion · pump spray	citronella oil, 10%	aloe vera gel, 89%
**	**Off! Deep Woods for Maximum Protection** S. C. Johnson	pump spray	n,n-diethyl-meta-toluamide, 95%	related isomers, 5%
	Off! Deep Woods Formula S. C. Johnson	aerosol spray	n,n-diethyl-meta-toluamide, 28.5%	other isomers, 1.5% · inert ingredients, 70%
**	**Off! Deep Woods Formula for Sportsmen** S. C. Johnson	aerosol spray	n,n-diethyl-meta-toluamide, 38%	other isomers, 2% · inert ingredients, 60%
** PE	**Off! Skintastic for Kids** S. C. Johnson	pump spray	n,n-diethyl-meta-toluamide, 4.75%	related isomers, 0.25% · inert ingredients, 95% · fragrance
	Off! Skintastic, Fresh Scent or Unscented S. C. Johnson	lotion	n,n-diethyl-meta-toluamide, 7.125%	related isomers, 0.375% · inert ingredients, 92.5%
	Off! Skintastic, Unscented S. C. Johnson	pump spray	n,n-diethyl-meta-toluamide, 6.65%	related isomers, 0.35% · inert ingredients, 93%
	Off!, Spring Fresh or Unscented S. C. Johnson	aerosol spray	n,n-diethyl-meta-toluamide, 14.25%	other isomers, 0.75% · inert ingredients, 85%
**	**Repel Family Formula Scented IPF 15** Wisconsin Pharmacal	aerosol spray	n,n-diethyl-meta-toluamide, 14.25%	other isomers, 0.75% · inert ingredients, 85%
**	**Repel Scented IPF 18** Wisconsin Pharmacal	pump spray	n,n-diethyl-meta-toluamide, 16.62%	other isomers, 0.88% · n-octylbicycloheptene dicarboximide, 5% · di-n-propyl isocinchomeronate, 2.5% · inert ingredients, 75%
**	**Repel Scented IPF 7** Wisconsin Pharmacal	gel	n,n-diethyl-meta-toluamide, 6.65%	related toluamides, 0.35% · n-octylbicycloheptene dicarboximide, 2.5% · inert ingredients, 90.5%

See Chapter 33, "Insect Sting and Bite Products," for more information about these products.

INSECT REPELLENT PRODUCTS - continued

	Product Manufacturer/Supplier	Dosage Form	Active Ingredients	Other Ingredients
**	**Repel Sportsmen Formula Unscented IPF 27** Wisconsin Pharmacal	aerosol spray	n,n-diethyl-meta-toluamide, 25.5%	other isomers, 1.35% · n-octylbicycloheptene dicarboximide, 7.67% · di-n-propyl isocinchomeronate, 3.84% · inert ingredients, 61.64%
**	**Repel Unscented IPF 20** Wisconsin Pharmacal	lotion	n,n-diethyl-meta-toluamide, 19%	other isomers, 1% · inert ingredients, 80%

** New listing

See Chapter 33, "Insect Sting and Bite Products," for more information about these products.

CALLUS, CORN, AND WART PRODUCTS

	Product Manufacturer/Supplier	Dosage Form	Salicylic Acid	Other Ingredients
	Clear Away One Step Wart Remover System Schering-Plough HealthCare	disc	40%	
	Clear Away Plantar Wart Remover System Schering-Plough HealthCare	disc	40%	
	Compound W Wart Remover Whitehall-Robins Healthcare	gel	17%	alcohol, 67.5% · camphor · castor oil · collodion · colloidal silicon dioxide · hydroxypropyl cellulose · hypophosphorous acid · polysorbate 80
	Compound W Wart Remover Whitehall-Robins Healthcare	liquid	17%	ether, 63.5% · alcohol, 21.2% · camphor · castor oil · collodion · ethylcellulose · hypophosphorous acid · menthol · polysorbate 80
	Corn Fix Alvin Last	liquid	12%	ether, 65.5% · alcohol, 33% · collodion
**	**Dr. Scholl's Advanced Pain Relief Callus Removers** Schering-Plough HealthCare	disc	40%	
	Dr. Scholl's Advanced Pain Relief Corn Removers Schering-Plough HealthCare	disc · pad	40% (disc)	
	Dr. Scholl's Callus Removers Schering-Plough HealthCare	disc · pad	40% (disc)	
	Dr. Scholl's Corn Removers, Regular or Waterproof Schering-Plough HealthCare	disc · pad	40% (disc)	
	Dr. Scholl's Corn/Callus Remover Schering-Plough HealthCare	liquid	12.6%	ether, 55% · alcohol, 18% (from SD alcohol 32)
	Dr. Scholl's Moisturizing Corn Remover Kit Schering-Plough HealthCare	cream · disc	40% (disc)	
**	**Dr. Scholl's One Step Callus Remover** Schering-Plough HealthCare	disc	40%	
	Dr. Scholl's One Step Corn Removers Schering-Plough HealthCare	strip	40%	
	Dr. Scholl's Wart Remover Kit Schering-Plough HealthCare	liquid	17%	ether, 52% · alcohol, 17% (from SD alcohol 32)
	DuoFilm Liquid Wart Remover Schering-Plough HealthCare	liquid	17%	ether, 42.6% · alcohol, 15.8%
	DuoFilm Patch System Wart Removers Schering-Plough HealthCare	disc	40%	
	DuoPlant Plantar Wart Remover Schering-Plough HealthCare	gel	17%	alcohol, 57.6% · ether, 16.42%
	Freezone Corn and Callus Remover Whitehall-Robins Healthcare	liquid	13.6%	ether, 64.8% · alcohol, 20.5% · balsam oregon · castor oil · hypophosphorous acid · zinc chloride
	Fung-O S.S.S. Company	liquid	17%	acetone collodion · camphor · menthol · castor oil

See Chapter 34, "Foot Care Products," for more information about these products.

CALLUS, CORN, AND WART PRODUCTS - continued

	Product Manufacturer/Supplier	Dosage Form	Salicylic Acid	Other Ingredients
**	**Gordofilm** Gordon Labs	solution	16.7%	flexible collodion
	Mosco Corn & Callus Remover Medtech Labs	liquid	17%	alcohol, 23% · flexible collodion
**	**Mosco-Cain** Medtech Labs	liquid		SDA alcohol, 40-60% · benzocaine, 20% · PEG-6
	Occlusal HP GenDerm	liquid	17%	ethyl acetate · isopropyl alcohol · butyl acetate · polyvinyl butyl · dibutyl phthalate · acrylates copolymer · nitrocellulose
	OFF·Ezy Corn and Callus Remover Kit Del Ph'cals	liquid	17%	
	OFF·Ezy Wart Remover Kit Del Ph'cals	liquid	17%	flexible collodion
	Sal-Acid Wart Remover Pedinol Pharmacal	plaster	40%	
	Sal-Plant Pedinol Pharmacal	gel	17%	
	Salactic Film Pedinol Pharmacal	liquid	17%	
**	**Trans-Ver-Sal 12mm "Adult Patch" Wart Remover Kit** Doak Dermatologics	patch	15%	karaya gum base
**	**Trans-Ver-Sal 20mm "PlantarPatch" Wart Remover Kit** Doak Dermatologics	patch	15%	karaya gum base
**	**Trans-Ver-Sal 6mm "PediaPatch" Wart Remover Kit** Doak Dermatologics	patch	15%	karaya gum base
	Wart Fix Alvin Last	liquid	12%	ether, 65.5% · alcohol, 33% · collodion
	Wart-Off Pfizer Consumer	liquid	17%	flexible collodion · alcohol · ether · propylene glycol dipelargonate

** New listing

See Chapter 34, "Foot Care Products," for more information about these products.

ATHLETE'S FOOT PRODUCTS

	Product Manufacturer/Supplier	Dosage Form	Antifungal	Other Ingredients
	Absorbine Jr. Antifungal Foot W. F. Young	cream · powder	tolnaftate, 1%	methylparaben · propylparaben · propylene glycol · diazolidinyl urea (powder)
	Absorbine Jr. Antifungal Foot W. F. Young	aerosol spray powder	miconazole nitrate, 2%	alcohol, 10% · propellant A-46 · sorbitan sesquioleate · stearalkonium hectorite · talc
	Absorbine Jr. Antifungal Foot Spray Liquid W. F. Young	pump spray	tolnaftate, 1%	acetone · polysorbate 80 · chloroxylenol · menthol · wormwood oil · FD&C blue#1
	Athlete's Foot Antifungal Goldline Labs	cream	miconazole nitrate, 2%	
	Desenex Foot & Sneaker Deodorant Plus Ciba Self-Medication	powder	calcium undecylenate, 10%	fragrance · talc
	Dr. Scholl's Athletes Foot Schering-Plough HealthCare	powder	tolnaftate, 1%	talc
	Dr. Scholl's Athletes Foot Schering-Plough HealthCare	aerosol spray powder	tolnaftate, 1%	SD alcohol 40, 14% · BHT · propellants · talc
	Dr. Scholl's Athletes Foot Spray Liquid Schering-Plough HealthCare	aerosol spray	tolnaftate, 1%	SD alcohol, 36% · BHT · propellants
**	**Johnson's Odor-Eaters** Johnson & Johnson Consumer	aerosol spray powder	tolnaftate, 1%	ethanol, 14.9% · isobutane · isopropyl myristate · talc
	Odor-Eaters Antifungal Combe	aerosol spray powder	tolnaftate, 1%	
	Rid-Itch Thomas & Thompson	liquid	benzoic acid, 2% · chlorothymol, 1% · resorcinol, 1%	salicylic acid, 7% · boric acid, 5% · alcohol · glycerin

** New listing

See Chapter 34, "Foot Care Products," for more information about these products.

HERBAL AND PHYTOMEDICINAL PRODUCTS

	Product Manufacturer/Supplier	Dosage Form [a]	Ingredients
	Bilberry (Vaccinium myrtillus)		
**	**Bilberry** Herbal Choice-Botalia	40 mg capsule	anthocyanidins, 25% (standardized extract)
**	**Bilberry Extract** PhytoPharmica	80 mg capsule	anthocyanosides, 25% (standardized extract)
**	**Bilberry Extract** Source Natural	50 mg tablet	anthocyanosides, 25% (standardized extract)
**	**Bilberry-Power** Nature's Herbs	440 mg capsule	anthocyanosides, 25% (40mg standardized extract) · quercitin · citrus bioflavinoids · rutin
**	**Optimum Bilberry** Nature's Way	300 mg capsule	anthocyanosides, 25% (60mg standardized extract)
	Capsicum (Capsicum species)		
**	**Cayenne** Nature's Resource	450 mg capsule	capsaicin, not less than 0.25%
**	**Cayenne Extract** Herb Pharm	tincture	alcoholic extract of dried mature fruit
	Chaste Tree Berry (Vitex agnus-castus)		
**	**Femaprin-Vitex** Nature's Way	290 mg capsule	agnuside, 0.15% (175mg standardized extract)
	Cranberry (Vaccinium macrocarpon)		
**	**Cranberry Extract** Herbal Choice-Botalia	400 mg capsule	quinic acid, 11-12% (standardized extract)
**	**Natural Cranberry Concentrate** Herbal Harvest	softgel capsule	cranberry, 140mg (extract) · vitamin E, 3 IU · vitamin C, 100mg
**	**Optimum Cranberry** Nature's Way	530 mg capsule	juice concentrate, 90% (380mg)
	Echinacea (Echinaeca species)		
**	**1st Sneeze** Trout Lake Farm	tincture	Echinacea angustifolia and Echinacea purpurea, 10% (extract of whole plants, including roots, in 55% alcohol)
**	**EchinaCare** PhytoPharmica	tincture	fresh juice of Echinacea purpurea stems, leaves, and flowers in 22% alcohol (not less than 2.4% soluble beta-1,2-D-fructofuranosides calculated on basis of juice solids)
**	**Echinacea** Herbal Choice-Botalia	125 mg capsule	echinacosides, 4% (standardized Echinacea angustifolia extract)
**	**Echinacea Complex** Shaklee	tablet	Echinacea angustifolia root and Echinacea purpurea root and herb, 335mg · additional herbal ingredients include: hyssop · peppermint · thyme
**	**Echinacea Extract** Botalia Gold	125 mg capsule	echinacosides, 4% (standardized Echinacea angustifolia extract)
**	**Echinacea-Power** Nature's Herbs	550 mg capsule	echinacoside, 4% (125mg Echinacea angustifolia) · un-standardized Echinacea angustifolia and Echinacea purpurea roots · prairie dock
**	**EchinaGuard** Nature's Way	355 mg capsule	herbal extract powder, 85mg

See Chapter 35, "Herbs and Phytomedicinal Products," for more information about these products.

HERBAL AND PHYTOMEDICINAL PRODUCTS - continued

	Product Manufacturer/Supplier	Dosage Form [a]	Ingredients
**	**Florammune** Flora Laboratories	tincture	Echinacea angustifolia and Echinacea purpurea, 10% (extract of whole plants, including roots, in 55% alcohol)
**	**Super Echinacea Extract Tablets** Herb Pharm	500 mg tablet	juice of root, leaf, and flower with dried root and seed of Echinacea purpurea and Echinacea angustifolia
**	**Super Echinacea Liquid Extract** Herb Pharm	tincture	fresh juice of seed, plant, and root of Echinacea purpurea and Echinacea angustifolia in alcohol
	Eleuthro (Eleutherococcus senticosus)		
**	**Siberian Ginseng** NaturaLife	410 mg capsule	eleutheroside E, not less than 0.08%
**	**Siberian Ginseng** Herbal Harvest	500 mg capsule	powdered root
**	**Siberian Ginseng** Herbal Choice-Botalia	100 mg capsule	eleutheroside E, 0.5% (standardized extract)
**	**Siberian Ginseng Extract** Herb Pharm	tincture	extract of dried root (2:1)
	Evening Primrose Oil (Oenothera biennis)		
**	**Efamol Evening Primrose Oil** Nature's Way	500 mg capsule	cis-linoleic acid, 365mg · gamma-linoleic acid, 45mg
**	**Royal Brittany Evening Primrose Oil** American Health	500 mg capsule	cis-linoleic acid, 365mg · gamma-linoleic acid, 45mg
	Feverfew (Tanacetum parthenium)		
**	**Feverfew** Herbal Choice-Botalia	125 mg capsule	parthenolide, 0.2% (standardized extract)
**	**Feverfew Extract** Herb Pharm	tincture	alcohol extract of dried leaf and flower
**	**MygraFew** Nature's Way	152 mg tablet	parthenolide, 400mcg
**	**Natural Feverfew** Herbal Harvest	380 mg capsule	dried herb containing parthenolide
**	**Standardized Feverfew Extract** Botalia Gold	125 mg capsule	parthenolide, 0.2% (standardized extract)
**	**Tanacet 125** Herbal Laboratories	125 mg tablet	parthenolide, 0.2% (standardized leaf powder)
	Garlic (Allium sativum)		
**	**Garlic** Shaklee	tablet	garlic equivalent to 0.5 fresh clove · additional herbal ingredients include: rosemary · spearmint
**	**Garlic** Herbal Choice-Botalia	300 mg capsule	standardized garlic containing allicin, 10000ppm · sulfur, 8000ppm · allicin, 1500ppm
**	**Garlicin Enteric Coated** Nature's Way	550 mg tablet	allicin yield, 2500mcg
**	**Garlique Enteric Coated** Sunsource	400 mg tablet	allicin yield, 1800mcg

See Chapter 35, "Herbs and Phytomedicinal Products," for more information about these products.

HERBAL AND PHYTOMEDICINAL PRODUCTS - continued

	Product Manufacturer/Supplier	Dosage Form [a]	Ingredients
**	**Garlitrin 4000 Enteric Coated** PhytoPharmica	320 mg tablet	allicin yield, 5000mcg
**	**Kwai Coated** Lichtwer	100 mg tablet	allicin yield, 600mcg
**	**One-A-Day Extras Garlic** Bayer Consumer	600 mg softgel	oil macerate standardized to yield allicin, not less than 1440mcg
	Ginger (Zingiber officinale)		
**	**Ginger** Herbal Choice-Botalia	250 mg capsule	essential oil, 0.8% (standardized extract)
**	**Ginger Extract** Herb Pharm	tincture	alcoholic extract of dried rhizome
**	**Ginger Root** Nature's Resource	550 mg capsule	essential oil, 1.5%
	Ginkgo (Ginkgo biloba)		
**	**Ginkgo** Herbal Choice-Botalia	60 mg capsule	ginkgo flavon glycosides, 24% (standardized extract)
**	**Ginkgo Biloba** Thompson Nut'l	360 mg capsule	ginkgo flavon glycosides, 24% (60mg standardized extract) · ginkgo leaf powder
**	**Ginkgo Biloba** Hudson	30 mg tablet	ginkgo flavon glycosides, 24% (as quercetin and kaempferol; standardized extract)
**	**Ginkgo Biloba Extract** NaturaLife	420 mg capsule	ginkgo flavon glycosides, 24% (40mg standardized extract)
**	**Ginkgo Biloba Extract** Botalia Gold	60 mg capsule	ginkgo flavon glycosides, 24% (standardized extract) · ginkgolides, 6%
**	**Ginkgo Biloba Leaf Extract** Nature's Resource	40 mg capsule	ginkgo flavon glycosides, 24% (standardized extract)
**	**Ginkgo Extract** Herb Pharm	tincture	alcoholic extract of fresh leaf
**	**Ginkgo Phytosome** PhytoPharmica	80 mg capsule	ginkgoheterosides bound to phosphatidylcholine, 24% (standardized extract)
**	**Ginkgold** Nature's Way	260 mg tablet	ginkgo flavon glycosides, 24% (40mg standardized extract)
**	**Ginkgolidin** PhytoPharmica	40 mg capsule	ginkgoheterosides, 24% (standardized extract)
	Ginseng (Panax ginseng)		
**	**Asian Ginseng Complex** Shaklee	tablet	blend of red and white Asian ginseng, 335mg · additional herbal ingredients include: licorice root · red jujube date
**	**Ginsai** Lichtwer	100 mg capsule	ginsenosides, 7% (standardized extract)
**	**Ginsana** Sunsource	100 mg capsule	ginsenosides, 4% (standardized extract)
**	**Ginseng Root - Korean White** Nature's Resource	560 mg capsule	ginsenoside, 1.5%

See Chapter 35, "Herbs and Phytomedicinal Products," for more information about these products.

HERBAL AND PHYTOMEDICINAL PRODUCTS - continued

	Product Manufacturer/Supplier	Dosage Form [a]	Ingredients
**	**Ginseng-7** Herbal Choice-Botalia	100 mg capsule	ginsenosides, 7% (standardized extract; Rg1:Rb1 = 2:1)
**	**Ginsun** Nature's Way	324 mg softgel	ginsenosides, 5% (110mg standardized extract)
**	**Korean White Ginseng** NaturaLife	560 mg capsule	ginsenosides, 2% (not less than)
**	**Natural Korean Ginseng** Herbal Harvest	500 mg capsule	ginsenosides, 0.7-3% (standardized product)
**	**Panax Ginseng Extract** Botalia Gold	100 mg capsule	ginsenosides, 7% (standardized extract, Rg1:Rb1 = 2:1)
**	**Panaxin** PhytoPharmica	100 mg capsule	saponins, 17% (calculated as ginsenoside Rg1; standardized extract)
	Lemon Balm (Melissa officinalis)		
**	**Herpalieve** PhytoPharmica	cream	melissa (70:1 extract) · allantoin, 1%
	Milk Thistle (Silybum marianum)		
**	**Milk Thistle** Herbal Choice-Botalia	100 mg capsule	silymarin, 80% (calculated as silibin; standardized extract)
**	**Milk Thistle** NaturaLife	310 mg capsule	silymarin, 140mg; including 60mg of silybinin and isosilybinin (180mg standardized extract)
**	**Milk Thistle Extract** Herb Pharm	tincture	alcoholic extract of dried mature seed
**	**Milk-Thistle Power** Nature's Herbs	535 mg capsule	silymarin, 80% (175mg standardized extract) · turmeric · artichoke
**	**Sib-150** PhytoPharmica	150 mg capsule	silymarin, 70% (standardized extract)
**	**Thisilyn** Nature's Way	310 mg capsule	silymarin, 140mg; including 60mg of silybinin and isosilybinin (180mg standardized extract)
	Oligomeric Proanthocyanidins		
**	**Grape Seed Extract** Herbal Choice-Botalia	25 mg tablet	procyanidolic value 95 (standardized extract from Vitis vinifera seed coat)
**	**Hawthorn HC** Nature's Way	160 mg softgel	oligomeric proanthocyanadins, 14.5mg (from Crataegus species)
**	**PCO Phytosome** PhytoPharmica	50 mg tablet	procyanidolic oligomers (from Vitis vinifera seed coat bound to phosphatidylcholine)
**	**Pycnogenol** Agrolabs	25 mg tablet	proanthocyanidin complex, 85% (from Pinus pinaster bark)
	St. John's Wort (Hypericum perforatum)		
**	**Hypericum Extract** PhytoPharmica	300 mg capsule	hypericin, 0.3% (standardized extract)
**	**St. John's Wort** Nature's Way	545 mg capsule	hypericin, 0.15% (standardized extract)

See Chapter 35, "Herbs and Phytomedicinal Products," for more information about these products.

HERBAL AND PHYTOMEDICINAL PRODUCTS - continued

	Product Manufacturer/Supplier	Dosage Form [a]	Ingredients
**	**St. John's Wort** Herbal Choice	150 mg capsule	hypericin, 0.14% (standardized extract)
**	**St. John's Wort Extract** Botalia Gold	150 mg capsule	hypericin, 0.3% (standardized extract)
**	**St. John's Wort Extract** Herb Pharm	tincture	alcoholic extract of fresh flowering and budding top
	Saw Palmetto (Serenoa repens)		
**	**Saw Palmetto** NaturaLife	160 mg softgel · 320 mg softgel	sabal extract (12:1 concentration)
**	**Saw Palmetto** Herbal Choice	80 mg capsule	fatty acids and sterols, 85-95% (standardized extract)
**	**Saw Palmetto Extract** Botalia Gold	80 mg capsule	fatty acids, 85-95% · fatty alcohols, 0.15-0.3% · total sterols, 0.2-0.4% · beta-sitosterol, 0.3% (standardized extract)
**	**Saw Palmetto Extract** Herb Pharm	tincture	alcoholic extract of dried mature berry
**	**Super Saw Palmetto-160** PhytoPharmica	160 mg capsule	fatty acids and sterols, 85-95% (standardized extract)
	Valerian (Valeriana officinalis)		
**	**Florased** Flora Laboratories	tincture	alcoholic root extract, 10%
**	**Rest Easy** Trout Lake Farm	tincture	alcoholic root extract, 10%
**	**Valer-A-Som** PhytoPharmica	150 mg capsule	valerenic acids, 0.2-0.8% (standardized extract)
**	**Valerian** Herbal Choice-Botalia	150 mg capsule	valerenic acids, 0.8% (standardized extract)
**	**Valerian Extract** Botalia Gold	150 mg tablet	valerenic acid, 0.8% (standardized extract)
**	**Valerian Extract** Herb Pharm	tincture	alcoholic extract of fresh rhizome and roots
**	**Valerian Nighttime Tablets** Nature's Way	495 mg tablet	160mg valerian root (extract; 4.5:1 concentration) · lemon balm, 80mg (extract)
**	**Valerian Plus** Shaklee	tablet	valerenic acid, 0.8% (75mg standardized valerian root extract) · additional herbal ingredients include: passion flower · German chamomile

** New listing
[a] Quantities specified in this column refer to the total weight of the solid dosage form, not the weight of the active ingredient.

See Chapter 35, "Herbs and Phytomedicinal Products," for more information about these products.

SMOKING CESSATION PRODUCTS

	Product Manufacturer/Supplier	Dosage Form	Active Ingredient	Other Ingredients
**	**Nicorette** SmithKline Beecham	gum	nicotine polacrilex, 2mg	flavors · glycerin · gum base · sodium carbonate · sorbitol · sodium bicarbonate
**	**Nicorette DS** SmithKline Beecham	gum	nicotine polacrilex, 4mg	flavors · glycerin · gum base · sodium carbonate · sorbitol · sodium bicarbonate

** New listing

See Chapter 36, "Smoking Cessation Products," for more information about these products.

Nonprescription Drug Manufacturers/Suppliers

The following companies are manufacturers and/or suppliers of products listed in *Nonprescription Products: Formulations & Features*. Although this directory is a comprehensive listing of the companies that produce or supply nonprescription products, it should not be considered an all-inclusive listing of such companies.

A

Abbott Laboratories
Pharmaceutical Products Div.
1 Abbott Park Rd.
Abbott Park, IL 60064-3500
800-633-9110

Advanced Care Products
Div. of Ortho Pharmaceutical Corp.
1001 U.S. Hwy. 202
P.O. Box 610
Raritan, NJ 08869-0610
800-582-6097

Advanced Nutrition Foods Co.
P.O. Box 3345
W. Palm Beach, FL 33401

Aero Assemblies, Inc.
Dist. for CPC (United Kingdom) Ltd.
Esher, Surrey, KT109PN
800-932-0177

Agrolabs
215 Rte. 22 W.
Hillside, NJ 07205

Akorn, Inc.
100 Akorn Dr.
Abita Springs, LA 70420
800-535-7155

AkPharma Inc.
P.O. Box 111
Pleasantville, NJ 08232
800-257-8650

Aladan Corp.
4725 Peachtree Corners Cir.
Norcross, GA 30092
770-840-9665

Alcon Laboratories, Inc.
P.O. Box 6600
Fort Worth, TX 76115
817-293-0450

Allergan Inc.
2525 Dupont Dr.
Irvine, CA 92715
800-347-4500

Allergan Optical
Div. of Allergan Inc.
2525 Dupont Dr.
P.O. Box 19534
Irvine, CA 92713-9534
800-347-5005

Alva-Amco Pharmacal Companies, Inc.
6625 Avondale Ave.
Chicago, IL 60631
312-792-0200

Alvin Last, Inc.
19 Babcock Pl.
Yonkers, NY 10701-2714
914-376-1000

American Health
4320 Veterans Memorial Hwy.
Holbrook, NY 11741

Andrew Jergens Co.
P.O. Box 145444
Cincinnati, OH 45250-5444
800-222-3553

Apothecon
Div. of Bristol-Myers Squibb Co.
P.O. Box 4500
Princeton, NJ 08543-4500
609-897-2470

Apothecus Pharmaceutical Corp.
20 Audrey Ave.
Oyster Bay, NY 11771-1532
516-624-8200

APS/Premier Products
Greenwich Office Park One
Greenwich, CT 06831
800-827-9283

Atwater Carey Ltd.
5505 Central Ave.
Boulder, CO 80301
800-359-1646

B

B. F. Ascher & Company, Inc.
P.O. Box 717
Shawnee Mission, KS 66201-0717
913-888-1880

Baker Cummins Dermatologicals
Div. of Baker Norton Pharmaceuticals
8800 N.W. 36th St.
Miami, FL 33178
305-590-2200

Bard Patient Care
Div. of C.R. Bard, Inc.
8195 Industrial Blvd.
Covington, GA 30209
800-526-4930

Barre-National, Inc.
7205 Windsor Blvd.
Baltimore, MD 21244-2654
800-638-9096

Bausch & Lomb Personal Products
Div. of Bausch & Lomb, Inc.
1400 N. Goodman St.
Rochester, NY 14692-0450
800-553-5340

Bausch & Lomb Pharmaceutical
Div. of Bausch & Lomb, Inc.
8500 Hidden River Pkwy.
Tampa, FL 33637
813-975-7700

Bayer Corp., Consumer Care Div.
Subs. of Bayer AG
99 Cherry Hill Rd.
Parsippany, NJ 07054
800-331-4536

Bayer Corp., Diagnostics Div.
Subs. of Bayer AG
511 Benedict Ave.
Tarrytown, NY 10591-5097
800-431-1970

BDI Pharmaceuticals, Inc.
P.O. Box 78610
Indianapolis, IN 46278-0610
800-428-1717

Becton Dickinson and Co.
Consumer Products Div.
1 Becton Dr.
Franklin Lakes, NJ 07417-1883
800-526-4650

Beiersdorf Inc.
360 Dr. Martin Luther King Dr.
P.O. Box 5529
Norwalk, CT 06856-5529
800-233-2340

Beutlich, L.P. Pharmaceuticals
1541 Shields Dr.
Waukegan, IL 60085-8304
800-238-8542

Biofilm, Inc.
3121 Scott St.
Vista, CA 92083-8323
800-848-5900

Biomerica, Inc.
1533 Monrovia Ave.
Newport Beach, CA 92663
714-645-2111

BIRA Corp.
2525 Quicksilver Rd.
McDonald, PA 15057
412-796-1820

Bird Products Corp.
1100 Bird Center Dr.
Palm Springs, CA 92262
619-778-7200

Blaine Company, Inc. Pharmaceuticals
1465 Jamike Ln.
Erlanger, KY 41018
606-283-9437

Blair Laboratories, Inc.
Div. of The Purdue Frederick Co.
(see **The Purdue Frederick Co.**)

Blairex Laboratories, Inc.
3240 N. Indianapolis Rd.
Columbus, IN 47202-2127
800-252-4739

Blanchard Ostomy Products
1510 Raymond Ave.
Glendale, CA 91201
818-242-6789

Blistex Inc.
1800 Swift Dr.
Oak Brook, IL 60521-1574
800-837-1800

Block Drug Co., Inc.
257 Cornelison Ave.
Jersey City, NJ 07302-3198
800-365-6500

Bock Pharmacal
P.O. Box 419056
St. Louis, MO 63141-9056
314-579-0770

Boehringer Mannheim Corp.
9115 Hague Rd.
P.O. Box 50100
Indianapolis, IN 46250-0100
800-428-5074

Botalia Pharmaceutical
Div. of Celestial Seasonings
4600 Sleepy Time Drive
Boulder, CO 80301-3292
800-468-1991

Bradley Pharmaceuticals, Inc.
383 Rte. 46 W.
Fairfield, NJ 07004-2402
800-929-9300

Breckenridge Pharmaceutical
Subs. of Breckenridge, Inc.
P.O. Box 206
Boca Raton, FL 33429
407-367-8512

Brimms Laboratories
Div. of Brimms Inc.
425 Fillmore Ave.
Tonawanda, NY 14150
800-828-7669

Bristol-Myers Products
Div. of Bristol-Myers Squibb Co.
345 Park Ave.
New York, NY 10154
800-468-7746

Buffington
Div. of Otis Clapp & Son, Inc.
(see **Otis Clapp**)

C

C & M Pharmacal, Inc.
1721 Maplelane Ave.
Hazel Park, MI 48030-1215
800-423-5173

C. B. Fleet Co., Inc.
4615 Murray Pl.
P.O. Box 11349
Lynchburg, VA 24506-1349
800-999-9711

C. S. Dent & Co.
Div. of Grandpa Brands Co.
317 E. 8th St.
Cincinnati, OH 45202
513-241-1677

Campbell Laboratories Inc.
700 W. Hillsboro Blvd. (# 2-201)
Deerfield Beach, FL 33441-1612
800-458-2681

Can-Am Care Corp.
Cimetra Industrial Park, Box 98
Chazy, NY 12921-0098
800-461-7448

CareCard Corp.
5604 Bonnell Vista, Ste. 3
Austin, TX 78731
800-452-0911

Cases Plus, Inc.
7757 Bell Rd.
Windsor, CA 95492
800-982-1880

Care-Tech Laboratories
3224 S. Kingshighway Blvd.
St. Louis, MO 63139-1183
314-772-4610

Carma Laboratories, Inc.
5801 W. Airways Ave.
Franklin, WI 53132
414-421-7707

Carnation Nutritional Products
Div. of Nestle Food Co.
800 N. Brand Blvd.
Glendale, CA 91203
818-549-6000

Carnrick Laboratories, Inc.
65 Horse Hill Rd.
Cedar Knolls, NJ 07927
201-267-2670

Carter Products
Div. of Carter-Wallace, Inc.
1345 Ave. of the Americas
New York, NY 10105
212-339-5000

Cascade Medical
10180 Viking Dr.
Eden Prairie, MN 55344
800-525-6718

CCA Industries, Inc.
200 Murray Hill Pkwy.
E. Rutherford, NJ 07073
201-330-1400

Central Pharmaceuticals, Inc.
120 E. Third St.
Seymour, IN 47274-0328
Telephone: 800-457-9856

Century Pharmaceuticals, Inc.
10377 Hague Rd.
Indianapolis, IN 46256-3399
317-849-4210

Chattem, Inc.
1715 W. 38th St.
Chattanooga, TN 37409-1248
800-366-6833

ChemTrak
929 E. Arques Ave.
Sunnyvale, CA 94086-4520
800-927-7776

Chesebrough-Pond's USA Co.
40 Merritt Blvd.
Trumbull, CT 06611
203-377-8300

Chronimed, Inc.
13911 Ridgedale Dr.
Minnetonka, MN 55305
800-444-5951

Church & Dwight Co., Inc.
469 N. Harrison St.
Princeton, NJ 08543-5297
609-683-5900

Ciba Self-Medication, Inc.
Div. of Ciba-Geigy Corp.
581 Main St.
Woodbridge, NJ 07095
908-602-6600

Ciba Vision Corp.
Div. of Ciba-Geigy Ltd.
11460 Johns Creek Pkwy.
Duluth, GA 30155-1518
800-227-1524

Ciba Vision Ophthalmics
Div. of Ciba-Geigy Ltd.
(see **Ciba Vision Corp.**)

Clear Mountain Laboratories
St. Charles, IL 60175
800-789-1515

Clement Clarke, Inc.
A Haag-Streit Co.
3128-D 17th Ave.
Columbus, OH 43219
800-848-8923

Colgate-Palmolive Co.
300 Park Ave.
New York, NY 10022
800-221-4607

Columbia Laboratories, Inc.
2665 S. Bayshore Dr.
Miami, FL 33133
305-860-1670

Combe, Inc.
1101 Westchester Ave.
White Plains, NY 10604
914-694-5454

ConvaTech
Div. of Bristol-Myers Squibb Co.
P.O. Box 5254
Princeton, NJ 08543-5254
800-422-8811

Copley Pharmaceutical Inc.
Canton Commerce Center
25 John Rd.
Canton, MA 02021-2897
617-821-6111

D

Del Pharmaceuticals, Inc.
Subs. of Del Laboratories, Inc.
565 Broad Hollow Rd.
Farmingdale, NY 11735
516-844-2020

Den-Mat Corp.
2727 Skyway Dr.
Santa Maria, CA 93455
805-922-8491

Dental Concepts Inc.
Dental Concepts
Elmsford, NY 10523
914-592-1860

Dentco, Inc.
Subs. of Block Drug Co., Inc.
(see **Block**)

Dep Corp.
2101 E. Via Arado
Rancho Dominguez, CA 90220
800-326-2855

Dermik Laboratories, Inc.
A Rhône-Poulenc Rorer Co.
500 Virginia Dr.
P.O. Box 1727
Fort Washington, PA 19034
800-523-6674

Dey Laboratories
A Lipha Americas Co.
2751 Napa Valley Corp. Dr.
Napa, CA 94558
800-755-5560

Direct Access Diagnostics
Div. of Ortho Pharmaceutical Corp.
440 Rt. 22 E.
Bridgewater, NJ 08807
908-218-7300

Doak Dermatologics
Subs. of Bradley Pharmaceuticals, Inc.
(see **Bradley**)

Dover Pharmaceutical, Inc.
P.O. Box 809
Islington, MA 02090
617-821-5400

Dr. G. H. Tichenor Antiseptic Co.
1700 Baronne St.
P.O. Box 53374
New Orleans, LA 70153
504-588-9131

E

The E. E. Dickinson Co.
2 Enterprise Dr.
Shelton, CT 06484-4666
203-929-1197

E. Fougera & Co.
Div. of Altana Inc.
60 Baylis Rd.
Melville, NY 11747-3816
800-645-9833

E. T. Browne Drug Co., Inc.
Englewood Cliffs, NJ 07632
201-947-3050

Edwards Pharmaceuticals, Inc.
111 Mulberry St.
Ripley, MS 38663
800-543-9560

Effcon Laboratories, Inc.
P.O. Box 7499
Marietta, GA 30065-1499
800-722-2428

Eli Lilly and Co.
Lilly Corp. Center
Indianapolis, IN 46285
800-545-5979

Entry 21 Ltd.
209 E. Baseline Rd., Ste. 107
Tempe, AZ 85283
800-400-5027

F

The Female Health Co.
875 N. Michigan Ave., Ste. 3660
Chicago, IL 60611
800-635-0844

Ferndale Laboratories, Inc.
780 W. Eight Mile Rd.
Ferndale, MI 48220-1218
313-548-0900

Fibertone Co.
14851 N. Scottsdale Rd.
Scottsdale, AZ 85254
800-899-4499

The Fielding Co.
94 Weldon Pkwy.
Maryland Heights, MO 63043
314-567-5462

Fischer Pharmaceuticals Inc.
165 Gibraltar Ct.
Sunnyvale, CA 94089
800-782-0222

Flanders, Inc.
Northbridge Station
P.O. Box 39143
Charleston, SC 29414
803-571-3363

Fleming & Co.
1600 Fenpark Dr.
Fenton, MO 63026
314-343-8200

Flora Laboratories
151 Little Mountain Rd.
Trout Lake, WA 98650
800-395-6093

Forest Pharmaceuticals, Inc.
Subs. of Forest Laboratories, Inc.
13622 Lakefront Dr.
St. Louis, MO 63045
800-678-1605

Fox Pharmacal, Inc.
6420 N.W. 5th Way
Ft. Lauderdale, FL 33309-6112
954-772-7487

Freeda Vitamins, Inc.
36 E. 41st St.
New York, NY 10017-6203
800-777-3737

Furst-McNess Co.
120 E. Clark St.
Freeport, IL 61032
815-235-6151

G

G & W Laboratories, Inc.
111 Coolidge St.
S. Plainfield, NJ 07080
800-922-1038

Gainor Medical USA Inc.
P.O. Box 353
McDonough, GA 30253-0353
800-825-8282

Galderma Laboratories, Inc.
P.O. Box 331329
Ft. Worth, TX 76163-1329
817-263-2600

Gebauer Co.
9410 St. Catherine Ave.
Cleveland, OH 44104-5599
800-321-9348

GenDerm Corp.
600 Knightsbridge Pkwy.
Lincolnshire, IL 60069-3657
800-533-3376

Generation Software Corp.
P.O. Box 363
Bloomingdale, IL 60108-9931
800-455-4GSC

Gerber Products Co.
445 State St.
Freemont, MI 49413-0001
800-828-9119

Glenwood Inc.
83 N. Summit St.
Tenafly, NJ 07670
201-569-0050

Goldline Laboratories
Subs. of Zenith Goldline Pharmaceuticals
1900 W. Commercial Blvd.
Ft. Lauderdale, FL 33309
800-327-4114

Goldware
P.O. Box 22335
San Diego, CA 92192
800-669-7311

Goody's Pharmaceuticals, Inc.
Div. of Block Drug Co., Inc.
(see **Block**)

Gordon Laboratories
6801 Ludlow St.
Upper Darby, PA 19082
800-356-7870

Graham-Field, Inc.
400 Rabro Dr. E.
Hauppauge, NY 11788
800-645-1023

Grandpa Soap Co.
Div. of Grandpa Brands Co.
317 E. 8th St.
Cincinnati, OH 45202
513-241-1677

H

Halsey Pharmaceutical
Subs. of Halsey Drug Co., Inc.
1827 Pacific St.
Brooklyn, NY 11233
800-252-5230

Harold Pharmacal
Div. of Allergan Inc.
1701 Touchstone Rd.
Colonial Heights, VA 23834
800-253-9499

Hawaiian Tropic
Div. of Tanning Research Laboratories
P.O. Box 5111
Daytona Beach, FL 32118-5111
904-677-9559

Health Care Products
Div. of Hi-Tech Pharmacal Co., Inc.
369 Bayview Ave.
Amityville, NY 11701
800-899-3116

HealthScan Products Inc.
908 Pompton Ave.
Cedar Grove, NJ 07009-1292
800-962-1266

HealthWare
P.O. Box 1693
Idyllwild, CA 92549-1693
800-682-9375

Helena Laboratories
1530 Lindbergh Dr.
Beaumont, TX 77704
800-231-5663

Herb Pharm
P.O. Box 116
Williams, OR 97544
800-348-4372

Herbal Harvest
(see **The Hudson Corp**.)

Hershey Chocolate
Div. of Hershey Foods Corp.
Hershey, PA 17033-0815
800-468-1714

Hogil Pharmaceutical Corp.
2 Manhattanville Rd.
Purchase, NY 10577-2118
914-696-7600

Hollister Inc.
2000 Hollister Dr.
Libertyville, IL 60048
847-680-1000

Home Diagnostics, Inc.
2300 N.W. 55th Ct.
Ft. Lauderdale, FL 33309
800-342-7226

The Hudson Corp.
Div. of NBTY
90 Orville Dr.
Bohemia, NY 11716-2599
516-567-9500

Hydrosal Company
Div. of Merchandise, Inc.
5929 State Rt. 128
P.O. Box 10
Miamitown, OH 45041-0010
513-353-2200

Hyrex Pharmaceuticals
3494 Democrat Rd.
Memphis, TN 38118-1542
800-238-5282

I

ICN Pharmaceuticals, Inc.
3300 Hyland Ave.
Costa Mesa, CA 92626
800-322-1515

Identifind
P.O. Box 567
Canton, NC 28716
704-648-6768

ITA Software, Inc.
11005 Township Rd.
Live Oak, CA 95953
800-510-1024

J

J. B. Williams Co., Inc.
65 Harrison Rd.
Glen Rock, NJ 07452
800-254-8656

J. K. Pharmaceuticals, Inc.
1645 Oak St.
Lakewood, NJ 08701
908-905-5252

Johnson & Johnson Consumer Products, Inc.
199 Grandview Rd.
Skillman, NJ 08558-9418
800-526-3967

Johnson & Johnson·Merck Consumer Pharmaceuticals Co.
Div. of Johnson & Johnson
7050 Camp Hill Rd.
Ft. Washington, PA 19034
215-233-7700

Jones Medical Industries, Inc.
P.O. Box 46903
St. Louis, MO 63146-6903
314-576-6100

Jordan Medical Enterprises, Inc.
202 Oaklawn Ave.
S. Pasadena, CA 91030
800-541-1193

K

Kaufman Associates, Inc.
513 Vienna Ave.
Radford, VA 24141
800-472-2080

Kenwood Laboratories
Div. of Bradley Pharmaceuticals, Inc.
(see **Bradley**)

Kimberly-Clark Corp.
Neenah, WI 54956
800-558-6423

Kingswood Laboratories, Inc.
10375 Hague Rd.
Indianapolis, IN 46256-3316
317-849-9513

Kiwi Brands, Inc.
Rt. 662 N.
Douglassville, PA 19518
215-385-3041

KLI Corp.
1119 Third Ave., S.W.
P.O. Box 567
Carmel, IN 46032
317-846-7452

Konsyl Pharmaceuticals, Inc.
4200 S. Hulen St.
Ft. Worth, TX 76109
817-763-8011

Kramer Laboratories, Inc.
8778 S.W. 8th St.
Miami, FL 33174-9990
800-824-4894

L

Lake Consumer Products
Subs. of Columbia Laboratories
625 Forst Edge Dr.
Vernon Hills, IL 60061
800-635-3696

Laser, Inc.
2200 W. 97th Pl.
P.O. Box 905
Crown Point, IN 46307
219-663-1165

Lavoptik Company, Inc.
661 Western Ave. N.
St. Paul, MN 55103
612-489-1351

Lederle Consumer Health
Div. of Whitehall-Robins Healthcare
401 N. Middletown Rd.
Pearl River, NY 10965
800-282-8805

Lee Pharmaceuticals
1444 Santa Anita Ave.
S. El Monte, CA 91733
800-950-5337

Legere Pharmaceuticals
7326 E. Evans Rd.
Scottsdale, AZ 85260
800-528-3144

Lemmon Co.
Div. of Teva Pharmaceutical Industries, Inc.
1510 Delp Dr.
Kulpsville, PA 19443
800-545-8800

Lichtwer Pharma
Foster Plaza 10
680 Andersen Drive
Pittsburgh, PA 15220
800-837-3203

LifeScan, Inc.
Subs. of Johnson & Johnson
1000 Gilbraltar Dr.
Milpitas, CA 95035-6312
800-227-8862

LLW Enterprises
P.O. Box 591353
Houston, TX 77259-1353
713-480-1506

Lobana Laboratories
Div. of Ulmer Pharmacal Co.
2440 Fernbrook Ln.
Plymouth, MN 55447
800-848-5637

London International U.S. Holdings Inc.
1819 Main St.
Sarasota, FL 34236
941-365-1600

Lumiscope Co., Inc.
400 Raritan Center Pkwy.
Edison, NJ 08837
800-422-LUMI

M

Martin Himmel Inc.
P.O. Box 5479
Lake Worth, FL 33466-5479
800-535-3823

McCue Labs
Div. of Quaker House Products
P.O. Box 21088
Houston, TX 77026
713-526-1248

McNeil Consumer Products Co.
Div. of McNeil-PPC, Inc.
7050 Camp Hill Rd.
Fort Washington, PA 19034-2299
800-962-5357

Mead Johnson Nutritionals
Div. of Bristol-Myers Squibb Co.
2400 W. Lloyd Expwy.
Evansville, IN 47721-0001
800-222-9123

Medco Lab, Inc.
716 W. 7th
P.O. Box 864
Sioux City, IA 51102-0864
712-255-8770

Medic Alert Foundation
P.O. Box 1009
Turlock, CA 95381-1009
800-432-5378

MediCheck International Foundation, Inc.
8320 Ballard Rd.
Niles, IL 60714
847-299-0620

Medicis Dermatologics, Inc.
4343 Camelback Rd., Ste. 250
Phoenix, AZ 85018
800-550-5115

Medicool, Inc.
23761 Madison St.
Torrance, CA 90505
800-433-2469

Medicore, Inc.
2647 W. 81st St.
P.O. Box 4826
Hialeah, FL 33014
800-327-8894

Med-I-Dent
Div. of The ELA Corp.
225 Stevens Ave., Ste. 207
Solana Beach, CA 92075-2059
800-942-7555

MediSense, Inc.
Subs. of Abbott Laboratories
266 Second Ave.
Waltham, MA 02154
800-527-3339

Meditec, Inc.
3322 S. Oneida Way
Denver, CO 80224
303-758-6978

Medport Inc.
23 Acorn St.
Providence, RI 02903
800-368-7248

Medtech Laboratories, Inc.
3510 N. Lake Creek Dr.
P.O. Box 1108
Jackson, WY 83001
800-443-4908

Menley & James Laboratories, Inc.
Commonwealth Corp. Center
100 Tournament Dr.
Horsham, PA 19044-3697
215-441-6500

Mentholatum Co., Inc.
1360 Niagara St.
Buffalo, NY 14213
716-882-7660

Mericon Industries, Inc.
8819 N. Pioneer Rd.
Peoria, IL 61615-1561
800-242-6464

Merrick Medicine Co.
P.O. Box 1489
Waco, TX 76703
817-753-3461

MetaMedix, Inc.
735 E. Ohio Ave., Ste. 202
Escondido, CA 92025
800-455-4105

Milex Products, Inc.
5915 Northwest Hwy.
Chicago, IL 60631
312-631-6484

Mission Pharmacal Co.
P.O. Box 786099
San Antonio, TX 78278-6099
800-531-3333

Modern Products, Inc.
3015 W. Vera Ave.
P.O. Box 09398
Milwaukee, WI 53209-9398
414-352-3333

Muro Pharmaceutical, Inc.
890 East St.
Tewksbury, MA 01876
800-225-0974

Mustang Enterprises, Inc.
1917 South St.
P.O. Box 748
Geneva, IL 60134-2548
708-232-1373

N

Natural White, Inc.
Buffalo, NY 14207
905-841-9229

NaturaLife
Murdock Madaus Schwabe Group
10 Mountain Springs Pkwy.
P.O. Box 4000
Springville, UT 84663
800-926-8883

Nature's Herbs
Twinlab Co.
600 E. Qality Dr.
American Fork, UT 84003
800-437-2257

Nature's Resource Products
Mission Hills, CA 91346-9606
818-837-3633

Nature's Way
(see **NaturaLife**)

Neutrogena Dermatologics
Div. of Neutrogena Corp.
5760 W. 96th St.
Los Angeles, CA 90045
800-421-6857

Nion Laboratories
15501 First St.
Irwindale, CA 91706
800-227-8526

Nomax, Inc.
40 N. Rock Hill Rd.
St. Louis, MO 63119-2242
800-255-6161

Northampton Medical, Inc.
(see **UCB Pharma**)

Novo Nordisk Pharmaceuticals Inc.
Subs. of Novo Nordisk A/S
100 Overlook Center, Ste. 200
Princeton, NJ 08540-7810
800-727-6500

Nu-Hope Laboratories, Inc.
P.O. Box 331150
Pacoima, CA 91333-1150
800-899-5017

Numark Laboratories, Inc.
P.O. Box 6321
Edison, NJ 08818
800-331-0221

O

Omron Healthcare, Inc.
300 Lakeview Pkwy.
Vernon Hills, IL 60061
847-680-6200

Optimox Corp.
P.O. Box 3378
Torrance, CA 90510-3378
800-223-1601

Oral-B Laboratories
Div. of Gillette Company, Inc.
1 Lagoon Dr.
Redwood City, CA 94065-1561
800-446-7252

Otis Clapp & Son, Inc.
P.O. Box 9160
Canton, MA 02021-9160
617-821-5400

Owen Mumford, Inc.
849 Pickens Industrial Dr., Ste. 14
Marietta, GA 30062-3165
800-421-6936

P

Paddock Laboratories, Inc.
3101 Louisiana Ave. N.
P.O. Box 27286
Minneapolis, MN 55427
800-328-5113

Palco Labs
8030 Soquel Ave.
Santa Cruz, CA 95062-2032
800-346-4488

Parnell Pharmaceuticals, Inc.
P.O. Box 5130
Larkspur, CA 94977-5130
800-45-PHARM

The Parthenon Co., Inc.
3311 W. 2400 South
Salt Lake City, UT 84119
800-453-8898

Pascal Company, Inc.
P.O. Box 1478
Bellevue, WA 98009-1478
206-827-4694

Pedinol Pharmacal, Inc.
30 Banfi Plaza N.
Farmingale, NY 11735
516-293-9500

Perio Products
6156 Wilcox Rd.
Dublin, OH 43017
614-791-1207

Perry Products
Div. of Health Care Marketing, Inc.
3803 E. Lake St.
Minneapolis, MN 55406-2298
612-722-4783

Person & Covey, Inc.
616 Allen Ave.
P.O. Box 25018
Glendale, CA 91221-5018
800-423-2341

Pfeiffer Pharmaceuticals, Inc.
Subs. of S.S.S. Company
(see **S.S.S. Company**)

Pfizer Inc
Consumer Health Care Group
235 E. 42nd St.
New York, NY 10017-5755
212-573-3131

Pharmaceutical Associates, Inc.
201 Delaware St.
Greenville, SC 29605
800-845-8210

Pharmacia & Upjohn, Inc.
7000 Portage Rd.
Kalamazoo, MI 49001
800-253-8600

Pharmacy Counter
2655 W. Central Ave.
Toledo, OH 43606
800-984-1137

PhytoPharmica
825 Challenger Drive
Greenbay, WI 54311
800-553-2370

PolyMedica Pharmaceuticals (USA), Inc.
2 Constitution Way
Woburn, MA 01801
617-933-2020

Polymer Technology
Div. of Wilmington Partners L. P.
100 Research Dr.
Wilmington, MA 01887
800-877-2343

The Procter & Gamble Co.
1 Procter & Gamble Plaza
P.O. Box 599
778Cincinnati, OH 45201
800-262-1637

The Purdue Frederick Co.
100 Connecticut Ave.
Norwalk, CT 06850-3590
203-853-0123

Q

Quality Health Products, Inc.
P.O. Box 31
Yaphank, NY 11980
800-233-7672

Quidel Corp.
10165 McKellar Ct.
San Diego, CA 92121
619-552-1100

R & D Laboratories, Inc.
4094 Glencoe Ave.
Marina del Rey, CA 90292
800-338-9066

R

Randob Laboratories, Ltd.
12 Grand St.
P.O. Box 440
Cornwall, NY 12518
914-534-2197

Reckitt & Colman, Inc.
1 Philips Pkwy.
Montvale, NJ 07645-1810
800-228-4722

Recsei Laboratories
330 S. Kellog Ave., Ste. M
Goleta, CA 93117
805-964-2912

Reese Chemical Co.
10617 Frank Ave.
P.O. Box 1957
Cleveland, OH 44106
800-321-7178

Republic Drug Company, Inc.
175 Great Arrow
Buffalo, NY 14027
716-874-5060

Requa, Inc.
1 Seneca Pl.
P.O. Box 4008
Greenwich, CT 06830
203-869-2445

Rexall Sundown, Inc.
851 Broken Sound Pkwy., N.W.
Boca Raton, FL 33487
800-344-8482

Rhône-Poulenc Rorer Pharmaceuticals, Inc.
500 Arcola Rd.
P.O. Box 1200
Collegeville, PA 19426-0107
800-340-7502

Ricola USA, Inc.
51 Gibraltar Dr.
Morris Plains, NJ 07950
201-984-6811

Roberts Pharmaceutical Corp.
4 Industrial Way W.
Eatontown, NJ 07724-2274
800-828-2088

Ross Products/Abbott Laboratories
625 Cleveland Ave.
Columbus, OH 43215-1724
614-624-7677

Roxane Laboratories, Inc.
Div. of Boehringer Ingelheim Corp.
1809 Wilson Rd.
P.O. Box 16532
Columbus, OH 43216-6532
614-276-4000

Rydelle Laboratories
Div. of S. C. Johnson & Son, Inc.
(see **S. C. Johnson**)

S

S. C. Johnson & Son, Inc.
1525 Howe St.
Racine, WI 53403-5011
800-558-5252

S.S.S. Company
P.O. Box 4447
Atlanta, GA 30302-4447
404-521-0857

Sandoz North American Consumer Pharmaceuticals
Div. of Sandoz Pharmaceuticals Corp.
59 Rte. 10
E. Hanover, NJ 07936-1080
201-503-7500

Sandoz Nutrition Corp.
5320 W. 23rd St.
P.O. Box 370
Minneapolis, MN 55440
800-999-9978

Savage Laboratories
Div. of Altana Inc.
60 Baylis Rd.
Melville, NY 11747
800-231-0206

Schein Pharmaceutical, Inc.
100 Campus Dr.
Florham Park, NJ 07932
800-548-6236

Scherer Laboratories, Inc.
Subs. of Scherer Healthcare, Inc.
2301 Ohio Dr., Ste. 234
Plano, TX 75093
214-612-6225

Schering-Plough HealthCare Products
Div. of Schering-Plough Corp.
3030 Jackson Ave.
Memphis, TN 38151
901-320-2998

Schwarz Pharma
A Kremers Urban Co.
P.O. Box 2038
Milwaukee, WI 53201
800-558-5114

Science Products
Box 888
Southeastern, PA 19399
800-888-7400

Scot-Tussin Pharmacal Co., Inc.
P.O. Box 8217
Cranston, RI 02920-0217
800-638-7268

Selfcare, Inc.
Waltham, MA 02154
800-899-SELF

Shaklee Corp.
Div. of Yamanovchi Pharmaceutical Co.
444 Market St.
San Francisco, CA 94111-5325
415-954-2080

Smith & Nephew United, Inc.
11775 Starkey Rd.
P.O. Box 1970
Largo, FL 34649-1970
800-876-1261

SmithKline Beecham Consumer Healthcare, L.P.
1500 Littleton Rd.
Parsippany, NJ 07054-3884
800-245-1040

Solvay Pharmaceuticals
901 Sawyer Rd.
Marietta, GA 30062
404-578-5540

Source Natural
P.O. Box 2118
anta Cruz, CA 95063
800-815-2333

Spectrum
Div. of United Industries, Corp.
P.O. Box 15842
St. Louis, M778O 63114-0842
800-767-9927

Stanback Co.
1500 S. Main St.
P.O. Box 1669
Salisbury, NC 28144-1669
800-338-5428

Stevens Skin Softener, Inc.
Div. of Stevens Products Corp.
4406 S. Century Dr.
Salt Lake City, UT 84123
800-678-7546

Stiefel Laboratories, Inc.
255 Alhambra Cir., Ste. 1000
Coral Gables, FL 33134
305-443-3807

Storz Ophthalmics
Div. of American Home Products Corp.
401 N. Middletown Rd.
Pearl River, NY 10965
800-533-3753

Summers Labs, Inc.
103 G.P. Clement Dr.
Collegeville, PA 19426
800-533-SKIN

Summit Industries, Inc.
839 Pickens Industrial Dr.
P.O. Box 7329
Marietta, GA 30065
404-590-0600

Sun Pharmaceuticals Corp.
Div. of Playtex Family Products Corp.
P.O. Box 2260
Del Ray Beach, FL 33447
800-SAFESUN

Sunbeam-Oster Household Products
1501 Woodfield Rd., Ste. 400N
Schaumburg, IL 60173
847-995-8900

Sunsource Health Products, Inc.
535 Lipoa Pwy., Ste. 110
Kihei, Maui, HI 96753
800-666-6505

T

T. N. Dickinson Co.
P.O. Box 319
E. Hampton, CT 06424
860-267-2279

Tec Laboratories
P.O. Box 1958
Albany, OR 97321
800-ITCHING

Tender Corp.
Littleton Industrial Park
P.O. Box 290
Littleton, NH 03561-0290
800-258-4696

Terumo Medical Co.
Consumer Products Div.
2100 Cottontail Ln.
Somerset, NJ 08873
800-283-7866

Thomas & Thompson Co.
3927 Falls Rd.
Baltimore, MD 21211
410-889-2960

Thompson Medical Company, Inc.
222 Lakeview Ave.
W. Palm Beach, FL 33401
407-820-9900

Thompson Nutritional Products
(see **Rexall Sundown**)

3M Health Care
3M Center
St. Paul, MN 55144-1000
800-328-0255

3M Pharmaceuticals
(see **3M Health**)

Tom's of Maine, Inc.
Lafayette Center
P.O. Box 710
Kennebunk, ME 04043
207-985-2944

Torbot Group Inc.
1185 Jeffferson Blvd.
P.O. Box 6008
Warwick, RI 02887-6008
800-545-4254

Transfer-Ease, Inc.
P.O. Box 108
Emerson, NJ 07630-0108
201-357-0114

Triton Consumer Products, Inc.
561 W. Golf Rd.
Arlington Heights, IL 60005
800-942-2009

Trout Lake Farm
149 Little Mountain Rd.
Trout Lake, WA 98650
800-395-6093

U

UCB Pharma, Inc.
1950 Lake Park Dr.
Atlanta, GA 30080
800-477-7877

Ulmer Pharmacal Co.
2440 Fernbrook Ln.
Plymouth, MN 55447
800-848-5637

Ulster Scientific, Inc.
83 S. Putt Corners Rd.
P.O. Box 819
New Paltz, NY 12561
800-431-8233

Unico Holding Co.
2920 N.W. Boca Raton Blvd., Ste. 1
Boca Raton, FL 33431
800-367-4477

Upsher-Smith Laboratories, Inc.
14905 23rd Ave. N.
Minneapolis, MN 55447-4709
800-654-2299

V

Vangard Labs, Inc.
890 No. L. Rogers Wells Blvd.
P.O. Box 1268
Glasgow, KY 42142-1268
502-651-6188

Vetco, Inc.
105 Baylis Rd.
Melville, NY 11747
800-754-8853

Vitaline Corp.
385 Williamson Way
Ashland, OR 97520
800-648-4755

VPI
P.O. Box 266
Spencer, IN 47460-0266
800-843-4851

W

W. F. Young, Inc.
111 Lyman St.
P.O. Box 14
Springfield, MA 01102-0014
413-737-0201

Walker, Corp. and Co., Inc.
P.O. Box 1320
Syracuse, NY 13201
315-463-4511

Warner Wellcome Consumer Health Care
(see **Warner-Lambert**)

Warner-Lambert Co.
201 Tabor Rd.
Morris Plains, NJ 07950
201-540-2000

Westwood-Squibb Pharmaceuticals
Div. of Bristol-Myers Squibb Co.
100 Forest Ave.
Buffalo, NY 14213-1091
800-333-0950 x7667

Whitehall-Robins Healthcare
Div. of American Home Products Corp.
5 Giralda Farms
Madison, NJ 07940-0871
800-322-3129

Whittier Medical, Inc.
865 Turnpike St.
N. Andover, MA 01845
800-645-1115

Wisconsin Pharmacal Co., Inc.
1 Repel Rd.
P.O. Box 198
Jackson, WI 53037
414-677-4121

Wyeth-Ayerst Laboratories
Div. of American Home Products Corp.
555 E. Lancaster Ave.
St. Davids, PA 19087
800-99-WYETH

Z

Zeneca Pharmaceuticals
A Business Unit of Zeneca Inc.
1800 Concorde Pike
P.O. Box 15437
Wilmington, DE 19850-5437
302-886-3000

Zila Pharmaceuticals Inc.
5227 N. 7th St.
Phoenix, AZ 85014-2817
602-266-6700

Index

Boldface entries designate product table titles.

Entries in regular lightface type designate product ingredients, therapetic drug classes, or product categories.

Italic entries in which all major words are capitalized designate product trade names, including phytomedicinal products.

Other italic entries designate the genus and species of plants from which phytomedicinal products are derived.

A

C

E

F

G

N

O

P

Q

R

S

T

U

V

W

X

Y

Z